Essential Enrolled Nursing Skills

FOR PERSON-CENTRED CARE
3RD EDITION

Essential Enrolled Nursing Skills

FOR PERSON-CENTRED CARE
3RD EDITION

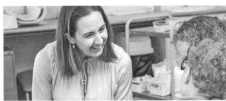
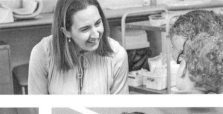
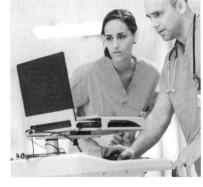
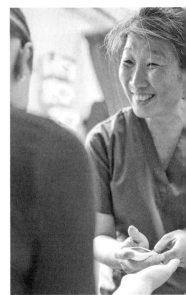
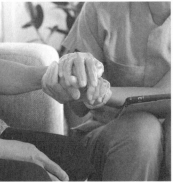
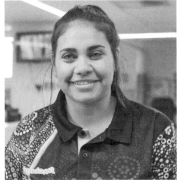

Gabrielle Koutoukidis

EdD(Research), MPH, BN(Mid), DipAppSci(Nurs), AdvDipN(Ed), DipBus,
VocGradCertBus(Transformational Management),
International Specialised Skills Institute Fellow
Dean, Faculty Health Science, Community & Social Studies, Holmesglen,
Vic, Australia

Kate Stainton

MHS(Nurs), GDipNurs(Ed), BN(Mid), DipAppSci(Nurs), Cert IV TAE, MACN
Strategy & Innovation Consultant, BaptistCare, NSW, Australia
Sessional Academic, School of Nursing & Midwifery, University of Newcastle,
NSW, Australia

ELSEVIER

Elsevier Australia. ACN 001 002 357
(a division of Reed International Books Australia Pty Ltd)
475 Victoria Avenue, Chatswood, NSW 2067

ISBN: 978-0-7295-4485-6

Notice

This publication has been carefully reviewed and checked to ensure that the content is as accurate and current as possible at time of publication. We would recommend, however, that the reader verify any procedures, treatments, drug dosages or legal content described in this book. Neither the author, the contributors, nor the publisher assume any liability for injury and/or damage to persons or property arising from any error in or omission from this publication.

National Library of Australia Cataloguing-in-Publication Data

 A catalogue record for this
book is available from the
National Library of Australia

Content Strategist: Elizabeth Coady
Content Project Manager: Fariha Nadeem
Edited by Lynn Watt
Proofread by Annabel Adair
Copyrights Coordinator: Regina Remigius
Cover Designer: Georgette Hall
Index by Innodata
Typeset by GW Tech
Printed in Singapore by Markono Print Media Pte Ltd

Last digit is the print number: 9 8 7 6 5 4 3 2 1

Contents

Contributors

Louise Baldwin BEd(Sec), MHSc(Health Prom), PhD
Senior Research Fellow, Queensland University
of Technology,
Qld, Australia

Ann Bolton RN, BN, MCN, GradDipAdNurs
(Management), GDipMid, GradDipCritCare,
GradDipVET, Cert IV TAE
Casual Educator, Batchelor Institute of Indigenous
Tertiary Education, NT, Australia
Partners in Training, Vic, Australia

Philippa Borjanov RN
Nursing Teacher/Diploma of Nursing,
Holmesglen Institute, Vic, Australia

Janine Bothe RN, BaEdSt, MaEdSt, DN
CNC Surgery, St George Hospital
Adjunct Research Fellow, Curtin University
Visiting Academic, Fiji National University
NSW, Australia

Megan Christophers RN, GCertYMH,
GDipMtlHlthN, DipInt,
Diploma of Auslan, Cert IV TAE
Nurse Lecturer, Holmesglen Institute,
Melbourne CBD Campus, Vic, Australia

Ashleigh Djachenko RN, BN, GradCertComm
&PrimHlthCare, GradDipHlthResearch, DipTrainDesDev
Nursing Teacher, TAFE Queensland,
Qld, Australia

Meagan Gaskett RN, BN, BHSc, Cert IV TAE,
GradDipVET(Adult Ed), MNursSci
Trainer & Assessor Nursing, GOTAFE,
Vic, Australia

Laura Healey MN(NP), MCN(Onc), GradDipN(Onc)
Nurse Practitioner, Medical Oncology
NSW, Australia

Gabrielle Koutoukidis EdD(Research), MPH,
BN(Mid), DipAppSci(Nurs), AdvDipN(Ed), DipBus,
VocGradCert Business(Transformational Management),
International Specialised Skills Institute Fellow
Dean, Faculty Health Science, Community & Social
Studies, Holmesglen,
Vic, Australia

Marie V Long RN, RM
Teacher, University of Wollongong, Charles Sturt
University, NSW, Australia

Anne MacLeod RN, BN, MA Ad Ed & Training,
DipVocEd, GradCert Simulation & Flexible Delivery,
AdDip Leadership and Management, Dip Business, Acute
Care Cert, Neuroscience Cert
Head Teacher Health Wellbeing and Community Services,
TAFE NSW Newcastle Campus,
NSW, Australia

Lise Martin RN, BNSc, TAE
RN/Educator, TAFE Queensland, Qld, Australia

Michelle McKay BN, BVoc ED, Grad Cert(Paeds &
Oncology), DipAppSc(Nurs), Dip TAE, Cert IV TAE
Nursing Teacher, TAFE NSW North Region,
NSW, Australia

Deepu Ponnappan RN, MHPE, GradCertClinEd,
GradDip NsgCardiacCare AssocDegVET,
DipLeadrshp&Mgt, Cert IV TAE
Education Manager, Holmesglen Institute,
Vic, Australia

Kylie Porritt BN, GradDipNursSc(Cardiac), MNSc, PhD
Director Transfer Science, JBI, School of Public Health,
University of Adelaide, SA, Australia

Kalpana Raghunathan RN, FACN, PhD, MN,
MHRMgt, MDevStudies, GradDipDevStudies, BN,
BASociology, DipBusMgt, DipComDev, Cert IV TAE
Nurse Education Consultant/Research Assistant,
Caramar Educational Design/La Trobe University,
Vic, Australia

Heather Redmond RN, BN, BNHon, MN, GradDip Critical Care, GradCert High Dependency Nursing, DipVET, Cert IV TAE
Program Manager, TAFE Gippsland Vic, Australia

Jasmin Rigby-Day RN, MCN, GradDipN(Community Health Nursing), GradCertN(Clinical Nursing and Teaching), TAE40116
Lecturer in Nursing, Holmesglen Institute,
Vic, Australia

Antony Robinson RN, BN, MN, GradCertIntCareNursing, GCertClinTeach
Acting Director of Nursing and Operations,
Division of Emergency Medicine, Royal Darwin and Palmerston Hospitals, NT, Australia

Kate Stainton MHS(Nurs), GDipNurs(Ed), BN(Mid), DipAppSci(Nurs), Cert IV TAE, MACN
Strategy & Innovation Consultant, BaptistCare,
NSW, Australia
Sessional Academic, School of Nursing & Midwifery, University of Newcastle, NSW, Australia

Christine Standley RN, MN
Lecturer Bachelor of Nursing, Holmesglen Institute,
Vic, Australia

Heather Wakefield RN, BN, MN(Ed), GradDipClinNursEd, PostGradDipAdvClinNurs (Crit Care), Cert IV TAE, DipVET
Education Manager, Diploma of Nursing, Health Science, Community and Social Studies, Holmesglen Institute,
Vic, Australia

Jing Wan (Persephone Wan) RN, GradDip, GradCert TAE
Nursing Teacher, Holmesglen Institute of TAFE,
Vic, Australia

Rachel Wassink RN, MBA, GradCertEd, BN, DipVET, DipTDD, Cert IV TAE
Director, Social Care and Health, RMIT University, City/Bundoora Campus, Vic, Australia

Andrea Zivin RN, BNurs(Psych), GCertAdNurs(Periop), GDipPsych(Adv), TAE40116
Lecturer in Nursing, Holmesglen Institute,
Vic, Australia

Acknowledgements

I was delighted to be invited as an editor for the third edition of *Essential Enrolled Nursing Skills for Person-Centred Care Workbook 3E* and to have the opportunity to do this again alongside one of my closest friends—Kate. This third edition is the culmination of work by many experienced nursing educators and writers with expertise in the chapter content they have contributed, and I would like to thank all contributors for their enthusiasm and support for Enrolled Nurse education.

I would also like to acknowledge all the nursing students and teams I have worked with over the years, who have inspired in me a passion for education and ensuring that evidence-based nursing practice is implemented. I have also been inspired by all the nurses (educators, students, frontline workers) who have continued working during unprecedented and challenging times.

Gabby Koutoukidis

Essential Enrolled Nursing Skills for Person-Centred Care Workbook 3E reflects the accumulated knowledge and expertise of all past and present contributors. Thank you for your hard work in preparing Enrolled Nurses for their future practice, and understanding the importance of providing them with contemporary evidence-based relevant information on which to base this practice.

This edition would not have been possible if it were not for my colleagues, friends, students, family and partners. To my co-editor and friend Gabby, my husband Anthony and children Ben, Alex and Maddy, thank you so much for joining me on the journey and your ongoing encouragement and support. For the team at Elsevier, as always, your knowledge and hard work to make the publication of this new edition possible is appreciated.

Kate Stainton

Credits for Cover Images:

Introduction

Essential Enrolled Nursing Skills for Person-Centred Care Workbook 3E supports learners to develop the confidence to undertake and perform all skills they need to successfully complete their Diploma of Nursing qualification and graduate to become safe, knowledgeable and competent Enrolled Nurses (ENs). This title aligns with *Tabbner's Nursing Care: Theory and Practice 9E* and provides an essential and up-to-date resource, reflecting current best practice and including the new changes to practice and guidelines.

Essential Enrolled Nursing Skills is specifically designed for enrolled nursing students and provides learners with the evidence-based practical skills and rationale for each skill activity, to enable them to work with the Registered Nurse (RN) as part of the multidisciplinary healthcare team. This resource will help learners strengthen critical thinking and problem-solving skills, and develop proficiency in providing person-centred care. The workbook also provides an observation checklist to accompany each skill. A key feature of the workbook are the NMBA *Decision-making Framework* (2020) considerations in each skill.

As a whole, the book is designed to be learner-focused, providing the foundation necessary for learning success through demonstration of practical skills and reflection. The book can be used in classroom lectures, skill laboratories, simulation and clinical practice.

It is recommended that to provide context to the learner, the educator/facilitator develops a scenario/case study in relation to each skill and case studies and critical-thinking exercises to assist learners to build skills, confidence and competence.

TEXT FEATURES

Each chapter includes an overview that focuses on what the student will learn from each set of skills.

Skills

The skills include the following:
- **Decision-making Framework considerations**—scope of practice in which nurses are educated, competent and permitted by law to perform. Each skill asks the student to consider:
  1. Am I educated?
  2. Am I authorised?
  3. Am I competent?

If the learner answers 'no' to any of these questions, they should not perform that activity. They are asked to seek guidance and support from their teacher/a nurse team leader/clinical facilitator/educator. In addition, learners are asked to refer to the NMBA Decision-making Framework for Nursing and Midwifery (2020).
- **Equipment**—lists the essential tools required to carry out the skill.
- **Skill Activity**—step-by-step instructions outlining each action that needs to be undertaken, to assist learners translate theory to practice.
- **Rationale**—provides the logic behind each step.
- **References**—each skill is referenced from fundamental nursing texts and various databases including government, medical and health-related websites using recent evidence-based material.

Observation checklist

The observation checklist that follows each skill allows learners to track their skill development progress as well as providing educators with a teaching and learning resource.

The checklists include the following:
- **Competency Elements**—indicate the steps the student must include while carrying out the skill. These include:
  > preparation for the activity
  > performs activity informed by evidence
  > applies critical thinking and reflective practice
  > practises within safety and quality assurance guidelines
  > documentation and communication.
- **Performance Criteria/Evidence**—lists the specific steps required to perform that particular skill.
- **The five-point Bondy Rating Scale**—provides the framework to clearly indicate the level of competence achieved (see p. xii). If the observation checklist is being used as an assessment tool, the learner will need to obtain a scale of independence for each of the performance criteria/evidence.
- **Student Reflection**—provides room for the learner to describe their experience, whether they master the skill on the first attempt or wish to record notes to assist in a future attempt.
- **Educator/Facilitator Feedback**—provides the opportunity for immediate feedback, allowing the assessor to indicate how the learner has performed or how they need to improve.

The five-point Bondy Rating Scale

The five-point Bondy Rating Scale is a tool used to assess professional competency and, subsequently, the amount of supervision needed to successfully master the nursing skills included in this workbook. The scale is also a useful indicator of learners' ability to carry out these skills with accuracy, safety and satisfactory effect.

Note: If the observation checklist is being used as an assessment tool, the learner will need to obtain a scale of independence for each of the performance criteria/evidence.

Scale label	Score	Standard of procedure	Quality of performance	Level of assistance required
Independent	5	Safe Accurate Achieved intended outcome Behaviour is appropriate to context	Proficient Confident Expedient	No supporting cues required.
Supervised	4	Safe Accurate Achieved intended outcome Behaviour is appropriate to context	Proficient Confident Reasonably expedient	Required occasional supportive cues.
Assisted	3	Safe Accurate Achieved most objectives for intended outcome Behaviour generally appropriate to context	Proficient throughout most of performance when assisted	Required frequent verbal and occasional physical directives in addition to supportive cues.
Marginal	2	Safe only with guidance Not completely accurate Incomplete achievement of intended outcome	Unskilled Inefficient	Required continuous verbal and frequent physical directive cues.
Dependent	1	Unsafe Unable to demonstrate behaviour Lack of insight into behaviour appropriate to context	Unskilled Unable to demonstrate behaviour/procedure	Required continuous verbal and continuous physical directive cues.
X	0	Not observed		

(Adapted from Bondy, K N 1983. Criterion-referenced definitions for rating scales in clinical evaluation. Journal of Nursing Education 22(9), 376–382)

Standard steps for all Clinical Skills

These are the essential steps that must be performed consistently to deliver responsible and safe nursing care.

Note: Apply critical thinking to determine the applicability of the standard steps. Not all the components of the standard steps will be applicable to all skills.

PREPARE FOR THE SKILL

STEP	SKILL ACTIVITY	RATIONALE
1	• Mentally review the steps of the skill. • Discuss the skill with your instructor/supervisor/team leader, if required. • Confirm correct facility/organisation policy/safe operating procedures.	• It is important to identify any gaps in knowledge, seek assistance/supervision as required and adequately prepare for the skill. • Abides by organisation policy and procedures and ensures that skill is within scope of practice.
2	• Validate the order in the individual's record. • Identify indication and rationale for performing the activity. • Assess for any contraindications. • Locate and gather equipment. If using a procedure trolley, ensure it is cleaned and place all equipment to be used on the bottom shelf. • Perform hand hygiene.	• Ensures that the procedure has been ordered. • Provides information about the individual's treatment, equipment/supplies needed. • It is important to understand why the skill is being performed. • Ensures correct procedure is about to take place for the correct person and promotes safety. Promotes time management and ensures efficiency. Prevents spread of microorganisms and cross-infection.

3	• Ensure therapeutic interaction. This may include but is not limited to:
	  > introducing yourself
	  > explaining why the skill has been ordered and the frequency, including what is involved
	  > listening to the individual's concerns or questions about the skill and confirming their understanding before the skill is undertaken
	  > ensuring the individual is aware of any requirements related to the skill
	  > identifying any opportunities for health education
	  > maintaining professional boundaries.
		• Reduces anxiety/apprehension and gains trust and cooperation.
		• Promotes participation in care and understanding of health status in relation to the skill.
		• Reduces the incidence of performing the skill on the incorrect individual.
		• Ensures informed consent.
		• Promotes individual comfort.

PREPARE FOR THE SKILL

STEP	SKILL ACTIVITY	RATIONALE
	• Identify the individual using three individual identifiers. This may include but is not limited to identifying the individual's: > identification-allocated healthcare number on hospital bracelet/band > given and family name, confirmed verbally > date of birth > gender > address > medical record number. • Gain consent to perform the skill. • Assess for pain relief.	
4	• Prepare the environment: > Raise the bed to appropriate working height. > Provide adequate lighting for the skill. > Arrange supplies and equipment. • Provide and maintain privacy. • Assist the individual to assume an appropriate position of comfort.	• Follows safe work practices. • Facilitates performance of the skill and promotes functional alignment and body mechanics. • Allows observation. • Prepares supplies and equipment ready for use. • Maintains individual's dignity and privacy. • Promotes individual comfort.

PERFORM THE SKILL

STEP	SKILL ACTIVITY	RATIONALE
5	• Perform hand hygiene. • Apply PPE: gloves, eyewear, mask and gown as appropriate.	• Prevents exposure to/spread of microorganisms and cross-infection.
6	• Ensure the individual's safety and comfort throughout skill. • Promote independence and involvement of the individual if possible and/or appropriate. • Assess the individual's tolerance to the skill throughout.	• It is important to measure for any changes in level of comfort. • Promotes a sense of control and participation in care.
7	• Dispose of used supplies, equipment, waste and sharps appropriately. • Remove PPE and discard or store appropriately. • Perform hand hygiene.	• Correct disposal prevents an unsafe working environment and sharps injury. • Prevents spread of microorganisms and cross-infection.

AFTER THE SKILL

STEP	SKILL ACTIVITY	RATIONALE
8	• Communicate outcome to the individual, any ongoing care and to report any complications. • Restore the environment: > Lower the bed and assist the individual to reassume a comfortable position. > Place call bell and personal items within reach. > Clean used equipment and store appropriately.	• Effective communication ensures person-centred care. • Promotes individual comfort and safety, monitors for adverse effects. • Prevents cross-infection.

Continued

AFTER THE SKILL

STEP	SKILL ACTIVITY	RATIONALE
9	• Report, record and document assessment findings, details of the skill performed and the individual's response. • Report, record and document any abnormalities and/or inability to perform the skill. • Reassess the individual to ensure there are no adverse effects/events from the skill.	• Maintains legal document of care and interventions provided. • Ensures that all members of the healthcare team are aware of changes in the individual's condition. • Appropriate care can be planned and implemented. • Any adverse effects can be managed promptly.

UNDERSTANDING AND PROMOTING HEALTH

Louise Baldwin

Overview

Promoting health is an integral part of the role of the nurse. As an Enrolled Nurse, this may be achieved with the consultation and collaboration of the Registered Nurse. As the complexity of individuals being discharged from hospitals increases, especially with early-discharge models and the financial constraints of healthcare providers, it is imperative that Enrolled Nurses understand the many conceptions of health, illness and wellbeing. Equally important is understanding what determines health to ensure individuals and their carers are partners in their healthcare in order to promote independence and better quality of life.

The World Health Organization's (WHO) definition of health is that **health** is 'a state of complete physical, social and mental well-being and not merely the absence of disease' (WHO 1946). Wellbeing is defined as 'the combination of feeling good and functioning well; the experience of positive emotions such as happiness and contentment as well as the development of one's potential, having some control over one's life, having a sense of purpose, and experiencing positive relationships' (Ruggeri et al 2020). People may possess a sense of personal wellbeing even when they are in very deprived situations, during stressful life events or confronted with acute or chronic disease. **Illness** is defined as a disease or period of sickness that affects an individual's body or mind and prevents the individual achieving his or her optimal outputs (Wills 2023).

An examination of health promotion theory and practice leads us to consider the definitions and descriptions from what has been called a socioenvironmental perspective. Notable efforts to do this have come not only from the World Health Organization (1946) but also from the environmental and Aboriginal and Torres Strait Islander peoples' health movements where recognition of the importance of ecological sustainability and cultural health is also woven into the descriptions of health.

Health promotion and education practice incorporates the current philosophies of health and wellness and understandings of what determines health. When working with communities, families and individuals the aim is to understand the sociocultural, environmental and behavioural factors, which will influence a cue for action.

In particular, an Enrolled Nurse can utilise knowledge and skills through adequate health promotion and education via the hospital or community settings, enabling individuals and their carers to be better informed and prepared for any complications that may arise from their illness, preventing multiple admissions into hospital.

Teaching and learning need not be a formal process as nurses are constantly reinforcing and informing individuals and their carers of relevant information pertaining to their health. However, formal teaching techniques are a large part of a nurse's role. Individuals and/or their carers have a right to understandable and relevant information about their or their loved one's health, ensuring a person-centred approach to health management and care.

Types of health education, promotion and wellness include:
- Performing clinical skills (e.g. taking blood pressure, blood glucose level, administering insulin)
- Information on medication
- General information on medical conditions
- Stressing the importance of exercise
- Encouraging people to stop smoking
- Asthma management
- Outlining signs and symptoms of medical conditions
- Particular treatments (e.g. chemotherapy, radiotherapy).

Health promotion and education involves developing personal skills that will enable the individual to continue to maintain as much independence as possible and stay as well as they possibly can.

Teaching and learning is a very complex process and requires thorough assessment prior to commencement of the teaching. Not all individuals and/or carers will be ready to make changes to improve their health.

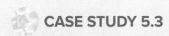 **CASE STUDY 5.3**

Individual assessment

Mary, 52, has recently been diagnosed with type 2 diabetes mellitus. She states, 'I have always loved my food—in many ways it is my only enjoyment in life and now my doctor says I have to give up all the things I love to eat. I'm finding it just too hard on the diet he has given me and I think I'll just give up.'

Health promotion should start from the existing knowledge and beliefs of the individual. To plan the individual care needed for Mary and to begin the nursing process, it will be helpful for the nurse to first determine Mary's health beliefs and her understanding of the diagnosis she has been given. This will require building up trust and obtaining a detailed social and medical history. This part of the nursing process is the assessment phase and basically requires the gathering of subjective and objective data.

Subjective data are the individual's, or other significant person's, perceptions, ideas and sensations about a health problem. For example, Mary has stated that she is finding it too hard and wants to give up. Objective data are the information observed or measured by the nurse. For example, the nurse has observed that Mary does not appear to have altered her lifestyle, or have an understanding about nutrition needs and planning meals.

In considering this case study—how might you consider the social determinants of health? Think about assumptions on availability and affordability of fresh food, access to fruit and vegetables and access to services like food shops and food delivery. Also consider determinants such as housing, transport, education and income. What strategies might the nurse use to facilitate a teaching–learning situation with Mary on type 2 diabetes mellitus?

CRITICAL THINKING EXERCISE 5.3

Applying the health belief model

Use the health belief model as a basis to develop a plan for one session of health education for refugees who attend the community health facility where you work. This is designed to encourage them to have their children fully immunised at the free public sessions that are available.

A detailed assessment phase will be essential and the success of the program will depend on whether the program meets the issues identified in the assessment. Because of the different cultural characteristics of the potential participants, you cannot assume that a successful program offered to one immigrant group will automatically be relevant to a different group.

CLINICAL SKILL 5.1 Health teaching

Make sure you adhere to the policy and procedures of the facility/organisation prior to undertaking the skill. Ensure this skill is in your scope of practice.

NMBA Decision-making framework considerations (refer to NMBA Decision-making framework for nursing and midwifery 2020):	Equipment
1. Am I educated? 2. Am I authorised? 3. Am I competent? If you answer 'no' to any of these, do not perform that activity. Seek guidance and support from your teacher, a nurse team leader, clinical facilitator or educator.	Audiovisual material or aids. If teaching a skill, ensure correct equipment, pen and paper and any published written material.

 PREPARE FOR THE SKILL

(Please refer to the Standard Steps on p. xii for related rationales.)
- Mentally review the steps of the skill.
- Discuss the skill with your instructor/supervisor/team leader if required.
- Confirm correct facility/organisation policy/safe operating procedures.
- Validate the order in the individual's record.
- Identify indication and rationale for performing the activity.
- Assess for any contraindications.
- Locate and gather equipment.
- Perform hand hygiene.
- Ensure therapeutic interaction.
- Identify the individual using three individual identifiers.
- Gain the individual's consent.
- Assess for pain relief.
- Prepare the environment.
- Provide and maintain privacy.
- Assist the individual to assume an appropriate position of comfort.

Skill activity	Rationale
Assess the individual's ability and willingness to learn—determine baseline knowledge, their cognitive status and ability to understand and speak English and culture. Establish a suitable time for the health teaching to take place.	Ensures a baseline assessment of the individual. Enables resources to be organised prior to commencing any formal health teaching (interpreter, family member or carer, language/visual/hearing aids). Ensures cooperation and involvement of the individual.

 PERFORM THE SKILL

(Please refer to the Standard Steps on p. xii for related rationales.)
- Perform hand hygiene.
- Apply PPE: gloves, eyewear, mask and gown as appropriate.
- Ensure the individual's safety and comfort throughout the skill.
- Promote independence and involvement of the individual if possible and/or appropriate.
- Assess the individual's tolerance to the skill throughout.
- Dispose of used supplies, equipment, waste and sharps appropriately.
- Remove PPE and discard or store appropriately.
- Perform hand hygiene.

Skill activity	Rationale
When conducting the health teaching	
Ensure the individual is away from any distractions (this may be in a room away from the individual's bed area or, if in their bedroom, ensure the curtains are closed or the door is closed). Ensure only the relevant people are present. Explain the purpose of the health teaching.	Maintains focus and avoids distractions, enabling better retention of information. Too many people in the room can distract the individual and cause interruptions to the process. Alleviates anxiety and reiterates the purpose of the education.

Continued

CLINICAL SKILL 5.1 Health teaching—cont'd

Demonstration of a skill

Demonstrate the skill from beginning to end with no interruptions. Demonstrate the skill again, breaking it down into steps, explaining each step as clearly and simply as possible. Explain the rationale of the skill and the reason for each step being performed in the way demonstrated.	Shows the skill in its entirety so that the individual and/or carer can see what is involved. Alleviates anxiety and makes the skill easier to learn. Reinforces the need for accuracy and ensures the skill is learnt correctly to eliminate error.
Ask the individual and/or carer to handle the equipment and go through each step with the nurse coaching them through it. If the individual/carer feels confident, ask them to demonstrate again, this time coaching themselves.	Gives the individual/carer the opportunity to demonstrate the skill and build their confidence with support from the nurse. The individual/carer may require another demonstration by the nurse if they are struggling to master the skill.
Run through any troubleshooting issues that may occur with the equipment. Go through the manufacturer's guidelines with the individual/carer. Provide feedback.	Allows the individual/carer to become familiar with some of the error readings or any issues with the equipment and what to do, care of the equipment and proper disposal of any waste. Promotes confidence in being able to perform the skill and may require further sessions.

General health teaching

Go through the areas of health teaching pertaining to the session with the individual and/or carer using any aids or written materials. Ask the individual and/or carer to repeat any information in their own words and ask any questions. Do not overload them with information.	Outlines the purpose of the health teaching and demonstrates efficiency. Determines a level of understanding and allows for repetition of any information. Too much information can confuse the individual and/or carer, making the learning harder. The nurse may need to follow through with another session.

 AFTER THE SKILL

(Please refer to the Standard Steps on p. xii for related rationales.)
- Communicate outcome to the individual, any ongoing care and to report any complications.
- Restore the environment.
- Report, record and document assessment findings, details of the skill performed and the individual's response.
- Report, record and document any abnormalities and/or inability to perform the skill.
- Reassess the individual to ensure there are no adverse effects/events from the skill.

(Burgess et al 2020; Crisp et al 2021; Tollefson et al 2022)

OBSERVATION CHECKLIST: HEALTH TEACHING

STUDENT NAME: _____

CLINICAL SKILL 5.1: Health teaching

DEMONSTRATION OF: The ability to effectively engage in health teaching/education

If the observation checklist is being used as an assessment tool, the student will need to obtain a scale of independence for each of the performance criteria/evidence.

Independent (I)
Supervised (S)
Assisted (A)
Marginal (M)
Dependent (D)

COMPETENCY ELEMENTS	PERFORMANCE CRITERIA/EVIDENCE	I	S	A	M	D
Preparation for the activity	Identifies indications and rationale for performing the activity Checks facility/organisation policy Identifies the individual using three individual identifiers Ensures therapeutic interaction Gains the individual's consent Assesses any cultural/language barriers Checks information required for teaching/education Provides a private area or room away from distractions for session to take place Ensures any carers also present Locates and gathers equipment Ensures individual and/or carer comfortable					
Performs activity informed by evidence	Goes through the equipment with the individual and/or their carers Ensures instruction and troubleshooting sheet available for individual's use					
Applies critical thinking and reflective practice	Is able to link theory to practice Demonstrates current best practice in the care provided Assesses the individual's clinical status and their ability to learn Monitors the individual's anxiety related to the health teaching/education Encourages feedback from the individual and/or carer Assesses the individual's ability to cooperate with the procedure and become independent Assesses own performance					
Practises within safety and quality assurance guidelines	Reviews against facility/organisation policy					
Documentation and communication	Explains and communicates the activity clearly to the individual Communicates outcome and ongoing care to individual and significant others Communicates abnormal findings to appropriate personnel Reports and documents all relevant information and any complications correctly in the healthcare record Reports any complications and/or inability to perform the procedure to the RN and/or medical officer Asks the individual and/or carer to report any concerns regarding performing the procedure					

Educator/Facilitator Feedback:

Educator/Facilitator Score: Competent Needs further development

How would you rate your overall performance while undertaking this clinical activity? (use a ✓ & initial)

Unsatisfactory Satisfactory Good Excellent

Student Reflection: (discuss how you would approach your practice differently or more effectively)

EDUCATOR/FACILITATOR NAME/SIGNATURE:

STUDENT NAME/SIGNATURE: DATE:

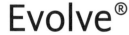 **Evolve**® Answer guide for the Critical Thinking Exercises and Critical Thinking Questions in Case Studies is hosted on Evolve: http://evolve.elsevier.com/AU/Koutoukidis/Tabbner/

References

Burgess, A., van Diggele, C., Roberts, C., et al., 2020. Tips for teaching procedural skills. *BMC Med Educ* 20(2), 458. Available at: <https://doi.org/10.1186/s12909-020-02284-1>.

Crisp, J., Taylor, C., Douglas, C., et al. (eds.), 2021. *Potter and Perry's fundamentals of nursing*, 6th ed. Elsevier, Sydney.

Nursing and Midwifery Board of Australia (NMBA), 2020. Decision-making framework for nursing and midwifery. Available at: <https://www.nursingmidwiferyboard.gov.au/Codes-Guidelines-Statements/Frameworks.aspx>.

Ruggeri, K., Garcia-Garzon, E., Maguire, Á., et al., 2020. Well-being is more than happiness and life satisfaction: A multidimensional analysis of 21 countries. *Health Qual Life Outcomes* 18, 192. Available at: <https://doi.org/10.1186/s12955-020-01423-y>.

Tollefson, J., Watson, G., Jelly, E., et al., 2022. *Essential clinical skills: Enrolled nurses*, 5th ed. Cengage Learning, Melbourne.

Wills, J., 2023. *Foundations of health promotion*, 5th ed. Elsevier Limited.

World Health Organization (WHO), 1946. Preamble to the Constitution of the World Health Organization. Available at: <https://apps.who.int/gb/bd/PDF/bd47/EN/constitution-en.pdf?ua51>.

DOCUMENTATION, HEALTH INFORMATICS AND TECHNOLOGY

Kalpana Raghunathan

Overview

DOCUMENTATION

Documentation is a core nursing competency and is important for the provision of effective and efficient care of individuals and to ensure their safety. Effective documentation reflects on the level of care given by health professionals and is both a legal requirement and a professional responsibility (Crisp et al 2021; Staunton & Chiarella 2020). The main purpose of documentation is to communicate information between the multidisciplinary team members caring for the individual. Other purposes of documentation include ensuring professional accountability, legislative requirements, quality improvement, research and resource management and funding. Documentation makes up the individual's health record; it allows contemporaneous information from multiple sources to be recorded by numerous health professionals to complete a historical account of the individual's health history. Nursing documentation encompasses all written and electronic or computerised recordings of data made by nurses or used by nurses to communicate information regarding individuals' care (Crisp et al 2021). For this clinical skill (Clinical Skill 8.1), we will be focusing on documentation in the form of charting an individual's progress notes.

There are many different types of healthcare records used depending on the healthcare facility and the reason for the individual's admission or the episode of care. These include flowcharts, assessment tools, incident forms, risk assessment tools, discharge forms, care pathways and nursing care planning forms (Tollefson et al 2022). To achieve safe, efficient and individualised care, documentation must be objective, consistent and an accurate statement of fact about the ongoing account of the person's healthcare experience (Staunton & Chiarella 2020). High-quality documentation requires the following attributes: factual, accuracy, completeness, currency and organisation (Crisp et al 2021).

Factual

For a report to be factual it must contain descriptive and objective information about what the nurse sees, hears, feels and smells. It needs to clearly explain the nurse's observations without the use of inferences such as 'appears' or 'seems', and in the recording of subjective data the nurse must document the individual's exact words, in addition to any objective findings which support their statements (Crisp et al 2021).

Accuracy

To determine whether an individual's condition has changed, exact measurements are essential. It is also important that documentation is concise and demonstrates correct spelling, correct entry and legible writing. Deviations in accuracy can contribute to potential adverse deviations in individual care (Crisp et al 2021).

Completeness

All documentation needs to be complete. It must contain concise, appropriate and thorough information about the individual's care and treatment. This makes it easier to understand and gives essential information without unnecessary words and irrelevant data (Crisp et al 2021).

Currency

Currency refers to timely entries within the individual's documentation. This is often made easier with the use of bedside records that facilitate immediate documentation of information collected from the individual, such as vital signs (Crisp et al 2021). Nursing documentation should be written as it occurs, allowing it to be presented in a logical and contemporaneous way.

Organisation

Organisation ensures the nurse communicates information in a logical order within the report while ensuring that it is easy to understand (Crisp et al 2021). Organisation improves communication and consequently leads to more efficient and effective care for the individual (Perry et al 2020).

Nursing documentation should also be individually centred and contain the actual work of the nurse completing the documentation. The method of reporting and documenting should be appropriate according to the preference of the department and include any variances in care (Perry et al 2020). A variety of formats can be used for documenting in progress notes; these include SOAP (Subjective data, Objective data, Assessment and Plan), PIE (Problem, Intervention and Evaluation), a narrative approach or a charting by exception (CBE) system (Perry et al 2020). Any health professional caring for the individual needs to be able to read a progress note and understand the individual's problems, the level of care provided, the result of the intervention and the nurse who is responsible (Perry et al 2020).

There are many legal and ethical considerations that nurses must consider regarding nursing documentation. These include ensuring the individual's privacy, confidentiality and consent, as well as fulfilling professional documentation guidelines (Staunton & Chiarella 2020). Nursing documentation is a legal document and as such may be used for evidence within a coroner's investigation, disciplinary hearing and lawsuits; therefore, it is important that it follows professional guidelines and fulfils any necessary legal requirements. In a legal situation, documentation is essential and poor documentation can be detrimental. According to the legal system, 'if it is not documented, then it was not done' (Tollefson & Hillman 2022). Legal requirements that nursing documentation must adhere to include the correct identification of individuals' details, legible entries, recorded facts, only care that is personally delivered recorded, charted in chronological order, identification of the individual documenting, no obliterated records and minimal use of abbreviations, and the organisational policy for maintaining accountability must be observed.

HEALTH INFORMATICS

Health informatics is the interdisciplinary science of how to use data, information and knowledge to improve human health and delivery of healthcare, focusing on the use of health information technologies, and involves computers, analytical and social sciences (American Medical Informatics Association [AMIA] 2011; Nelson & Staggers 2018). Nursing informatics is a specialty within health informatics that integrates nursing science with multiple information management and analytical systems to identify, define, manage and communicate data, information, knowledge and wisdom in nursing practice and support decision-making (AMIA 2018). Essentially, it involves the use of computers, and information and communication technologies (ICT) to support nursing practice (McGonigle & Mastrian 2022). Given the rapid digital advancements and pervasive use of ICT in healthcare, an essential minimum standard of informatics knowledge and skills is necessary for all nurses to support nursing care activities and to operate effectively as clinicians in the digitally enabled work environment. Being equipped with core informatics competencies will assist nurses in the delivery of safer, better integrated and evidence-based care, resulting in positive health outcomes for the community (Australian Nursing and Midwifery Federation [ANMF] 2015; Hebda et al 2018). A basic level of knowledge of informatics concepts and principles, and digital capability, is vital for nursing students to be prepared for clinical placement settings and transitioning to professional practice (Raghunathan & Tomkins 2019).

Informatics competency is essential for all health professionals to be able to engage and interact with the different point-of-care technologies and information systems used to support clinical workflows, decision-making tools, health data management, and safety and quality improvements. Informatics skills and technology ability are critical to navigate the workplace information technologies and participate in decision-making to support safe and informed person-centred care (Nelson & Staggers 2018).

Information management and use of technology in delivery of care

Health information technologies (health IT) are a necessary and critical part of the evolving healthcare landscape with the advancement of 'digital health'—the use of sophisticated information and communication technology (ICT) for health (Rowlands 2019). Computerised health information systems such as electronic medical records (EMRs) are being implemented to improve access to health data, reduce healthcare costs, result in better integrated and safer care and improve overall care outcomes (McBride & Tietze 2019). EMRs are digital systems created and utilised within a single healthcare organisation such as a clinic, medical centre or hospital (Nelson & Staggers 2018). These health IT systems are the core of information management in the health setting. They incorporate many levels of health data that inform integrated clinical databases, workflows and clinical information and decision support systems used by clinicians. They are informatics tools designed to collect, store and make available important health data to facilitate individual care planning and clinical decision-making by clinicians (Hebda et al 2018).

Healthcare organisations rely on EMR systems for data gathering, communication and decision-making by clinicians, which involve interdisciplinary engagement, with nurses having an integral role in the collection, recording and managing of health data (McBride & Tietze 2019). Nurses need to be proficient in not only point-of-care technology skills, but also in utilising the various workplace health IT to support clinical decision-making and deliver high-quality and safe healthcare at the same time (Honey et al 2018; Hunter et al 2013; Raghunathan et al 2022).

In the clinical environment, a range of information systems are in use, and their functionality and applications vary between providers and the different care contexts. As frontline users of health IT, it is expected that nurses have some basic ICT skills, as well as informatics capabilities, to manage and use the technology and data applications at the point of care and in a variety of practice environments to deliver safe and competent person-centred care (Kleib & Nagle 2018; Rahman 2015). Competent use of ICT and related hardware and software underpins nursing informatics competencies. This includes actual psychomotor skills to use computer tools and devices confidently and specific informatics knowledge and skills, which require working with health data, processing information and contributing to knowledge development for nursing practice. Proficiency in the use of computing devices and workplace health IT systems used to manage clinical data and quality care is vital to support safe and informed clinical practice for health professionals.

Applying nursing informatics in practice

The application of nursing informatics knowledge and skill in everyday nursing practice processes involves active engagement with information technologies and computerised health information management systems in the practice environment. Informatics and technology skills are necessary for direct and indirect care processes. The way nurses use informatics skills in daily routine nursing care practice is through:

- The effective use of ICT to access, record, retrieve and manage health data
- Interpretation and organisation of health information for decision support and nursing care
- Synthesising the health data to generate new knowledge for nursing practice (McGonigle & Mastrian 2022).

Nurses play a significant role in health information processes, being at the frontline in the delivery of care, and informatics skills are essential for nurses in the ubiquitous IT-enhanced healthcare environment. With increasing adoption of digital information systems, such as EMRs by healthcare organisations, it is important that nurses are equipped with adequate informatics capabilities to engage with the hardware and software of health IT and critically manage the health data to support person-centred safe and quality care for the individual (Hebda et al 2018; McBride & Tietze 2019). Knowledge of clinical data systems and informatics competencies will assist nurses to not only support effective care delivery, but also improve healthcare outcomes for individuals through informed and evidence-based clinical decisions at the point of care.

Nursing informatics standards and digital health capabilities

In Australia, the *National Informatics Standards for Nurses and Midwives* (ANMF 2015), developed with funding from the Australian government, provide a framework and a set of essential and minimum informatics competencies that nurses should possess to operate in the technology-dependent healthcare contexts. The standards serve as a detailed resource and a valuable tool for practising nurses, educators and nursing students to build informatics capability to support practice (Reeves 2016).

Three domains of practice for nursing informatics education and competence for nurses at all levels are identified in these standards; they include computer literacy, information literacy and information management. There are technical, cognitive and application-based competencies necessary to support routine daily nursing practice activities and processes in the digital work environment described within these informatics standards. Adherence to professional practice requirements, legal and ethical parameters and compliance with local policies and procedures are essential criteria within each domain of the standards.

Aligned with the nursing informatics standards is the Australian *National Nursing and Midwifery Digital Health Capabilities Framework*, which provides guidance for individuals and organisations towards developing digital health knowledge and skills in an increasingly ICT-embedded work environment (Australian Digital Health Agency [ADHA] 2020). Five key domains broadly set within the context of roles, workplace settings and the professional standards informing practice are identified: digital professionalism, leadership and advocacy, data and information quality, information-enabled care and technology. Three progressive achievement levels, from novice to expert, are also described for each capability area: formative, intermediate and proficient, which relate to the role and practice setting of the professional (ADHA 2020). The informatics standards and digital health capability framework should be used by nurses to evaluate own individual capability, which can then be used to inform continuing professional development needs.

Nursing informatics competencies

In the practice setting, the required level of work-related informatics proficiency among health professionals will vary depending on the clinician's specific work area and role, which can be viewed along a continuum from basic to advanced competencies as informatics specialists (Nelson & Staggers 2018). Clinical Skill 8.2, presented in this chapter, describes the core informatics competencies necessary to support beginning-level nurses in everyday routine nursing activities in the delivery of healthcare, no matter where they work.

The level of performance identified within the skill (Clinical Skill 8.2) is a basic level of proficiency. It outlines essential professional practice requirements and fundamental computer technology and information management skills needed to use informatics tools utilised in the healthcare setting. The aim is to facilitate a key set of transferable knowledge and skills for students to be comfortable and confident to manage encounters with the health IT used in different clinical environments during placements, as well as preparation for entering the health workforce. On entry to practice, it will be necessary to develop a more specific and advanced understanding of health informatics concepts and processes depending on context, the nurse's role and different ICT applications in the work setting. As with all nursing competencies, a commitment to lifelong learning and ongoing continuing education is necessary to keep up to date with evolving health IT advancements to support practice.

The skill has been developed based on the three domains of practice identified by the *National Informatics Standards for Nurses and Midwives* (ANMF 2015). It is aligned to the *National Nursing and Midwifery Digital Health Capability Framework* (ADHA 2020), as well as the *Code of Conduct for Nurses* (Nursing and Midwifery Board of Australia [NMBA] 2018), and *Enrolled Nurse Standards for Practice* (NMBA 2016) (currently under review at the time of print). It is also informed by Australian and international perspectives on nursing informatics competency within the nursing education curriculum.

The following four areas of competence can assist to facilitate a basic level of knowledge and skills to guide quality, safety and informed practice. The nursing informatics competencies to support beginning-level practice include:

- *Digital literacy:* the application of basic knowledge and skills in ICT to support work practice
- *Professional practice:* working in accordance with the legal and regulatory requirements, professional standards, and ethical principles for all uses of ICT used in work practice
- *Information literacy:* application of fundamental knowledge and skills to identify, locate, access, evaluate and apply information to support work practice
- *Information management:* application of fundamental knowledge and skills in collection, use, management, storage of data and information, and ICT systems to support safe and informed practice.

 CASE STUDY 8.2

Documenting progress notes

Mr Q returned from operating theatre at 1600 hrs post right video-assisted thoracotomy (VAT) and wedge biopsy for diagnosis of right lung pathology. He returned to the ward with oxygen 6 L/min via a Hudson mask (HM) maintaining oxygen saturations (SpO$_2$) greater than 94%. Intravenous 1L 0.9% sodium chloride infusing at 80 mL/hour. Tolerating ice only orally. Fentanyl patient-controlled analgesia (PCA) providing effective pain relief, pain score as per patient 2/10. Indwelling urinary catheter (IDC) output 50 mL–110 mL/hour. Two chest drains (ICC) are combined into one underwater seal drain (UWSD) with 300 mL of haemoserous fluid drained, 10 cm H$_2$O suction, swing and air leak are present. Cutifilm dressing is intact to right thoracotomy wound, clean and dry. Vital signs: blood pressure 100/84 mmHg, respiratory rate 12 breaths/minute, pulse rate 88 beats/min.

Use this information to write a nursing progress note using the following formats: SOAPIE, PIE and DAR.

CRITICAL THINKING EXERCISE 8.8

You are a nurse working in a medical–surgical ward. The EMR system implemented at the hospital is relatively new. You have been assigned a new client, an 80-year-old man with multiple heath issues including diabetes, hypertension and chronic kidney disease requiring multidisciplinary care. He has a history of falls and impaired skin integrity. You complete a nursing assessment including vital signs, physical assessment, current medications and relevant medical history. Based on the admission assessment, identify the information (key components) that should be recorded in the EMR system. Consider the potential consequences of inaccurate or incomplete documentation for this individual's care.

CLINICAL SKILL 8.1 Documentation

Please adhere to the policy and procedures of the facility/organisation prior to undertaking the skill. Ensure this skill is in your scope of practice.

NMBA Decision-making Framework considerations (refer to NMBA Decision-making framework for nursing and midwifery 2020):	Equipment:
1. Am I educated? 2. Am I authorised? 3. Am I competent? If you answer 'no' to any of these, do not perform that activity. Seek guidance and support from your teacher/a nurse team leader/clinical facilitator/educator.	Individual care profile/individual history Progress note Pen (blue or black) for handwritten notes Computer (if electronic records)

 PREPARE FOR THE SKILL

(Please refer to the Standard Steps on p. xii for related rationales.)
Mentally review the steps of the skill.
Discuss the skill with your instructor/supervisor/team leader, if required.
Confirm correct facility/organisation policy/safe operating procedures.
Validate the order in the individual's record.
Identify indication and rationale for performing the activity.
Assess for any contraindications.
Locate and gather equipment.
Perform hand hygiene.
Ensure therapeutic interaction.
Identify the individual using three individual identifiers.
Gain the individual's consent.
Assess for pain relief.
Prepare the environment.
Provide and maintain privacy.
Assist the individual to assume an appropriate position of comfort.

 PERFORM THE SKILL

(Please refer to the Standard Steps on p. xii for related rationales.)
Perform hand hygiene.
Apply PPE: gloves, eyewear, mask and gown as appropriate.
Ensure the individual's safety and comfort throughout skill.
Promote independence and involvement of the individual if possible and/or appropriate.
Assess the individual's tolerance to the skill throughout.
Dispose of used supplies, equipment, waste and sharps appropriately.
Remove PPE and discard or store appropriately.
Perform hand hygiene.

Skill activity	Rationale
Documenting in progress notes	
Review individual's assessment data and problems identified (e.g. nursing diagnosis, goals, expected outcomes, interventions and individual's responses during each contact).	Makes it easier to document in an organised/structured manner and decreases errors.
After contact with the individual, identify information that needs to be documented. Consider abnormal findings, changes in individual's status and any new problem identification.	Ensures quality. Ensures accurate and timely information and continuity of information. Ensures completion of documentation in a timely manner. Therefore, the record is contemporaneous.
Obtain necessary forms or access appropriate computer for documentation depending on hospital protocol.	In accordance with legal requirements for documentation. Charting on the correct form ensures the information can be accessed efficiently by other health professionals.

CLINICAL SKILL 8.1 Documentation—cont'd

Ensure the documentation is correctly identifiable with the individual's details: full name, date of birth and gender. Generally, this will be with an identification label attached to the healthcare record.	In accordance with legal requirements for documentation and to reduce the risk of errors in documentation.
Use a blue or black pen. Ensure your writing is legible, free of blank areas, comprehensible and contemporaneous.	In accordance with legal requirements for documentation. Makes the reporting more legible and ensures the correct sequence of events and that correct treatment is provided to the individual. Blank spaces should be eliminated to ensure no incorrect information is added into the space.
Record date and time using the dd/mm/yy system and 24-hour clock for each entry.	In accordance with legal requirements for documentation. This ensures the correct sequence of events is recorded.
In conjunction with facility/organisation policy and recommended format, document in chronological order the following: • Pertinent, factual, objective data • Selected subjective data that validates and clarifies (avoid subjective statements) • Nursing actions taken • Evaluation of the individual's responses to nursing actions • Any additional nursing actions needed • To whom information has been reported, including name and status.	Ensures high-quality documentation is attained in order to enhance efficient and individualised care and that documentation is completed to professional standards as for legal requirements.
Depending on the facility/organisation procedure, make a progress note entry using the SOAP format. The SOAP format consists of subjective data, objective data, assessment and plan and is usually based on a numbered list of problems or nursing diagnoses.	Written plans are developed to deal with each problem the individual has. As more problems develop, more plans are made, and additionally as more problems are resolved, the plans are completed and no longer addressed in the documentation.
Depending on the facility/organisation procedure, make a progress note using the PIE format. The PIE format consists of problem, intervention and evaluation. It is a problem-orientated system in which documentation is based on individual problems.	This format is used to address problems identified during baseline assessment and monitor during care. This tends to be more nursing-focused and flexible with specific information easier to find.
Depending on the facility/organisation procedure, make a progress note using a basic narrative note format. This is not using a problem list but tells a story/account of the individual's problem, interventions and outcomes in a chronological order.	Narrative documentation can tend to be repetitive, especially in long-term care.
Depending on facility/organisation procedure, make a progress note using a CBE: charting by exception format. This progress note will describe any deviations from the individual's normal assessment findings and can sometimes be described as a variance. This is usually completed in addition to care pathways.	Reduces the amount of time and documentation required. It relies on the nurses using the established flow sheets, graphic records, standard protocols and care plans or pathways that are already in place to ensure continuous appropriate care is provided.
Ensure your writing is error-free or if you make an error it is crossed out with a single line through it and 'error' plus your initials written above.	In accordance with legal requirements for documentation. Chart may become illegible and it can appear you were attempting to hide information. It is important that errors are corrected promptly to ensure no errors in treatment.
Only care that has been personally delivered is documented, with the exception being in an emergency situation, in which case a designated scribe is in control of all recording of information.	In accordance with legal requirements for documentation.
Record the individual's response to treatment.	Allows for ineffective treatment to be ceased and effective interventions to continue.

Continued

CLINICAL SKILL 8.1 Documentation—cont'd

Ensure appropriate medical/health terminology and approved abbreviations and acronyms are used.	In accordance with legal and facility requirements for documentation. Reduces the chance of errors and ineffective communication, therefore improving individual safety.
Sign the progress note with full name or first initial and last name and status according to healthcare organisation policy. If you are a student, you need to indicate your school affiliation and level of education.	In accordance with legal requirements for documentation. Documents who is accountable for the information written and care provided.
If documenting a late entry, this must follow the last entry and be noted as such: either 'addit' or 'late entry' written beside the time you actually wrote the notation. The time of the original occurrence must also be documented within the note.	In accordance with legal requirements for documentation.

Skill activity	**Rationale**
Use of electronic medical records (EMRs)	
Sign on to EMR using your password; never share passwords and keep your password private.	For accountability purposes, your user name and password become your electronic signature and therefore you are accepting accountability for your documentation. This ensures data security, and only authorised personnel access the health records.
Do not leave individual's information on the monitor/screen where others can view it.	The individual's privacy and confidentiality must be maintained.
Review assessment data, problems identified (e.g. nursing diagnosis, goals, expected outcomes, interventions and individual's responses during each contact).	Makes it easier to document in an organised manner and decreases errors.
Follow procedures for entering and updating information in all workflow areas or appropriate menu items or forms in the EMR.	Some programs will not allow pages to be entered until other forms or procedures are completed to ensure documentation is complete.
Review previously documented entries with those that you enter, identifying if there is any significant change in the individual's health status or care and report as needed.	Changes in medical, physical, emotional or psychological condition are documented to report and alert other healthcare professionals to potential complications.
Know and implement procedures to address documentation errors in the EMR.	This may be different across various computer programs and is important to be done promptly to ensure errors in individual's treatment and care do not occur.
Save information as you complete documentation.	Information may be lost if you do not save your documentation.
Log off when you leave the computer or finish using the system.	

Note: Documentation must be completed according to the facility/organisation's guidelines and policy. Therefore, it is important to become familiar with different formats of documentation and their best indications of use.
You need not document information that is already charted on flowcharts, unless that information is relevant to other pertinent information you are recording. Content of documentation will depend on the individual and their condition. But whatever the individual's condition, there should always be nursing interventions documented and the individual's response to these.
When documenting, remember the guidelines for quality documentation:
- Factual
- Accurate
- Complete
- Concise
- Current
- Organised.

CLINICAL SKILL 8.1 Documentation—cont'd

 AFTER THE SKILL

(Please refer to the Standard Steps on p. xii for related rationales.)

Communicate outcome to the individual, any ongoing care and to report any complications.

Restore the environment.

Report, record and document assessment findings, details of the skill performed and the individual's response.

Report, record and document any abnormalities and/or inability to perform the skill.

Reassess the individual to ensure there are no adverse effects/events from the skill.

(Crisp et al 2021; Perry et al 2020; Tollefson & Hillman 2022)

OBSERVATION CHECKLIST: DOCUMENTATION

STUDENT NAME: _____

CLINICAL SKILL 8.1: Documentation

DEMONSTRATION OF: The ability to accurately and appropriately record information about an individual in a timely manner

If the observation checklist is being used as an assessment tool, the student will need to obtain a scale of independence for each of the performance criteria/evidence.

Independent (I)

Supervised (S)

Assisted (A)

Marginal (M)

Dependent (D)

COMPETENCY ELEMENTS	PERFORMANCE CRITERIA/EVIDENCE	I	S	A	M	D
Preparation for the activity	Identifies indications and rationale for performing the activity Identifies the individual using three individual identifiers Ensures therapeutic interaction Checks facility/organisation policy Locates and gathers equipment Discusses documentation with instructor/supervisor/team leader if required Obtains necessary forms or computer access appropriate for documentation					
Performs activity informed by evidence	Documenting in progress notes: • Ensures the documentation is identifiable with individual's details • Ensures writing is legible, free of blank areas, comprehensible and contemporaneous • Records date and time • Documents information in conjunction with the facility/organisation policy • Documents according to facility/organisation policy and using one of the following formats: SOAP format, PIE format, basic narrative note format or charting by exception format • Only documents care that has been personally delivered • Records the individual's response to treatment • Ensures appropriate medical terminology and approved abbreviations are being used • Ensures writing is error free; if there is an error it is crossed out with a single line • Signs the progress note according to the facility/organisation policy • Reviews previous documented entries to identify any changes in the individual's health status Documenting with electronic medical records (EMR): • Signs on to EMR system using electronic signature (password, code or personal identification number) • Does not leave individual's information on the monitor/screen where others can see it • Reviews assessment data and problems identified • Follows procedures for entering information in all appropriate program functions • Reviews previous documented entries to identify any changes in the individual's health status • Knows and implements procedures to correct documentation errors					

COMPETENCY ELEMENTS	PERFORMANCE CRITERIA/EVIDENCE	I	S	A	M	D
	• Saves information as documentation is completed • Logs off when leaving the computer terminal or finishing using the system					
Applies critical thinking and reflective practice	Is able to link theory to practice Demonstrates current best practice in the care provided Reviews the individual's history and identifies any significant changes in the individual's condition Assesses own performance					
Practises within safety and quality assurance guidelines	Reviews against facility/organisation policy Ensures individual's documented information remains confidential Ensures documented content is relevant and accurate Adheres to legal requirements of documentation					
Documentation and communication	Reports and documents all relevant information and any complications correctly Reports any complications and/or inability to perform the procedure to the RN Explains and communicates the activity clearly to the individual Communicates outcome and ongoing care to individual and significant others Communicates abnormal findings to appropriate personnel					

Educator/Facilitator Feedback:

Educator/Facilitator Score: Competent   Needs further development

How would you rate your overall performance while undertaking this clinical activity? (use a ✓ & initial)

Unsatisfactory   Satisfactory   Good   Excellent

Student Reflection: (discuss how you would approach your practice differently or more effectively)

EDUCATOR/FACILITATOR NAME/SIGNATURE:

STUDENT NAME/SIGNATURE: DATE:

CLINICAL SKILL 8.2 Nursing informatics competency

Please adhere to the policy and procedures of the facility/organisation prior to undertaking the skill. Ensure this skill is in your scope of practice.

NMBA Decision-making Framework considerations (refer to NMBA Decision-making framework for nursing and midwifery 2020):	Equipment:
1. Am I educated? 2. Am I authorised? 3. Am I competent? If you answer 'no' to any of these, do not perform that activity. Seek guidance and support from your teacher/a nurse team leader/clinical facilitator/educator.	Computer (desktop, workstation or computers on wheels [COWs]) Tablets and handheld devices ICT external devices Multimedia tools Telecommunication tools Smartphones Internet web access Healthcare records Learning software/applications (e.g. simulated or academic EMR [electronic medication record]) Clinical information resources (e.g. drug reference, ClinicalKey) Evidence-based databases

PREPARE FOR THE SKILL

(Please refer to the Standard Steps on p. xii for related rationales.)
Mentally review the steps of the skill.
Discuss the skill with your instructor/supervisor/team leader, if required.
Confirm correct facility/organisation policy/safe operating procedures.
Validate the order in the individual's record.
Identify indication and rationale for performing the activity.
Assess for any contraindications.
Locate and gather equipment.
Perform hand hygiene.
Ensure therapeutic interaction.
Identify the individual using three individual identifiers.
Gain the individual's consent.
Assess for pain relief.
Prepare the environment.
Provide and maintain privacy.
Assist the individual to assume an appropriate position of comfort.

PERFORM THE SKILL

(Please refer to the Standard Steps on p. xii for related rationales.)
Perform hand hygiene.
Apply PPE: gloves, eyewear, mask and gown as appropriate.
Ensure the individual's safety and comfort throughout skill.
Promote independence and involvement of the individual if possible and/or appropriate.
Assess the individual's tolerance to the skill throughout.
Dispose of used supplies, equipment, waste and sharps appropriately.
Remove PPE and discard or store appropriately.
Perform hand hygiene.

Skill activity	Rationale
Digital literacy	
Application of basic knowledge and skills in information and communication technology (ICT) to support work practice	
Understand basic ICT terminology.	Knowledge of common ICT terminology such as web browser, website, cloud based, internet, intranet, interoperability, operating systems, home page, hypertext link, bookmark, URL (uniform resource locator) address, encryption, backing up.

CLINICAL SKILL 8.2 Nursing informatics competency—cont'd

Basic use of ICT to support work includes: • Computer system • Computer and device security • Electronic devices • Intranet, internet, the world wide web and Wi-Fi • Electronic communication tools • Electronic file management • Word processing • Spreadsheets • Databases • Presentation.	Demonstrates psychomotor skills as well as knowledge to use the software and device applications optimally. Able to use hardware (e.g. mouse, screen, workstation) and the software (primary operating systems, programs and applications) relevant to work; knows basic troubleshooting for checking power, rebooting and printing. Understands and respects legal and organisation policy guidelines to protect data privacy and confidentiality, login and logging out, suspending sessions and password protection. Protects against computer viruses and malware. Reports unauthorised use or breach to appropriate personnel. Knows how to use external/peripheral devices such as USBs, tablets and handheld devices, smartphones, apps and point of care (POC) digital devices, wearables. Able to use internal organisational (intranet, private networks, shared file servers) and external web-based (world wide web, cloud computing, internet browsers) systems. Able to use remote communication tools such as emails, facsimile, skype, online discussion forums, chat or other messaging applications and telehealth apps and tools. Able to navigate the computer operating systems to access installed applications such as Microsoft Windows to organise and manage information files and data. Able to use basic desktop software such as Microsoft Word and Excel to create, access, categorise and store reports and documents. Able to save, cut, copy, paste and delete information. Able to locate online search engines and electronic collections of data to research and search information. Able to use basic desktop software Microsoft PowerPoint and other web-based multimedia tools (e.g. videos, podcasts, YouTube, slideshow etc.).
Consider the workspace design, the environment and workstation safety.	Understands workplace health and safety requirements, to protect self and others in relation to equipment, body mechanics and safe work practices, and minimise risk of injury or harm. Includes bedside, workstation and portable technology.
Skill activity	**Rationale**
Professional practice	
Work in accordance with the legal and regulatory requirements, professional standards and ethical principles for all uses of ICT in work practice	
Uphold the legal, regulatory and ethical standards related to the use of digital health information.	Understands and respects legislation and policies. For example, data security, storage, disposal, protection of health information, privacy, confidentiality, individual's rights, impact on individual and community, harmful content, safety, social media, professional boundaries, passwords, information sharing, unauthorised or illegal use and breaches in data security. Standards for safe and appropriate use of ICT in health. For example, the Australian Council on Healthcare Standards (ACHS) (EQuIP) *Information Management Standard* includes: criteria for health records management; corporate records management; collection, use and storage of information; and information and communication technology.

Continued

CLINICAL SKILL 8.2 Nursing informatics competency—cont'd

Follow requirements for intellectual property, copyright and fair use of copyrighted material.	Understands and respects legislation and policies pertaining to patents, design, trademarks, authorship, publications, ownership of material etc. Aware of Australian *Copyright Act 1968*, statutes, fair dealings, provisions and exceptions.
Consider cultural, ethical and socioeconomic issues related to accessing and using the information.	Understands and respects legislation and policies. For example, protection of privacy and confidentiality, impact on individual and community, human rights, cultural safety, access and equity issues.
Proactive use of ICT to improve health outcomes, support professional practice and lifelong learning.	Actively promotes and engages in the use of educational, informatics and other ICT tools to build on digital capability to support work, professional development and ongoing learning.
Skill activity	**Rationale**
Information literacy	
Application of fundamental knowledge and skills to identify, locate, access, evaluate and apply information to support work practice	
Use the internet to search, locate and download relevant information.	Able to use basic online searching options through a search engine to locate organisations, services, websites etc. (e.g. Google, Ask.com, Bing).
Plan and use online search strategies for scholarly literature.	Knows how to conduct literature search and locate evidence-based resources and websites to support informed and safe practice. Knows how to use available proprietary search databases such as PubMed, MEDLINE, CINAHL, EBSCO, JBI, EMBASE etc.
Use multiple sources of data to retrieve information to support work.	Able to use various and additional services such as library resources, professional associations, government websites, research institutes, peak bodies, community resources, relevant experts and practitioners to obtain or retrieve information needed to support clinical judgment and evidence-based decision-making.
Use ICT and informatics tools to obtain information.	Able to use electronic records, POC databases, clinical applications and communication tools to assist workflow, evidence-based decision-making and care planning, and for health teaching. For example, digital systems for care plans, admission and discharge, clinical information systems (CIS), handovers, medication management and proprietary clinical decision solutions such as ClinicalKey and UpToDate.

CLINICAL SKILL 8.2 Nursing informatics competency—cont'd

Evaluate various sources of information.	Ensures information is evidence-based, best practice, current and supports safe and informed high-quality practice. Analyses and understands the available information by critically evaluating reliability, currency, validity, accuracy, authority, timeliness and point of view or bias in information for determining its suitability and appropriate use. For example, guidelines, policies, procedures and protocols, scholarly and best practice literature. Recognises specific cultural, physical or other context of information. Understands the background and specific nature or type of information, including its range and limitations, when interpreting and applying it to practice. For example, population health, demography, cultural safety, gender, specific health needs etc.
Manage information collected or generated.	Organises and documents data and information using ICT tools. Appropriate use of POC digital tools and CIS (e.g. vital signs, measurements, observations, progress notes, care plans, medication management), electronic record systems (e.g. EMRs, EHRs and personal health records [PHRs]) and other ICT tools used in healthcare.
Skill activity	**Rationale**
Information management	
Application of fundamental knowledge and skills in collection, use, management and storage of data, information and ICT to support safe and informed practice	
Recognise digital data storage methods and formats.	Knowledge of EHRs, EMRs, PHRs (e.g. My Health Record), including levels and types of POC applications. For example, practice management systems, patient administration systems, bed management systems, hospital management systems, aged-care and long-term care systems, clinical portals and patient acuity systems, digital monitoring systems, prescribing and medication administration systems, order entry systems, health and safety reporting, quality and audit systems, and clinical data repositories and POC decision tools.
Distinguish between data and information and how it can be used to support work.	Understands that data is raw, unorganised and unprocessed individual information (facts) that may not be useful by itself. When this data is organised, processed and given context to make it meaningful it becomes information. For example, by itself, a person's vital signs, measurements, pathology or diagnostic test results are raw data. When this data is organised and presented to obtain a picture of the person's health it is information about the individual.
Use of digital records and information systems appropriately.	Knows how to use digital health records, clinical databases and other informatics tools for accessing and investigating information to support safe and informed practice as per organisation policy (e.g. use of EMR, EHRs, PHRs, CIS and other data systems).

Continued

CLINICAL SKILL 8.2 Nursing informatics competency—cont'd

Integrate and use digital communication.	Communicates remotely with other healthcare professionals, services, colleagues and healthcare recipients/their families/carers in delivery and management of timely care. Knows how to use networks, intranets and internet for emails, messaging, referrals, reports, handovers, transfers, telehealth etc.
Use data and statistical reports for quality improvement.	Understands value and link between quality nursing care and health outcomes, which has the ability to influence policy, budgets, practice, allocation of resources, research and education. For example, episode of care outcomes and activities can be evaluated for improvements.
Recognise common informatics classifications, coding systems and languages.	Aware of technical and IT specific coding systems, classifications, standard terminology and language used to describe, standardise and collate the computer data or common set of data to make it meaningful. For example, application of data standards, minimum datasets, clinical dictionaries and clinical language systems such as Systemised Nomenclature of Medicine (SNOMED), International Classification of Diseases (ICD-10), the North American Nursing Diagnosis Association (NANDA), Nursing Interventions Classification (NIC) and Nursing Outcomes Classification (NOC) and the International Classification for Nursing Practice (ICNP).
Maintain accurate and up-to-date records and documentation.	Accurate, comprehensive, timely and up-to-date information enhances quality of data and increases reliability and validity of information to guide timely decisions and improve safety and health outcomes.
Interdisciplinary and stakeholder engagement relating to digital records.	Demonstrates interprofessional interdisciplinary and individual/family/carer collaboration for effective and efficient holistic and person-centred model of care. Uses digital applications and information methods for health teaching.

Note: There are several different information systems in the clinical environment. How each facility and healthcare agency use these information management and clinical support systems varies. With rapid technology developments and ICT constantly evolving, new POC and information management solutions to improve health services and delivery of care continue to emerge. In reality, it is not practical to learn the use of each and every individual ICT tool in the work environment. Therefore, the emphasis for developing nursing informatics competencies among nursing students is an understanding of the core principles and essential skills that can be built upon with ongoing exposure to health IT and professional experiences.

Due to liability for data entry errors, confidentiality and data security concerns, some facilities may restrict or only allow limited access to the digital systems during clinical placement for students. At some clinical facilities, students may be required to complete an orientation module before being allowed access to the system. In the clinical environment, all staff are required to complete user training modules before being allowed to use the health IT systems.

It is recommended that students optimise opportunities to master ICT and informatics skills through educational and communication technologies used in the course and the institution.

CLINICAL SKILL 8.2 Nursing informatics competency—cont'd

 AFTER THE SKILL

(Please refer to the Standard Steps on p. xii for related rationales.)
Communicate outcome to the individual, any ongoing care and to report any complications.
Restore the environment.
Report, record and document assessment findings, details of the skill performed and the individual's response.
Report, record and document any abnormalities and/or inability to perform the skill.
Reassess the individual to ensure there are no adverse effects/events from the skill.

(ANMF 2015; Honey et al 2018; Hunter et al 2013; Kleib & Nagle 2018; Rahman 2015; Yoon et al 2015)

OBSERVATION CHECKLIST: NURSING INFORMATICS COMPETENCY

STUDENT NAME: _____

CLINICAL SKILL 8.2: Nursing informatics competency

DEMONSTRATION OF: The ability to apply essential information and communication technology, and informatics knowledge and skills to guide quality, safety and informed practice

If the observation checklist is being used as an assessment tool, the student will need to obtain a scale of independence for each of the performance criteria/evidence.

Independent (I)
Supervised (S)
Assisted (A)
Marginal (M)
Dependent (D)

COMPETENCY ELEMENTS	PERFORMANCE CRITERIA/EVIDENCE	I	S	A	M	D
Preparation for the activity	Identifies indications and rationale for performing the activity Checks facility/organisation policy Locates and gathers equipment/resources Discusses activity with instructor/supervisor/team leader if required Obtains necessary instructions and computer/ICT access					
Performs activity informed by evidence	Information and communication technology (ICT): • Uses ICT hardware and peripheral devices appropriately • Uses ICT safely (data security, protection, password, login and log out, suspending sessions, work health and safety) • Demonstrates basic troubleshooting skills (power, rebooting and printing) • Uses computer operating systems • Uses the intranet, internet and Wi-Fi to support work • Uses digital/telecommunication tools and networks, and emails effectively • Navigates Microsoft Windows environment effectively • Uses word processing applications • Uses spreadsheet applications • Uses presentation tools and multimedia presentations Information literacy: • Searches and locates information online • Plans and conducts database literature searches • Accesses evidence-based sources of information related to nursing practice and care • Able to access multiple sources for information • Synthesises data from various sources • Organises and manages information collected					

COMPETENCY ELEMENTS	PERFORMANCE CRITERIA/EVIDENCE	I	S	A	M	D
	Information management: • Uses digital technology to enter health data (health history, assessments, vital signs, physiological data) • Uses digital clinical monitoring systems effectively (bedside, mobile, handheld, remote, wearables) • Accesses, enters and retrieves data from health information systems • Uses database applications to access, enter and retrieve data and information • Uses digital health records to document care • Uses computer applications for care planning and discharge planning • Uses decision support systems (alerts, workflow triggers, expert systems and other information supports) for clinical decision-making and care planning • Uses information systems to communicate and coordinate information flow with health team • Uses information systems to improve health outcomes and to assist in health teaching • Uses information systems to support professional practice and lifelong learning					
Applies critical thinking and reflective practice	Is able to link theory to practice Demonstrates current best practice Recognises relevance of health and nursing data for improving practice Awareness of limitations of digital systems Recognises factors for human–computer interface Recognises need for ongoing learning for informatics skills and knowledge development Assesses own performance					
Practises within safety and quality assurance guidelines	Reviews against facility/organisation policy Adheres to legal and regulatory requirements and ethical principles related to use of ICT and digital health information. Follows requirements for intellectual property, copyright and fair use of copyrighted material Uses ICT to improve health outcomes. Uses ICT to support professional practice and lifelong learning					
Documentation and communication	Reports and documents all relevant information and any problems correctly Reports any issues, complications or problems to appropriate personnel Explains and communicates the activity clearly to the person/s Communicates variances or problems to appropriate personnel					

Educator/Facilitator Feedback:

Educator/Facilitator Score: Competent   Needs further development

How would you rate your overall performance while undertaking this skill activity in the four areas? (use a ✓ & initial)

1. **Digital Literacy**

Unsatisfactory   Satisfactory   Good   Excellent

2. **Professional Practice**

Unsatisfactory   Satisfactory   Good   Excellent

3. **Information Literacy**

Unsatisfactory   Satisfactory   Good   Excellent

4. **Information Management**

Unsatisfactory   Satisfactory   Good   Excellent

Student Reflection: (discuss how you would approach your practice differently or more effectively)

EDUCATOR/FACILITATOR NAME/SIGNATURE:

STUDENT NAME/SIGNATURE: **DATE:**

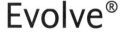 Answer guide for the Critical Thinking Exercises and Critical Thinking Questions in Case Studies is hosted on Evolve: http://evolve.elsevier.com/AU/Koutoukidis/Tabbner/

References

American Medical Informatics Association (AMIA), 2011. What is informatics? Fact Sheet. Online. Available at: <https://www.amia.org/fact-sheets/what-informatics>.

American Medical Informatics Association (AMIA), 2018. Nursing Informatics: IMIA Special Interest Group on Nursing Informatics 2009. Available at: <https://amia.org/communities/nursing-informatics>.

American Medical Informatics Association, 2018. Nursing Informatics: IMIA Special Interest Group on Nursing Informatics 2009. Available at: <https://amia.org/communities/nursing-informatics>.

Australian Digital Health Agency (ADHA), 2020. National Nursing and Midwifery Digital Health Capability Framework. Australian Government, Sydney. Available at: <https://www.digitalhealth.gov.au/sites/default/files/2020-11/National_Nursing_and_Midwifery_Digital_Health_Capability_Framework_publication.pdf>.

Australian Nursing and Midwifery Federation (ANMF), 2015. National Informatics Standards for Nurses and Midwives. Australian Government Department of Health and Ageing. Online. Available at: <https://anmf.org.au/documents/National_Informatics_Standards_For_Nurses_And_Midwives.pdf>.

Crisp, J., Douglas, C., Rebeiro, G., et al. (eds.), 2021. *Potter & Perry's fundamentals of nursing*, 6th ed. Elsevier, Chatswood.

Hebda, T.L., Hunter, K., Czar, P., 2018. *Handbook of informatics for nurses & healthcare professionals*. Pearson Higher Education, Boston, MA.

Honey, M., Collins, E., Britnell, S., 2018. Guidelines: Informatics for nurses entering practice 2018. Auckland, New Zealand. Available at: <http://doi.org/10.17608/k6.auckland.7273037>.

Hunter, K.M., McGonigle, D.M., Hebda, T.L., 2013. TIGER-based measurement of nursing informatics competencies: The development and implementation of an online tool for self-assessment. *Journal of Nursing Education and Practice* 3(12), 70–80. Available at: <https://doi.org/10.5430/jnep.v3n12p70>.

Kleib, M., Nagle, L., 2018. Development of the Canadian nurse informatics competency assessment scale and evaluation of Alberta's registered nurses' self-perceived informatics competencies. *Computers Informatics Nursing (CIN)* 36(7), 350–358. https://doi.org/10.1097/CIN.0000000000000435.

McBride, S., Tietze, M., 2019. *Nursing informatics for the advanced practice nurse: Patient safety, quality, outcomes, and interprofessionalism*, 2nd ed. Springer, New York.

McGonigle, D., Mastrian, K., 2022. *Nursing informatics and the foundation of knowledge*, 5th ed. Jones Bartlett Learning, Burlington, MA.

Nelson, R., Staggers, N., 2018. *Health informatics: An interprofessional approach*, 2nd ed. Elsevier, St Louis.

Nursing and Midwifery Board of Australia (NMBA), 2016. Enrolled Nurse Standards for Practice. Available at: <https://www.nursingmidwiferyboard.gov.au/Codes-Guidelines-Statements/Professional-standards.aspx#>.

Nursing and Midwifery Board of Australia (NMBA), 2018. Code of Conduct for Nurses. Available at: <https://www.nursingmidwiferyboard.gov.au/Codes-Guidelines-Statements/Professional-standards.aspx#>.

Nursing and Midwifery Board of Australia (NMBA), 2020. Decision-making framework for nursing and midwifery. Available at: <https://www.nursingmidwiferyboard.gov.au/Codes-Guidelines-Statements/Frameworks.aspx>.

Perry, A., Potter, P., Ostendorf, W., 2020. *Nursing interventions and clinical skills*, 7th ed. Elsevier, St Louis.

Raghunathan, K., Tomkins, Z., 2019. Preparing future nurses for the technology enabled work environment. The Hive. Australian College of Nursing (ACN) Publications, 28, Summer ed.

Raghunathan, K., McKenna, L. Peddle, M., 2022. Informatics competency measurement instruments for nursing students: A rapid review. *Computers, Informatics, Nursing (CIN)* 40(7) 466–477. DOI: 10.1097/CIN.0000000000000860.

Rahman, A., 2015. Development of a nursing informatics competency assessment tool (NICAT) (Order No. 3734182). Available from ProQuest One Academic; Social Science Premium Collection. (1732389458.)

Reeves, J., 2016. All things digital. *Australian Nursing & Midwifery Journal* 24(3), 13.

Rowlands, D., 2019. What is digital health? And why does it matter. Digital Health Workforce Academy and Health Informatics Society Australia (HISA). White Paper. Available at: <https://www.hisa.org.au/wp-content/uploads/2019/12/What_is_Digital_Health.pdf?x97063>.

Staunton, P.J., Chiarella, M., 2020. *Law for nurses and midwives*, 9th ed. Elsevier, Chatswood.

Tollefson, J., Hillman, E., 2022. *Clinical psychomotor skills*, 8th ed. Cengage Learning, Melbourne.

Tollefson, J., Watson, G., Jelly, E., et al., 2022. *Essential clinical skills: Enrolled nurses*, 5th ed. Cengage Learning, Melbourne.

Yoon, S., Shaffer, J.A., Bakken, S., 2015. Refining a self-assessment of informatics competency scale using Mokken scaling analysis. *Journal of Interprofessional Care*, 29(6) 579–586. Available at: <https://doi.org/10.3109/13561820.2015.1049340>.

COMMUNICATION AND CLINICAL HANDOVER

Michelle McKay

Overview

CLINICAL HANDOVER

Clinical handover is a core nursing skill and a critical procedure that occurs at transitions of care where all or part of an individual's care is transferred between clinicians, for example, change of shift and multidisciplinary rounds, healthcare locations or when discharged (Marin 2019; ACSQHC 2021). The process of clinical handover involves the nurse or healthcare professional providing an accurate, current and relevant summary of the individual's overall condition, care plan, interventions and outcomes. Handover preserves continuity of care by providing a current update of knowledge to the health professional taking accountability for the individual's care, builds rapport between health professionals, provides support and comfort, provides an opportunity for shared critical thinking, allows debriefing, clarifies information and can highlight the need for further action dependent on the efficiency of the transmission of the individual's health information (O'Toole 2020).

Clinical handover can be completed using a variety of methods, and locations may include in a private, quiet room or by the individual's bedside in the healthcare setting. It can be conducted orally in person or via a recorded medium; it can be done in a group or individually, depending on the healthcare facility protocol and the department. In each handover setting it is important that privacy and confidentiality are managed, especially when performing bedside handover (Perry et al 2019).

Clinical handover should be person-centred and encourage patient involvement. A structured and standardised process of individual handover is seen as key in improving individual safety (Porritt 2022; Burgess et al 2020), with organisations adopting a documented clinical handover checklist tool as well as bedside handover to increase individual safety. Nurses should discuss individuals and their families in a professional manner and ensure compliance with the national Nursing and Midwifery Board of Australia's (2016) *Enrolled nurse standards for practice* in regard to reports and the information contained within.

Poor communication during clinical handover can increase communication errors within and between health service organisations, increasing the risk of nursing care errors; therefore, accurate knowledge of the individual being handed over is imperative and crucial to the provision of the individual's comfort and safety (Perry et al 2019; Tollefson et al 2021). Clinical handover has been a focus of quality improvement in Australia since 2007, with recent focus being on structures and frameworks needed to improve quality and, therefore, individual safety (Crisp et al 2021; Marin 2019).

The Australian Commission on Safety and Quality in Health Care (ACSQHC) has developed National Safety and Quality Health Service (NSQHS) Standards aimed at achieving a nationally consistent set of standards for safety and quality in all areas of healthcare services. There are eight Standards, one of which is 'Communicating for safety', which includes clinical handover. The 'Communicating for safety' Standard ensures safe individual care by ensuring that timely and relevant clinical handover is attained in a structured manner (ACSQHC 2023).

Clinical handover methods can be unreliable and vary according to different clinicians, healthcare facilities and situations, which is why it is considered a high-risk area regarding the safety of individuals. There are six principles for clinical handover:

Principle 1: Preparing and scheduling clinical handover.

Principle 2: Having the relevant information at clinical handover.

Principle 3: Organising relevant clinicians and others to participate.

Principle 4: Being aware of the patient's goals and preferences.

Principle 5: Supporting patients, carers and families to be involved in clinical handover in accordance with the wishes of the patients.

Principle 6: Ensuring that clinical handover results in the transfer of responsibility and accountability for care.

(ACSQHC 2021; ACSQHC 2023)

ISBAR is an example of a structured clinical handover tool, allowing clinical handover information to be clear, focused and relevant. ISBAR follows the following structure:

- I —Identify
- S—Situation
- B —Background
- A —Assessment
- R —Recommendation.
  (ACSQHC 2021; ACSQHC 2023; Kaltoft et al 2021)

ISBAR can be used in a variety of clinical conversations and can be customised for the clinical context. It assists in the safe transfer of information and therefore ensures that an individual's safety and quality of care is maintained. This chapter will describe the skills needed for effective clinical handover (see Clinical Skill 10.1).

CASE STUDY 10.2

David Malcolm, 40 years old, was admitted to hospital with bilateral pneumonia after seeing his GP. The nurse told him to drink plenty of water and ambulate within his room as tolerated. David was not very mobile due to having multiple IV lines and a protracted cough with moderate pleuritic pain. The following morning, David reported a throbbing pain in his right leg and stated he was having trouble walking. The nurse replied that this was to be expected because he wasn't really mobilising so was probably stiff from lying in bed. He was encouraged to move more in bed and up to the toilet. David's sister arrived that evening and found him to be in severe pain from his right leg. She pulled back the sheets and saw that his right leg was twice the size of his left leg and promptly alerted the nurse. She told the nurse there was a family history of Factor V Leiden in their family and that David had this gene. The doctor was called, an urgent doppler was performed where the diagnosis of multiple deep vein thrombosis was made. David was commenced on an intravenous thrombolytic, compression stockings were applied, and David was told by the doctor he would need to be on oral anticoagulants for months.

It was not clear if information about David's Factor V Leiden and family history was communicated from the GP to the emergency department.

1. How would a handover using the ISBAR format, and a documented handover checklist have helped in this situation?
2. What would be the advantages of a structured clinical handover in this situation?

(NSW Department of Health 2019)

CRITICAL THINKING EXERCISE 10.2

Using the SBAR communication tool detailed in Table 10.8 in *Tabbner's Nursing Care: Theory and Practice* 9e, how would you hand over the details of the following situation? What recommendations would you make?

Maureen Smith, 73 years old, was admitted with nausea, vomiting, diarrhoea and lethargy following chemotherapy for breast cancer. She was commenced on IV fluids, IV antiemetics and placed in protective isolation. On entering her room to assess her vital signs you assess her blood pressure as 167/100 mmHg, heart rate as 120 beats/min and her temperature as 37.7°C. Her oxygen saturations are 92% on room air. She has shortness of breath and swelling of her face, hands and feet. You call the doctor for an urgent clinical, as indicated by the standard adult general observation chart. You position Maureen in the orthopneic position, apply oxygen at 4 litres/min via the nasal prongs and reassure Maureen that help is on the way. You decrease the IV fluids TKVO to maintain intravenous access.

On completion of this chapter, review Nursing Care Plan 10.1 in *Tabbner's Nursing Care: Theory and Practice* 9e. This sample demonstrates that effective communication was vital to developing appropriate nursing care.

CLINICAL SKILL 10.1 Clinical handover

Please adhere to the policy and procedures of the facility/organisation prior to undertaking the skill. Ensure this skill is in your scope of practice.

NMBA Decision-making Framework considerations (refer to NMBA Decision-making framework for nursing and midwifery 2020):	Equipment:
1. Am I educated? 2. Am I authorised? 3. Am I competent? If you answer 'no' to any of these, do not perform that activity. Seek guidance and support from your teacher/a nurse team leader/clinical facilitator/educator.	Handover sheet Care board/journey board Individual care charts as necessary (health record, observation charts, medication charts, fluid balance charts, care plan and risk assessment charts)

 PREPARE FOR THE SKILL

(Please refer to the Standard Steps on p. xii for related rationales.)
Mentally review the steps of the skill.
Discuss the skill with your instructor/supervisor/team leader, if required.
Confirm correct facility/organisation policy/safe operating procedures.
Validate the order in the individual's record.
Identify indication and rationale for performing the activity.
Assess for any contraindications.
Locate and gather equipment.
Perform hand hygiene.
Ensure therapeutic interaction.
Identify the individual using three individual identifiers.
Gain the individual's consent.
Assess for pain relief.
Prepare the environment.
Provide and maintain privacy.
Assist the individual to assume an appropriate position of comfort.

Skill activity	Rationale
All clinical handover	
Prepare for handover. Read the individual's medical record and check the individual's bedside charts to ensure accuracy. Plan what to say using a time planner guide or prompts as necessary. Gather all appropriate documentation.	Provides consistency and allows those who are receiving the report to listen and assimilate the material more easily. Ensuring that all required information is available will prevent interruptions and ensure smooth delivery of information.
Use the most current information regarding individual's condition and treatment. Information must be accurate, concise and complete—review the most recent recorded set of observations noting any trends, changes in condition, recent clinical review and/or rapid response calls and resultant management.	Inaccurate or incomplete information during handover can compromise the individual's comfort and safety. Use only the most current and relevant information about the individual. Missing or incorrect information can impact on the individual's recovery, delay diagnosis, decrease individual satisfaction, increase length of hospital stay and increase the risk of potential complications.
Inform the individual prior to starting handover that during the change of shift you will be informing the oncoming nurse about their progress and any updates to their care plan.	Prepares the individual for the clinical handover.

Continued

CLINICAL SKILL 10.1 Clinical handover—cont'd

 PERFORM THE SKILL

(Please refer to the Standard Steps on p. xii for related rationales.)
Perform hand hygiene.
Apply PPE: gloves, eyewear, mask and gown as appropriate.
Ensure the individual's safety and comfort throughout skill.
Promote independence and involvement of the individual if possible and/or appropriate.
Assess the individual's tolerance to the skill throughout.
Dispose of used supplies, equipment, waste and sharps appropriately.
Remove PPE and discard or store appropriately.
Perform hand hygiene.

Skill activity	Rationale
Use effective communication techniques in a timely manner.	Effective communication will help decrease the time for handover to be complete and ensures the information is communicated clearly and accurately.
Be interactive and engaged in communication.	The receiver of the information must be allowed to question the deliverer of the handover for clarification and more extensive information if needed. Active listening skills to be utilised.
Use medical terminology, clear language and avoid confusing abbreviations and jargon. Be sensitive to identifying pronouns used by the individual.	Allows a report to be complete and concise, demonstrates knowledge of the medical terminology and acknowledges the professional status of the person being handed over to, ensures inclusivity.
Limit interruptions during the handover process and conduct the handover in a private and safe environment.	To maintain privacy and confidentiality. If performing bedside handover and sensitive information may be overheard by other individuals or staff, voices must be kept low and personal comment refrained from, other than what is strictly necessary. If appropriate, uninvolved people may be asked to vacate the area.

General clinical handover format	
Confirm the individual's identity using three approved identifiers (name, age, DOB). State individual's demographics including room number, or indicate if they are off the ward and where, and attending medical officer's name. Introduce all team members by name and role.	Ensures the individual is identified and identifies the multidisciplinary team caring for the individual.
Summarise relevant clinical history and current clinical situation, including allergies, infectious status, diet/fluid/supervision requirements, invasive or implanted devices and medications.	Gives a general overview of the individual and allows a plan of nursing care to be implemented.
Describe the individual's response to treatment or medications. Include physical, psychological and emotional response to treatment initiated, alterations in medications ordered and response to medications.	The individual's response to treatment is imperative in ensuring the treatment is effective or ineffective, and in either continuing or changing the treatment plan.
State any tubes (IV, NGT) and include site, fluid, amount, rate and time to change. Also state any drains (IDC, wound) the individual has including location, type, and amount of drainage.	Any information regarding tubes and drains needs to be accurate to ensure any changes in the individual's condition are identified In a tImely manner.
Describe the individual's physical assessment, vital signs and pain assessment. Note any information that indicates a change in condition.	Important for prompt recognition of changes in condition.

CLINICAL SKILL 10.1 Clinical handover—cont'd

State any recent test results that require follow-up (e.g. scans, X-rays and blood tests).	Prompt reporting of results can ensure the individual's treatment is effective and, if ineffective, changes can be implemented.
Discuss the current treatment plan, include procedures scheduled, preparation done or needed, education, treatments, consents required, new orders and any concerns of staff about the individual.	Ensures continuity of and accountability for care provided to the individual.
State any consultations requested or completed including specialist physicians, physiotherapy, dietitian, or occupational therapy.	Provides the individual with effective holistic care; different health professionals may be needed to treat the individual.
Discuss any special needs such as aids (hearing, mobility etc.), equipment needed, family concerns, spiritual or cultural concerns, anything else important not yet mentioned.	Special needs of individuals need to be discussed to ensure the individual receives person-centred care.
Discuss any future plans or concerns about the individual including discharge planning, community referrals, expected date of discharge.	Discharge planning should be discussed with the individual throughout their admission to ensure they have continuity of care when they leave the department.
Bedside handover using ISBAR format (Identify, Situation, Background, Assessment, Recommendation)	
Prepare the individual's bedside environment. Determine if the individual wishes family to be present during the handover and ask non-family members to wait outside while handover is completed.	Ensures privacy and confidentiality is maintained and allows a quiet area for handover to be completed.
Exchange the information using the ISBAR format, which encompasses the following: • Identify—identify yourself, your role, your ward or location. Identify the name, role of the receiver/nurses who will be taking over care and call the individual by name, establishing their identity. Identify the individual: include name, individual ID number, date of birth, age, gender. • Situation—inform the receiver of the reason for the admission. State the individual's condition and severity. • Background—provide background information related to the situation. Include the following information: admitting diagnosis, date of admission, list of current medications, allergies, test results, vital signs, code status and any other pertinent clinical information. • Assessment—give assessment of the situation during the transfer of care. • Recommendation—discuss any recommendations/requests regarding the individual to the oncoming nurse.	The use of a standardised communication tool provides a predictable structure for communication between healthcare professionals and improves the individual's safety during handover from one nurse to another. It ensures the quality of the content and simplifies the communication of complex information.
Involve the individual; ask them if they have any concerns. If the oncoming nurse wishes to clarify information, they can do this with both the individual and the nurse who is handing over.	Person-centred care is the basis of nursing and by involving the individual in the handover process they can discuss their concerns and priorities, which may be different from that of the healthcare team.

Continued

CLINICAL SKILL 10.1 Clinical handover—cont'd

The oncoming nurse will need to perform a safety scan including checking the call bell is within the individual's reach, the suction and oxygen equipment are working and reviewing the bedside chart, ensuring accurate records are maintained. Assess for potential hazards.	A safety check is important for both the individual's and the nurse's safety within the room. It also ensures all equipment is in working order in case of emergency. By reviewing the bedside chart, the oncoming nurse is reviewing the individual's flowcharts and ensuring these are completed and they are prepared to take responsibility for the individual.
If there is sensitive information that needs to be handed over, this can be done outside the room in a private area.	Some information may be too sensitive to address within the individual's room; this may be due to their comfort, knowledge or wish to not discuss certain issues. To ensure privacy and confidentiality this must be completed in a private area.

 AFTER THE SKILL

(Please refer to the Standard Steps on p. xii for related rationales.)
Communicate outcome to the individual, any ongoing care and to report any complications.
Restore the environment.
Report, record and document assessment findings, details of the skill performed and the individual's response.
Report, record and document any abnormalities and/or inability to perform the skill.
Reassess the individual to ensure there are no adverse effects/events from the skill.

Skill activity	Rationale
Verify information received, including a read back or repeat back process. This is where a plan of ongoing care for the individual is confirmed.	Allows clarification of information and decreases the incidence of communication errors occurring.

Note: Reporting on an individual's condition during handover should be completed as per healthcare organisation policy; therefore, it is important for nurses to familiarise themselves with the relevant format and local policy and procedure before they provide the handover. All nursing change of shift handovers should include the use of a structured, standardised communication tool to preserve continuity of individual care and to ensure effective transfer of accountability and responsibility. The handover process should include a clear transfer of responsibility as this relates to the accountability of care for individuals and the transfer of this accountability of care from one nurse to another.

(Crisp et al 2021; NSW Health 2019; Rebeiro et al 2021; Tollefson & Hillman 2021; Tollefson et al 2021)

OBSERVATION CHECKLIST: CLINICAL HANDOVER

STUDENT NAME: _____

CLINICAL SKILL 10.1: Clinical handover

DEMONSTRATION OF: The ability to report on the condition of an individual clearly and concisely to other healthcare professionals

If the observation checklist is being used as an assessment tool, the student will need to obtain a scale of independence for each of the performance criteria/evidence.

Independent (I)

Supervised (S)

Assisted (A)

Marginal (M)

Dependent (D)

COMPETENCY ELEMENTS	PERFORMANCE CRITERIA/EVIDENCE	I	S	A	M	D
Preparation for the activity	Identifies indications and rationale for performing the activity Identifies the individual using three individual identifiers Ensures therapeutic interaction Checks facility/organisation policy Locates and gathers equipment Ensures all required individuals are present Asks non-family members to wait outside until handover is complete					

Performs activity informed by evidence	Interactive communication:
	  • Uses medical terminology and clear language
	  • Ensures information is given in a timely manner
	  • Uses accurate, current, and relevant information
	General clinical handover format:
	  • States individual demographics
	  • Describes the individual's complaint, treatment, and diagnosis
	  • States the individual's response to treatment
	  • States any tubes or drains present
	  • Describes the physical assessment, vital signs and pain assessment undertaken
	  • States any laboratory results or imaging
	  • Discusses the individual's current treatment plan
	  • States any consultations required or completed
	  • Discusses any special needs of the individual
	  • Discusses discharge planning of the individual					

Continued

COMPETENCY ELEMENTS	PERFORMANCE CRITERIA/EVIDENCE	I	S	A	M	D
	Clinical bedside handover using the ISBAR tool: • Introduces the nurse taking over care of the individual • Exchanges information using the SBAR format • States the individual's condition and severity • Provides background information related to the situation • Includes assessment information such as vital signs, clinical assessments, allergies and medications, and any further assessment findings as required • Discusses assessment of the situation during the transfer of care • Discusses recommendations regarding the individual's care • Allows the oncoming nurse to perform a safety scan of the room • If any sensitive information is to be handed over ensures this is done in a private area • On completion of handover, allows the oncoming nurse to verify information received and confirm a plan of ongoing care for the individual • Ensures the individual is comfortable					
Applies critical thinking and reflective practice	Reviews information pertinent to clinical handover prior to its commencement Is able to link theory to practice Demonstrates current best practice in the care provided Ensures only relevant information is transferred during clinical handover Assesses own performance					
Practises within safety and quality assurance guidelines	Ensures clinical handover is focused on the individual Ensures clinical handover is timely, relevant and structured Reviews against facility/organisation policy Disposes of equipment and waste appropriately					
Documentation and communication	Explains and communicates the activity clearly to the individual Communicates outcome and ongoing care to individual and significant others Communicates abnormal findings to appropriate personnel Reports and documents all relevant information and any complications correctly Reports any complications and/or inability to perform the procedure to the RN					

Educator/Facilitator Feedback:

Educator/Facilitator Score: Competent   Needs further development

How would you rate your overall performance while undertaking this clinical activity? (Use a ✓ & initial)

Unsatisfactory   Satisfactory   Good   Excellent

Student Reflection: (discuss how you would approach your practice differently or more effectively)

EDUCATOR/FACILITATOR NAME/SIGNATURE:

STUDENT NAME/SIGNATURE: **DATE:**

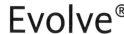 ® Answer guide for the Critical Thinking Exercises and Critical Thinking Questions in Case Studies is hosted on Evolve: http://evolve.elsevier.com/AU/Koutoukidis/Tabbner/

References

Australian Commission on Safety and Quality in Health Care (ACSQHC), 2021. National Safety and Quality Primary and Community Healthcare Standards, 2nd ed. Available at: <https://www.safetyandquality.gov.au/publications-and-resources/resource-library/national-safety-and-quality-health-service-standards-second-edition>.

Australian Commission on Safety and Quality in Health Care (ACSQHC), 2023. Communicating for safety standard. Communication at clinical handover. Available at: <https://www.safetyandquality.gov.au/standards/nsqhs-standards/communicating-safety-standard/communication-clinical-handover>.

Burgess, A., van Diggele, C., Roberts, C., Mellis, C., 2020. Teaching clinical handover with ISBAR. *BMC Medical Education* 20(2). Available at: <https://bmcmededuc.biomedcentral.com/articles/10.1186/s12909-020-02285-0>.

Crisp, J., Douglas, C., Rebeiro, G., et al. (eds.), 2021. *Potter and Perry's fundamentals of nursing*, 6th ed. Elsevier, Sydney.

Kaltoft, A., Jacobsen, Y.I., Tangsgaard, H.I.J., 2021. ISBAR as a structured tool for patient handover during post operative recovery. *Journal of Perianesthesia Nursing* 37(1), P34–39, Available at: <https://doi.org/10.1016/j.jopan.2021.01.002>.

Marin, T., 2019. Nursing: Clinical handover. JBI evidence summary. JBI1615. Available at: <https://jbi.global/ebp>.

Nursing and Midwifery Board of Australia (NMBA), 2016. Enrolled nurse standards for practice. Available at: <https://www.nursingmidwiferyboard.gov.au/Codes-Guidelines-Statements/Professional-standards.aspx>.

Nursing and Midwifery Board of Australia (NMBA), 2020. Decision-making framework for nursing and midwifery. Available at: <https://www.nursingmidwiferyboard.gov.au/Codes-Guidelines-Statements/Frameworks.aspx>.

NSW Health, 2019. Clinical Handover. Policy Directive. Available at: <https://www1.health.nsw.gov.au/pds/ActivePDSDocuments/PD2019_020.pdf>.

O'Toole, G., 2020. *Communication: Core interpersonal skills for health professionals*, 4th ed. Elsevier.

Perry, A., Potter, P., Ostendorf, W., 2019. *Nursing interventions and clinical skills*, 7th ed. Elsevier, St Louis.

Porritt, K., 2022. Clinical handover: Transfer between units within an acute care hospital. JBI evidence summary. Available at: <https://jbi.global/ebp>.

Rebeiro, G., Wilson, D., Fuller, S., 2021. *Potter and Perry's fundamentals of nursing workbook*, 4th ed. Elsevier, Chatswood.

Tollefson, J., Hillman, E., 2021. *Clinical psychomotor skills: Assessment tools for nurses*, 8th ed. Cengage Learning, Melbourne.

Tollefson, J., Watson, G., Jelly, E., et al., 2021. *Essential clinical skills: Enrolled nurses*, 5th ed. Cengage Learning, Australia.

HEALTH ASSESSMENT FRAMEWORKS

Deepu Ponnappan

Overview

A general health assessment serves as a vital tool for nurses to acquire and interpret data, enabling them to plan and deliver effective care to enhance an individual's overall health status. It is largely dependent on a nurse's ability to communicate effectively with the individual. By establishing clear and empathetic communication, nurses can gather crucial information and gain insights necessary for comprehensive care planning (McCormack & McCance 2017). It consists of a systematic and holistic collection of both subjective data (history obtained from the individual) and objective data (evidence collected through observation). A general health assessment includes evaluating an individual's physical and mental health, as well as their socioeconomic and financial statuses. The collected data help nurses focus on understanding how health and illnesses impact the quality of life (Jensen 2019).

A general health assessment generally consists of the following elements:
- Information collection, including an individual's history
- Arranging appropriate allied health staff for examinations that may be required
- Referring or undertaking ordered investigations as required
- Constructing an overall assessment of an individual
- Assessing, evaluating and recommending appropriate interventions
- Educating and providing advice and information to an individual
- Retaining a record of a health assessment of the individual in a written report
- Recommending an individual's family or carer for assistance and/or services.

Sometimes a more focused assessment may be necessary. Focused assessments are used to observe and monitor systems-related complications. A focused assessment is a more detailed assessment of a particular problem (Brown et al 2020; Lewis & Foley 2020).

Health assessments are an essential procedure where nurses gather intrinsic and extrinsic data to formulate a personalised care plan. Data collection primarily involves direct observation and verbal communication with the individual, but it is important for students to recognise other vital sources of information for a holistic assessment. This comprehensive data collection serves as a solid foundation for making and evaluating clinical judgments in collaboration with the interdisciplinary team.

As nurses are typically present with individuals for the majority of their time, it is crucial for them to possess the skills to promptly assess and address health needs or concerns. This is vital to prevent any deterioration in the individual's condition. Student Enrolled Nurses should acquire a solid understanding of assessment techniques, data collection, and how to make informed clinical judgments in collaboration with the broader allied health team.

This chapter will explore, describe and allow for the practice and consolidation of the skills required for screening for general health assessments to determine an individual's needs and requirements.

CASE STUDY 15.2

The following are details of Tom's health assessment.

General health assessment:

- A 64-year-old male with 4-year history of type 2 diabetes with non-compliance to medication
- Physical assessment: BMI 32.6 kg/m^2, BP 154/96 mmHg, RR 20 breaths/min, pulse 88 beats/min
- After a physical health assessment was conducted, a pressure injury was identified on one of Tom's right toes. Tom was not aware of this sore.

1. What education considerations may Tom need in relation to his diabetes?
2. What could you do to educate Tom about foot care?

CRITICAL THINKING EXERCISE 15.2

Sarah, a 75-year-old woman, is admitted to the hospital for evaluation. During the initial nursing assessment, it is observed that Sarah displays signs of cognitive impairment, such as forgetfulness and difficulty following instructions. Her daughter mentions that Sarah has been experiencing episodes of urinary incontinence, which is a new development for her. What assessments will you undertake as an Enrolled Nurse and why?

CLINICAL SKILL 15.1 Pressure injury risk assessment

Please adhere to the policy and procedures of the facility/organisation prior to undertaking the skill. Ensure this skill is in your scope of practice.

NMBA Decision-making Framework considerations (refer to NMBA Decision-making framework for nursing and midwifery 2020):	Equipment:
1. Am I educated? 2. Am I authorised? 3. Am I competent? If you answer 'no' to any of these, do not perform that activity. Seek guidance and support from your teacher/a nurse team leader/clinical facilitator/educator.	Assessment tool used in the clinical facility/organisation The individual's nursing care plan and history

 PREPARE FOR THE SKILL

(Please refer to the Standard Steps on p. xii for related rationales.)
- Mentally review the steps of the skill.
- Discuss the skill with your instructor/supervisor/team leader, if required.
- Confirm correct facility/organisation policy/safe operating procedures.
- Validate the order in the individual's record.
- Identify indication and rationale for performing the activity.
- Assess for any contraindications.
- Locate and gather equipment.
- Perform hand hygiene.
- Ensure therapeutic interaction.
- Identify the individual using three individual identifiers.
- Gain the individual's consent.
- Assess for pain relief.
- Prepare the environment.
- Provide and maintain privacy.
- Assist the individual to assume an appropriate position of comfort.

Skill activity	Rationale
Identify indications and rationale for performing the activity. This may include identifying: - past history of pressure injuries - intrinsic and extrinsic factors that may contribute to pressure injuries - understanding reasons why the pressure injury risk assessment needs to be performed or has been ordered.	Reduces unnecessary assessments performed on an individual.

 PERFORM THE SKILL

(Please refer to the Standard Steps on p. xii for related rationales.)
- Perform hand hygiene.
- Apply PPE: gloves, eyewear, mask and gown as appropriate.
- Ensure the individual's safety and comfort throughout skill.
- Promote independence and involvement of the individual if possible and/or appropriate.
- Assess the individual's tolerance to the skill throughout.
- Dispose of used supplies, equipment, waste and sharps appropriately.
- Remove PPE and discard or store appropriately.
- Perform hand hygiene.

Continued

CLINICAL SKILL 15.1 Pressure injury risk assessment—cont'd

Skill activity	Rationale
Assess and document the individual's sensory perception in the progress notes and facility/organisational chart: • by assessing the individual's ability to detect pain • in unconscious individuals, the ability to react to pain.	Assesses the individual's ability to verbalise pressure-related discomfort that will indicate skin damage. Prompts the EN to apply interventions and strategies on how often to replace and clean linen, incontinence aids. Assesses the unconscious individual's ability to react to pressure-related discomfort, which will indicate skin damage.
Assess and document the individual's degree of exposure to moisture in the progress notes and organisation chart by direct observation or assessment of turgor, dampness, excessive moisture loss affecting skin. Assess continence.	Assesses the individual's risk of skin damage and degeneration if exposed to excessive moisture. Prompts the EN to apply interventions and strategies on how often to replace and clean linen, incontinence aids.
Assess and document the individual's activity and mobility status in the progress notes and organisational chart: • by assessing the ability of the individual to move or the ability to be moved • in unconscious individuals, the ability to be moved • observing for any reddened skin that blanches white under light pressure; please note, darkly pigmented skin may not have visible blanching; its colour may differ from the surrounding area. The area may be painful, firm, soft, warmer or cooler as compared to adjacent tissue.	Assesses the individual's risk of skin damage and degeneration from the degree of physical mobility. Prompts the EN to apply interventions and strategies on how often to assist the individual in changing body position to relieve pressure on the skin. Prompts the EN to engage the use and expertise of an occupational therapist and physiotherapist.
Assess and document the individual's nutritional status in the progress notes and organisational chart. Nutritional data collection will include: • loss of appetite of an individual • unusual weight loss or gain in an individual • fluid intake of an individual.	Assesses the individual's risk of skin damage and degeneration caused by malnutrition or poor nutritional status. Prompts the EN to apply interventions and strategies on how often to assist the individual with meals. Prompts the EN to engage the use and expertise of a dietitian.
Assess and document vascular/perfusion status of lower limbs, heels and feet. If at risk of heel pressure injury, elevate the heels, ensuring weight of the leg is distributed along the calf without placing pressure on the Achilles tendon and popliteal vein.	May help to lower risk and incidence of pressure injuries. Prompts the EN to apply interventions and strategies on preventing pressure injuries.
Assess support surface and whether it is meeting the needs of the individual in terms of pressure redistribution.	May help to lower risk and incidence of pressure injuries. Prompts the EN to apply interventions and strategies on preventing pressure injuries.
Assess and document the individual's risk of friction and shear when moving in the progress notes and organisational chart by: • assessing and identifying any mechanical force that could occur when two surfaces rub together, creating resistance between the skin and a surface • identifying typical areas where this will occur (e.g. heels and elbows), resulting from repositioning • assessing and identifying any mechanical force created from parallel loads (e.g. movement on a bed sheet), which can create an occlusion or displacement of tissue.	Assesses the individual's risk of skin damage and degeneration from friction or shearing of the skin when moving. Prompts the EN to apply interventions and strategies on how often to assist the individual in changing body position to relieve pressure on the skin. Prompts the EN to engage the use and expertise of an occupational therapist and physiotherapist. Shear forces are a significant risk for pressure injury formation as blood flow is disrupted.

CLINICAL SKILL 15.1 Pressure injury risk assessment—cont'd

Undertake a head-to-toe assessment of the skin to identify any existing or new skin tears, especially over bony prominences such as sacrum, elbows, shoulder blades. This includes identifying: • intact skin or skin loss • blanchable or non-blanchable skin • areas that may be painful, warmer, cooler or oedematous. If skin breaks have been identified: • Skin break is measured and documented in depth and width on the pressure area risk tool. • Colour and/or ooze is documented on the pressure area risk tool. • Location is identified on the pressure area risk tool. • Treatment plan is documented on the pressure area risk tool in consultation with the Registered Nurse.	These are warning signs of impending skin damage. Ensures pressure areas are identified and treated early.
Determine the frequency of the pressure-risk monitoring by identifying and evaluating the individual's risk status, such as high, medium or low, according to the pressure injury chart.	Ensures a range of data is collected over different situations and times.

 AFTER THE SKILL

(Please refer to the Standard Steps on p. xii for related rationales.)
• Communicate outcome to the individual, any ongoing care and to report any complications.
• Restore the environment.
• Report, record and document assessment findings, details of the skill performed and the individual's response.
• Report, record and document any abnormalities and/or inability to perform the skill.
• Reassess the individual to ensure there are no adverse effects/events from the skill.

(Adapted from ACSQHC 2021; EPUAP et al 2019; Jensen & Smock 2022)

OBSERVATION CHECKLIST: PRESSURE INJURY RISK ASSESSMENT

STUDENT NAME: _____

CLINICAL SKILL 15.1: Pressure injury risk assessment

DEMONSTRATION OF: The ability to effectively and safely assess an individual's pressure risk status

Independent (I)
Supervised (S)
Assisted (A)
Marginal (M)
Dependent (D)

If the observation checklist is being used as an assessment tool, the student will need to obtain a scale of independence for each of the performance criteria/evidence.

COMPETENCY ELEMENTS	PERFORMANCE CRITERIA/EVIDENCE	I	S	A	M	D
Preparation for the activity	Identifies indications and rationale for performing the activity Identifies the individual using three individual identifiers Ensures therapeutic interaction Gains the individual's consent Checks facility/organisation policy Validates the order in the individual's record Locates and gathers equipment Assists the individual into an appropriate position					
Performs activity informed by evidence	Assesses the individual's sensory perception Assesses the individual's exposure to moisture Assesses the individual's activity and mobility status Assesses the individual's nutritional status Assesses the individual's risk of friction and shear when moving Undertakes a head-to-toe assessment of the skin					
Applies critical thinking and reflective practice	Is able to link theory to practice Demonstrates current best practice in the care provided Assesses own performance					
Practises within safety and quality assurance guidelines	Reviews against facility/organisation policy Performs hand hygiene Ensures provision of comfort measures after the assessment including repositioning of the individual Determines the frequency of the falls risk monitoring					
Documentation and communication	Explains and communicates the activity clearly to the individual Communicates outcome and ongoing care to individual and significant others Reports and documents all relevant information and any complications correctly in the healthcare record Reports any complications and/or inability to perform the procedure to the RN and/or medical officer Asks the individual to report any complications during and post procedure					

Educator/Facilitator Feedback:

Educator/Facilitator Score: Competent   Needs further development

How would you rate your overall performance while undertaking this clinical activity? (use a ✓ & initial)

Unsatisfactory   Satisfactory   Good   Excellent

Student Reflection: (discuss how you would approach your practice differently or more effectively)

EDUCATOR/FACILITATOR NAME/SIGNATURE:

STUDENT NAME/SIGNATURE: **DATE:**

CLINICAL SKILL 15.2 Mental health assessment

Please adhere to the policy and procedures of the facility/organisation prior to undertaking the skill. Ensure this skill is in your scope of practice.

NMBA Decision-making Framework considerations (refer to NMBA Decision-making framework for nursing and midwifery 2020):	Equipment:
1. Am I educated? 2. Am I authorised? 3. Am I competent? If you answer 'no' to any of these, do not perform that activity. Seek guidance and support from your teacher/ a nurse team leader/clinical facilitator/educator.	Assessment tool used in the clinical facility/organisation The individual's nursing care plan and history

 PREPARE FOR THE SKILL

(Please refer to the Standard Steps on p. xii for related rationales.)
- Mentally review the steps of the skill.
- Discuss the skill with your instructor/supervisor/team leader, if required.
- Confirm correct facility/organisation policy/safe operating procedures.
- Validate the order in the individual's record.
- Identify indication and rationale for performing the activity.
- Assess for any contraindications.
- Locate and gather equipment.
- Perform hand hygiene.
- Ensure therapeutic interaction.
- Identify the individual using three individual identifiers.
- Gain the individual's consent.
- Assess for pain relief.
- Prepare the environment.
- Provide and maintain privacy.
- Assist the individual to assume an appropriate position of comfort.

 PERFORM THE SKILL

(Please refer to the Standard Steps on p. xii for related rationales.)
- Perform hand hygiene.
- Apply PPE: gloves, eyewear, mask and gown as appropriate.
- Ensure the individual's safety and comfort throughout skill.
- Promote independence and involvement of the individual if possible and/or appropriate.
- Assess the individual's tolerance to the skill throughout.
- Dispose of used supplies, equipment, waste and sharps appropriately.
- Remove PPE and discard or store appropriately.
- Perform hand hygiene.

Skill activity	Rationale
Assess presenting problems. Assess history of presenting problems (onset, duration, course, severity). Assess current functioning (across domains [e.g. employment/education, family, social]). Assess previous assessments and interventions. Assess psychiatric history (personal and family history). Assess current medications. Assess medical history. Assess family history of mental health. Assess developmental history. Assess substance use. Assess forensic and legal history. Assess risk screen (e.g. suicide, self-harm, aggression, vulnerability, absconding risk, risks to dependent children).	Provides a baseline dataset and possible links to an individual's mental health.

CLINICAL SKILL 15.2 Mental health assessment—cont'd

Assess mental health status.	Gathers data on the individual's current status and highlights indications of the individual's mental health status.
Appearance: • Usual and unusual appearance (e.g. stature) • Grooming or any evidence of neglect • Apparent age vs real age • Facial features • Identifying features such as skin marks, moles	Provides a baseline dataset and possible links to an individual's mental health.
Behaviour: • Any physical signs of anxiety • Restlessness, relaxed • Hand or facial gestures • Eye contact	Provides a baseline dataset and possible links to an individual's mental health.
Speech: • Rate—slow, fast, normal • Logic • Ability to complete sentences • Absence	Provides a baseline dataset and possible links to an individual's mental health.
Mood and affect: • Responses to questions • Emotional status—crying, laughing inappropriately • Anger • Anxiety • Irritability	Provides a baseline dataset and possible links to an individual's mental health.
Form of thought, content of thought: • Hallucinations—visual or auditory • Hearing of voices • Concerns • Evidence of paranoia	Provides a baseline dataset and possible links to an individual's mental health.
Insight and cognition: • Orientation to time, place, person • Understanding of health issues • Understanding of medication therapy and treatment	Provides a baseline dataset and possible links to an individual's mental health.
Memory: • Long-term memory • Short-term memory	Provides a baseline dataset and possible links to an individual's mental health.

 AFTER THE SKILL

(Please refer to the Standard Steps on p. xii for related rationales.)
• Communicate outcome to the individual, any ongoing care and to report any complications.
• Restore the environment.
• Report, record and document assessment findings, details of the skill performed and the individual's response.
• Report, record and document any abnormalities and/or inability to perform the skill.
• Reassess the individual to ensure there are no adverse effects/events from the skill.

(Adapted from ACSQHC 2021; Chambers 2017; Jensen & Smock 2022)

OBSERVATION CHECKLIST: MENTAL HEALTH ASSESSMENT

STUDENT NAME: _____

CLINICAL SKILL 15.2: Mental health assessment

DEMONSTRATION OF: The ability to effectively and safely assess an individual's mental health status

If the observation checklist is being used as an assessment tool, the student will need to obtain a scale of independence for each of the performance criteria/evidence.

Independent (I)
Supervised (S)
Assisted (A)
Marginal (M)
Dependent (D)

COMPETENCY ELEMENTS	PERFORMANCE CRITERIA/EVIDENCE	I	S	A	M	D
Preparation for the activity	Identifies indications and rationale for performing the activity Identifies the individual using three individual identifiers Ensures therapeutic interaction Gains the individual's consent Checks facility/organisation policy Validates the order in the individual's record Locates and gathers equipment					
Performs activity informed by evidence	Assesses presenting problems Assesses history of presenting problems (onset, duration, course, severity) Assesses current functioning (across domains, e.g. employment/education, family, social) Assesses previous assessments and interventions Assesses psychiatric history (personal and family history) Assesses current medications Assesses medical history Assesses family history of mental health Assesses developmental history Assesses substance use Assesses forensic and legal history Assesses risk screen (e.g. suicide, self-harm, aggression, vulnerability, absconding risk, risks to dependent children) Assesses mental status: • Appearance (identifying features such as skin marks, moles) • Behaviour • Speech • Mood and affect • Irritability • Form of thought, content of thought • Evidence of paranoia • Insight and cognition Assesses understanding of medication therapy and treatment Assesses memory Identifies lifespan, cultural and language barriers Provides privacy Ensures therapeutic interaction Works in collaboration with other allied healthcare staff					
Applies critical thinking and reflective practice	Is able to link theory to practice Demonstrates current best practice in the care provided Assesses own performance					

COMPETENCY ELEMENTS	PERFORMANCE CRITERIA/EVIDENCE	I	S	A	M	D
Practises within safety and quality assurance guidelines	Reviews against facility/organisation policy Performs hand hygiene					
Documentation and communication	Explains and communicates the activity clearly to the individual Communicates outcome and ongoing care to individual and significant others Communicates abnormal findings to appropriate personnel Reports and documents all relevant information and any complications correctly in the healthcare record Reports any complications and/or inability to perform the procedure to the RN and/or medical officer					

Educator/Facilitator Feedback:

Educator/Facilitator Score: Competent   Needs further development

How would you rate your overall performance while undertaking this clinical activity? (use a ✓ & initial)

Unsatisfactory   Satisfactory   Good   Excellent

Student Reflection: (discuss how you would approach your practice differently or more effectively)

EDUCATOR/FACILITATOR NAME/SIGNATURE:

STUDENT NAME/SIGNATURE: **DATE:**

CLINICAL SKILL 15.3 Falls risk assessment

Please adhere to the policy and procedures of the facility/organisation prior to undertaking the skill. Ensure this skill is in your scope of practice.

NMBA Decision-making Framework considerations (refer to NMBA Decision-making framework for nursing and midwifery 2020):	Equipment:
1. Am I educated? 2. Am I authorised? 3. Am I competent? If you answer 'no' to any of these, do not perform that activity. Seek guidance and support from your teacher/ a nurse team leader/clinical facilitator/educator.	Assessment tool used in the clinical facility/organisation Appropriately fitted mobility aids if required The individual's nursing care plan and history

 PREPARE FOR THE SKILL

(Please refer to the Standard Steps on p. xii for related rationales.)
- Mentally review the steps of the skill.
- Discuss the skill with your instructor/supervisor/team leader, if required.
- Confirm correct facility/organisation policy/safe operating procedures.
- Validate the order in the individual's record.
- Identify indication and rationale for performing the activity.
- Assess for any contraindications.
- Locate and gather equipment.
- Perform hand hygiene.
- Ensure therapeutic interaction.
- Identify the individual using three individual identifiers.
- Gain the individual's consent.
- Assess for pain relief.
- Prepare the environment.
- Provide and maintain privacy.
- Assist the individual to assume an appropriate position of comfort.

 PERFORM THE SKILL

(Please refer to the Standard Steps on p. xii for related rationales.)
- Perform hand hygiene.
- Apply PPE: gloves, eyewear, mask and gown as appropriate.
- Ensure the individual's safety and comfort throughout skill.
- Promote independence and involvement of the individual if possible and/or appropriate.
- Assess the individual's tolerance to the skill throughout.
- Dispose of used supplies, equipment, waste and sharps appropriately.
- Remove PPE and discard or store appropriately.
- Perform hand hygiene.

Skill activity	Rationale

Undertake an assessment data collection and document this on the falls risk chart and progress notes by reading and researching the individual's:
- medical history:
  > past and current health history
  > medications
- social situation:
  > whether the individual lives alone or with family.
	Provides an understanding of any medical conditions on the individual's falls risk history. This assessment will include relevant medical history including medications. This data will provide an understanding of any family members requiring the need for education or assistance when planning care.
	If the individual is alone, this data will provide insight into the individual's need for assistance or aids. This assessment will include whether an individual lives alone or with a carer and carer/individual difficulty managing at home.

Continued

CLINICAL SKILL 15.3 Falls risk assessment—cont'd

Identify and document on the falls chart history past or recent falls by talking to the individual or identifying this in the past medical history of the individual: • when • where • any underlying cause of fall.	This data will provide insight into a pattern of recent or past falls by an individual that can be used in the planning of care.

Collect and document on the falls risk chart and in the individual's progress notes intrinsic assessment data (data collected from the individual, family or by direct observation):
• past and present medical history
• past or present vision impairments
• past or present nutritional impairments
• past or present mobility impairments including gait, balance and transfer
• past or present cognitive impairments
• past or present continence (faecal/urinary) impairments
• past or present medication history.
Medical history includes:
• past history of the individual
• relevant history of the individual
• symptoms of dizziness voiced by an individual
• any unsteadiness on standing by an individual
• any visible signs after a head-to-toe assessment of bleeding, bruising or skin breaks.
Vision data collection includes:
• visual aids used by an individual
• difficulty in seeing obstacles by an individual.
Nutritional data collection includes:
• loss of appetite of an individual
• unusual weight loss or gain in an individual
• fluid intake of an individual.
Mobility data collection includes:
• identifying concerns in an individual's gait such as swaying or holding onto furniture to assist with walking
• identifying an individual's concerns with limb weakness or reduced sensation
• identifying an individual's incorrect usage of previously prescribed mobility aids
• identifying ill-fitting footwear.
Cognitive data collection includes:
• identifying difficulties in an individual's ability to follow or interpret instructions.
Continence data collection includes:
• identifying an individual's concerns about urinary or faecal urgency, nocturia or incontinence that may be identified as risk factors in falls management.
Medication data collection includes:
• identifying an individual's emaciation management plan
• identifying if the individual is prescribed more than two of the following medications, which may be identified as risk factors in falls management:
  > diuretics
  > psychotropic medications
  > Parkinson's disease medications
  > antidepressants
  > antihypertensives
  > sedative medication.
	Intrinsic data collection provides insight into risk factors that may require invasive actions that will reduce or minimise falls of an individual.

CLINICAL SKILL 15.3 Falls risk assessment—cont'd

Collect and document on the falls risk chart and in the individual's progress notes extrinsic assessment data on past or present environmental hazards by direct observation or talking with the individual or family. This will include identifying: • an individual's reporting of difficulty with stairs. Observation or reporting of: • indoor and outdoor hazards • poor lighting • restricted traffic ways or cluttering • an individual's reporting of difficulty moving on and off the bed/toilet/chair.	Extrinsic data collection provides an insight into risk factors that may require invasive actions that will reduce or minimise falls of an individual.
Determine the frequency of the falls risk monitoring by identifying and evaluating the individual's risk status, such as high, medium or low, according to the falls risk chart.	Ensures a range of data is collected over different situations and times. The higher the falls risk the more frequent the individual's monitoring should be.
To link theory to practice, the Enrolled Nurse should understand the pathophysiology of the individual's health conditions and why this activity was undertaken.	An understanding of why the nurse is undertaking the assessment ensures a thorough collection of data and an understanding of the data collected.
Demonstrate current best practice in the care provided by understanding the current trends in falls risk management.	Ensures quality care is provided to the individual.
Collaborate with other allied healthcare staff by working with the Registered Nurse and identifying referral to allied health staff, if required.	Referral to other health professions ensures holistic care with appropriate interventions.

 AFTER THE SKILL

(Please refer to the Standard Steps on p. xii for related rationales.)
• Communicate outcome to the individual, any ongoing care and to report any complications.
• Restore the environment.
• Report, record and document assessment findings, details of the skill performed and the individual's response.
• Report, record and document any abnormalities and/or inability to perform the skill.
• Reassess the individual to ensure there are no adverse effects/events from the skill.

(Adapted from ACSQHC 2021; Department of Health, Government of Western Australia 2014; Jensen & Smock 2022)

OBSERVATION CHECKLIST: FALLS RISK ASSESSMENT

STUDENT NAME: _____

CLINICAL SKILL 15.3: Falls risk assessment

DEMONSTRATION OF: The ability to effectively and safely assess an individual's falls risk status

If the observation checklist is being used as an assessment tool, the student will need to obtain a scale of independence for each of the performance criteria/evidence.

Independent (I)
Supervised (S)
Assisted (A)
Marginal (M)
Dependent (D)

COMPETENCY ELEMENTS	PERFORMANCE CRITERIA/EVIDENCE	I	S	A	M	D
Preparation for the activity	Identifies indications and rationale for performing the activity Identifies the individual using three individual identifiers Ensures therapeutic interaction Gains the individual's consent Checks facility/organisation policy Validates the order in the individual's record Locates and gathers equipment					
Performs activity informed by evidence	Undertakes an assessment data collection and documents this on the falls risk chart and in the progress notes Identifies and documents on the falls chart history of past or recent falls Collects and documents on the falls risk chart and in the individual's progress notes intrinsic assessment data Collects and documents on the falls risk chart and in the individual's progress notes assessment data on activities of daily living Provides privacy Ensures provision of comfort measures prior to the assessment Identifies the individual's need for assistance and comorbidities Prepares the environment to ensure safety measures are addressed for the individual Determines the frequency of the falls risk monitoring					
Applies critical thinking and reflective practice	Is able to link theory to practice Demonstrates current best practice in the care provided Assesses own performance					
Practises within safety and quality assurance guidelines	Reviews against facility/organisation policy Performs hand hygiene					

COMPETENCY ELEMENTS	PERFORMANCE CRITERIA/EVIDENCE	I	S	A	M	D
Documentation and communication	Explains and communicates the activity clearly to the individual Communicates outcome and ongoing care to individual and significant others Communicates abnormal findings to appropriate personnel Reports and documents all relevant information and any complications correctly in the healthcare record Reports any complications and/or inability to perform the procedure to the RN and/or medical officer					

Educator/Facilitator Feedback:

Educator/Facilitator Score: Competent   Needs further development

How would you rate your overall performance while undertaking this clinical activity? (use a ✓ & initial)

Unsatisfactory   Satisfactory   Good   Excellent

Student Reflection: (discuss how you would approach your practice differently or more effectively)

EDUCATOR/FACILITATOR NAME/SIGNATURE:

STUDENT NAME/SIGNATURE: **DATE:**

CLINICAL SKILL 15.4 Venous thromboembolism assessment

Please adhere to the policy and procedures of the facility/organisation prior to undertaking the skill. Ensure this skill is in your scope of practice.

NMBA Decision-making Framework considerations (refer to NMBA Decision-making framework for nursing and midwifery 2020):	Equipment:
1. Am I educated? 2. Am I authorised? 3. Am I competent? If you answer 'no' to any of these, do not perform that activity. Seek guidance and support from your teacher/a nurse team leader/clinical facilitator/educator.	Assessment tool used in the clinical facility/ organisation The individual's nursing care plan and history

 PREPARE FOR THE SKILL

(Please refer to the Standard Steps on p. xii for related rationales.)
- Mentally review the steps of the skill.
- Discuss the skill with your instructor/supervisor/team leader, if required.
- Confirm correct facility/organisation policy/safe operating procedures.
- Validate the order in the individual's record.
- Identify indication and rationale for performing the activity.
- Assess for any contraindications.
- Locate and gather equipment.
- Perform hand hygiene.
- Ensure therapeutic interaction.
- Identify the individual using three individual identifiers.
- Gain the individual's consent.
- Assess for pain relief.
- Prepare the environment.
- Provide and maintain privacy.
- Assist the individual to assume an appropriate position of comfort.

 PERFORM THE SKILL

(Please refer to the Standard Steps on p. xii for related rationales.)
- Perform hand hygiene.
- Apply PPE: gloves, eyewear, mask and gown as appropriate.
- Ensure the individual's safety and comfort throughout skill.
- Promote independence and involvement of the individual if possible and/or appropriate.
- Assess the individual's tolerance to the skill throughout.
- Dispose of used supplies, equipment, waste and sharps appropriately.
- Remove PPE and discard or store appropriately.
- Perform hand hygiene.

Continued

CLINICAL SKILL 15.4 Venous thromboembolism assessment—cont'd

Skill activity	Rationale

Determine individual's reason for hospitalisation:
• Assess the likelihood of, for example, a surgical site bleed, an intracranial bleed or a gastrointestinal bleed, and the consequences of bleeding should it occur.
• Assess individual patient-related factors that may increase risk of bleeding:
  > procedures with potentially critical consequences of bleeding (such as a lumbar puncture, epidural or spinal anaesthesia)
  > abnormal renal function or liver disease
  > uncontrolled hypertension
  > active peptic ulcer or ulcerative gastrointestinal disease
  > thrombocytopenia (platelet count less than 50,000 mcg/L)
  > acute haemorrhagic stroke.
• Bleeding history:
  > family history of bleeding or personal history of bleeding disorders
  > recent bleeding (within the week) or active bleeding.
• Medication history:
  > use of other medicines known to either increase bleeding risk or to increase the risk of clotting, or that alter the metabolism of medicines used to prevent VTE
  > other medicine that may interact with medicines used to prevent VTE.
• Assess mobility:
  > Identify concerns in an individual's gait such as swaying or holding onto furniture to assist with walking.
  > Identify an individual's decrease in mobility.
  > Identify an individual's concerns with limb weakness or reduced sensation.
	The indication of VTE risk can be established by identifying if an individual is having a medical or surgical procedure.

Assess baseline risk (intrinsic factors) from the individual, family or by direct observation: • past and present medical history • past or present medication history • past or present nutritional impairments. Medical history includes: • past history of the individual • relevant history of the individual • symptoms of shortness of breath.	The indication of VTE risk can be established by identifying an individual's age, pregnancy status, previous history of VTE, obesity, varicose veins, active malignancy. This assessment helps establish the initial risk level and guide further evaluation and preventative measures.
Assess additional risk of VTE (extrinsic) by direct observation or talking with the individual or family: • dehydration status • surgical risk by type (pelvic, orthopaedic, joint surgery) • medical risk by type (stroke, heart failure, myocardial infarction).	The indication of additional VTE risk can allow for accurate evaluation of the individual's overall VTE risk level and early intervention.
Administer and document in the individual's medication chart pharmacological treatments as ordered by reviewing the individual's medication chart.	The administration of prescribed pharmacological treatments will decrease the VTE risk.

CLINICAL SKILL 15.4 Venous thromboembolism assessment—cont'd

Assess contraindications to pharmacological treatments by reviewing the individual's medication chart. This may include but is not limited to: • known hypersensitivity to agents used in pharmacological prophylaxis • active bleeding or risk of bleeding.	Understanding the contraindications of administering the pharmacological treatment and drug interactions will decrease the risk of bleeding or reaction. This must be reported to the Registered Nurse before the treatment is withheld.
Apply and document in the individual's progress notes mechanical VTE inventions as ordered: • anti-embolic stockings at correct size by measuring length and width of extremity and applying the appropriate size as indicated on the packaging.	The application of mechanical compression stockings will decrease the VTE risk. Bunching of the stockings from incorrect fitting could result in leg ulceration, pressure injuries, slipping and falling on mobilisation.
Assess any contraindications to mechanical prophylaxis treatment. This may include but is not limited to: • morbid obesity where correct fitting cannot be achieved • inflammatory conditions of the lower leg • severe peripheral arterial disease • diabetic neuropathy (there is a risk of injury due to decreased sensation and discomfort if there is a problem with the fitting) • severe oedema of the legs • unusual leg deformity • allergy to stocking material • cardiac failure.	Understanding the contraindications of administering mechanical treatment will decrease the risk of reduced blood flow, pressure ulcers or risk of falls. This must be reported to the Registered Nurse if a decision is made to withhold the treatment.
Discuss overall risk assessment and management with the Registered Nurse before treatment is applied.	Ensures that evidence-based decisions have been considered and are appropriately required (e.g. risk vs benefits of treatment).
Collaborate with other allied healthcare staff by working with the Registered Nurse and identifying referral to allied health staff, if required.	Referral to other health professions ensures holistic care with appropriate interventions.

 AFTER THE SKILL

(Please refer to the Standard Steps on p. xii for related rationales.)
• Communicate outcome to the individual, any ongoing care and to report any complications.
• Restore the environment.
• Report, record and document assessment findings, details of the skill performed and the individual's response.
• Report, record and document any abnormalities and/or inability to perform the skill.
• Reassess the individual to ensure there are no adverse effects/events from the skill.

(Adapted from ACSQHC 2021; Jensen & Smock 2022; NSW Government 2019)

OBSERVATION CHECKLIST: VENOUS THROMBOEMBOLISM ASSESSMENT

Independent (I)	
Supervised (S)	
Assisted (A)	
Marginal (M)	
Dependent (D)	

STUDENT NAME: _____

CLINICAL SKILL 15.4: Venous thromboembolism assessment

DEMONSTRATION OF: The ability to effectively and safely assess an individual's venous thromboembolic status

If the observation checklist is being used as an assessment tool, the student will need to obtain a scale of independence for each of the performance criteria/evidence.

COMPETENCY ELEMENTS	PERFORMANCE CRITERIA/EVIDENCE	I	S	A	M	D
Preparation for the activity	Identifies indications and rationale for performing the activity Identifies the individual using three individual identifiers Ensures therapeutic interaction Gains the individual's consent Checks facility/organisation policy Validates the order in the individual's record Locates and gathers equipment					
Performs activity informed by evidence	Assesses all individuals for level of mobility Assesses baseline risk Assesses additional risk of VTE Administers and documents pharmacological treatments as ordered Assesses contraindications to pharmacological treatments Applies and documents mechanical VTE inventions as ordered Assesses any contraindications to mechanical prophylaxis treatment					
Applies critical thinking and reflective practice	Is able to link theory to practice Demonstrates current best practice in the care provided Assesses own performance					
Practises within safety and quality assurance guidelines	Reviews against facility/organisation policy					
Documentation and communication	Explains and communicates the activity clearly to the individual Communicates outcome and ongoing care to individual and significant others Communicates abnormal findings to appropriate personnel Reports and documents all relevant information and any complications correctly in the healthcare record Reports any complications and/or inability to perform the procedure to the RN and/or medical officer					

Educator/Facilitator Feedback:

Educator/Facilitator Score: Competent   Needs further development

How would you rate your overall performance while undertaking this clinical activity? (use a ✓ & initial)

Unsatisfactory   Satisfactory   Good   Excellent

Student Reflection: (discuss how you would approach your practice differently or more effectively)

EDUCATOR/FACILITATOR NAME/SIGNATURE:

STUDENT NAME/SIGNATURE: **DATE:**

CLINICAL SKILL 15.5 Nutritional assessment/weight, height and BMI

Please adhere to the policy and procedures of the facility/organisation prior to undertaking the skill. Ensure this skill is in your scope of practice.

NMBA Decision-making Framework considerations (refer to NMBA Decision-making framework for nursing and midwifery 2020): 1. Am I educated? 2. Am I authorised? 3. Am I competent? If you answer 'no' to any of these, do not perform that activity. Seek guidance and support from your teacher/a nurse team leader/clinical facilitator/educator.	**Equipment:** Assessment tool used in the clinical facility/organisation The individual's nursing care plan and history

 PREPARE FOR THE SKILL

(Please refer to the Standard Steps on p. xii for related rationales.)
- Mentally review the steps of the skill.
- Discuss the skill with your instructor/supervisor/team leader, if required.
- Confirm correct facility/organisation policy/safe operating procedures.
- Validate the order in the individual's record.
- Identify indication and rationale for performing the activity.
- Assess for any contraindications.
- Locate and gather equipment.
- Perform hand hygiene.
- Ensure therapeutic interaction.
- Identify the individual using three individual identifiers.
- Gain the individual's consent.
- Assess for pain relief.
- Prepare the environment.
- Provide and maintain privacy.
- Assist the individual to assume an appropriate position of comfort.

 PERFORM THE SKILL

(Please refer to the Standard Steps on p. xii for related rationales.)
- Perform hand hygiene.
- Apply PPE: gloves, eyewear, mask and gown as appropriate.
- Ensure the individual's safety and comfort throughout skill.
- Promote independence and involvement of the individual if possible and/or appropriate.
- Assess the individual's tolerance to the skill throughout.
- Dispose of used supplies, equipment, waste and sharps appropriately.
- Remove PPE and discard or store appropriately.
- Perform hand hygiene.

Skill activity	Rationale
Assess the individual's past and current history: • past medical and surgical history • medication history • alcohol and drug use • bowel habits.	Establishes data on past history that may contribute to weight loss or gain.
Assess the individual's psychosocial history: • economic status • occupation • education level • living and cooking arrangements • education level • mental health status.	Establishes a database that may identify any effects on nutritional status.

CLINICAL SKILL 15.5 Nutritional assessment/weight, height and BMI—cont'd

Undertake a nutritional history by asking and/or observing the individual: • nausea/vomiting (>3 days) • diarrhoea • dysphagia • usual adult weight—refer to normal BMI charts • current weight by weighing the individual • current height by measuring the individual • recent changes in appetite or food tolerance • oedema and/or abnormal swelling.	Provides data on appetite.
Undertake a nutritional intake history by asking and/or observing the individual: • diet restrictions • appetite • eating patterns and intakes • taste changes • dentition • dysphagia • feeding independence • vitamin/mineral intake • abdominal pain • nausea and vomiting • changes in bowel pattern (normal or baseline), diarrhoea (consistency, frequency, volume, colour, presence of cramps) • difficulty swallowing (solids vs liquids, intermittent vs continuous) • indigestion or heartburn • mouth sores (ulcers, tooth decay) • pain in swallowing • sore tongue or gums.	Establishes nutritional assistance and modality.
Assess unexplained weight loss or gain: • Undertake a current weight measurement. • Undertake a height measurement.	Collects data for possible undiagnosed medical conditions.
Assess other factors that may affect nutritional status: • age • level of physical activity.	Establishes other not-identified risk factors.
Work in collaboration with other allied healthcare staff.	Referral to other health professions ensures holistic care with appropriate interventions.

AFTER THE SKILL

(Please refer to the Standard Steps on p. xii for related rationales.)
• Communicate outcome to the individual, any ongoing care and to report any complications.
• Restore the environment.
• Report, record and document assessment findings, details of the skill performed and the individual's response.
• Report, record and document any abnormalities and/or inability to perform the skill.
• Reassess the individual to ensure there are no adverse effects/events from the skill.

(Adapted from ACSQHC 2021; Jensen & Smock 2022; NSW Government 2017)

OBSERVATION CHECKLIST: NUTRITION ASSESSMENT/ WEIGHT, HEIGHT AND BMI

Independent (I)

Supervised (S)

Assisted (A)

Marginal (M)

Dependent (D)

STUDENT NAME: _____

CLINICAL SKILL 15.5: Nutrition assessment/weight, height, BMI

DEMONSTRATION OF: The ability to effectively and safely assess an individual's nutritional status including weight, height and BMI

If the observation checklist is being used as an assessment tool, the student will need to obtain a scale of independence for each of the performance criteria/evidence.

COMPETENCY ELEMENTS	PERFORMANCE CRITERIA/EVIDENCE	I	S	A	M	D
Preparation for the activity	Identifies indications and rationale for performing the activity Identifies the individual using three individual identifiers Ensures therapeutic interaction Gains the individual's consent Checks facility/organisation policy Validates the order in the individual's record Locates and gathers equipment					
Performs activity informed by evidence	Assesses the individual's past and current history Assesses the individual's psychosocial history Undertakes a nutritional history by asking and/or observing the individual Undertakes a nutritional intake history Assesses unexplained weight loss or gain Undertakes a current weight measurement Undertakes a height measurement Assesses other factors that may affect nutritional status Identifies lifespan, cultural and language barriers Ensures therapeutic interaction					
Applies critical thinking and reflective practice	Is able to link theory to practice Demonstrates current best practice in the care provided Assesses own performance					
Practises within safety and quality assurance guidelines	Reviews against facility/organisation policy Performs hand hygiene					
Documentation and communication	Explains and communicates the activity clearly to the individual Communicates outcome and ongoing care to individual and significant others Communicates abnormal findings to appropriate personnel Reports and documents all relevant information and any complications correctly in the healthcare record Reports any complications and/or inability to perform the procedure to the RN and/or medical officer					

Educator/Facilitator Feedback:

Educator/Facilitator Score: Competent   Needs further development

How would you rate your overall performance while undertaking this clinical activity? (use a ✓ & initial)

Unsatisfactory   Satisfactory   Good   Excellent

Student Reflection: (discuss how you would approach your practice differently or more effectively)

EDUCATOR/FACILITATOR NAME/SIGNATURE:

STUDENT NAME/SIGNATURE: DATE:

CLINICAL SKILL 15.6 Mobility assessment

Please adhere to the policy and procedures of the facility/organisation prior to undertaking the skill. Ensure this skill is in your scope of practice.

NMBA Decision-making Framework considerations (refer to NMBA Decision-making framework for nursing and midwifery 2020):	Equipment:
1. Am I educated? 2. Am I authorised? 3. Am I competent? If you answer 'no' to any of these, do not perform that activity. Seek guidance and support from your teacher/a nurse team leader/clinical facilitator/educator.	Assessment tool used in the clinical facility/organisation The individual's nursing care plan and history Mobility aids

 ### PREPARE FOR THE SKILL

(Please refer to the Standard Steps on p. xii for related rationales.)
- Mentally review the steps of the skill.
- Discuss the skill with your instructor/supervisor/team leader, if required.
- Confirm correct facility/organisation policy/safe operating procedures.
- Validate the order in the individual's record.
- Identify indication and rationale for performing the activity.
- Assess for any contraindications.
- Locate and gather equipment.
- Perform hand hygiene.
- Ensure therapeutic interaction.
- Identify the individual using three individual identifiers.
- Gain the individual's consent.
- Assess for pain relief.
- Prepare the environment.
- Provide and maintain privacy.
- Assist the individual to assume an appropriate position of comfort.

 ### PERFORM THE SKILL

(Please refer to the Standard Steps on p. xii for related rationales.)
- Perform hand hygiene.
- Apply PPE: gloves, eyewear, mask and gown as appropriate.
- Ensure the individual's safety and comfort throughout skill.
- Promote independence and involvement of the individual if possible and/or appropriate.
- Assess the individual's tolerance to the skill throughout.
- Dispose of used supplies, equipment, waste and sharps appropriately.
- Remove PPE and discard or store appropriately.
- Perform hand hygiene.

Skill activity	Rationale
Assess the individual's cognitive status. This may include but is not limited to: • identifying the individual's conscious state • identifying if the individual has trouble remembering instructions • identifying if the individual understands instructions • identifying if the individual has trouble remembering conversations • identifying if the individual has difficulty finding the right word or often uses incorrect words.	Identifies the individual's ability to understand instructions and to mobilise safely.

CLINICAL SKILL 15.6 Mobility assessment—cont'd

Assess the individual's trunk strength. This may include but is not limited to: • identifying if the individual can stand from a sitting position • identifying if the individual can stand unsupported • identifying if the individual can sit from a standing position with or without support • identifying if an individual can pick up items from the floor safely without falling • identifying any symptoms or signs of paralysis.	Identifies the individual's ability to be seated safely.
Assess the individual's lower extremity for strength, symmetry and tone. This may include but is not limited to: • identifying the strength of both limbs as equal—this can be done by having the individual resist your force as you move the body part against the direction of pull • identifying the muscle bulk of both limbs is equal—this can be done by observation of symmetry of both limbs • identifying the coordination of both limbs is equal—this can be done by observation of a sequence of movements • identifying the abnormal movements of the limbs such as tremors, dystonia, weakness • identifying any symptoms or signs of paralysis.	Identifies the individual's lower extremity stability in order to stand.
Assess the individual's standing balance and gait. This may include but is not limited to: • identifying the symmetry of gait • identifying the length of stride • identifying walking at normal pace • identifying the ability to turn at normal pace using the least amount of steps • identifying the ability to walk in a straight line • identifying any symptoms or signs of paralysis.	Identifies the individual's ability to stand and mobilise safely.
Collaborate with other allied healthcare staff by working with the Registered Nurse and identifying referral to allied health staff, if required.	Referral to other health professions ensures holistic care with appropriate interventions.

 AFTER THE SKILL

(Please refer to the Standard Steps on p. xii for related rationales.)
• Communicate outcome to the individual, any ongoing care and to report any complications.
• Restore the environment.
• Report, record and document assessment findings, details of the skill performed and the individual's response.
• Report, record and document any abnormalities and/or inability to perform the skill.
• Reassess the individual to ensure there are no adverse effects/events from the skill.

(Adapted from ACSQHC 2021; Jensen & Smock 2022)

OBSERVATION CHECKLIST: MOBILITY ASSESSMENT

STUDENT NAME: _____

CLINICAL SKILL 15.6: Mobility assessment

DEMONSTRATION OF: The ability to effectively and safely assess an individual's mobility status

If the observation checklist is being used as an assessment tool, the student will need to obtain a scale of independence for each of the performance criteria/evidence.

Independent (I)
Supervised (S)
Assisted (A)
Marginal (M)
Dependent (D)

COMPETENCY ELEMENTS	PERFORMANCE CRITERIA/EVIDENCE	I	S	A	M	D
Preparation for the activity	Identifies indications and rationale for performing the activity Identifies the individual using three individual identifiers Ensures therapeutic interaction Gains the individual's consent Checks facility/organisation policy Validates the order in the individual's record Locates and gathers equipment					
Performs activity informed by evidence	Assesses the individual's cognitive status Assesses the individual's trunk strength Assesses the individual's lower extremity strength, symmetry and tone Assesses the individual's standing balance and gait Evaluates the presence of pain or discomfort during physical activity. Utilises pain scales or numeric rating scales as required to measure the intensity of pain Assesses environmental factors that could pose barriers or hazards impacting mobility					
Applies critical thinking and reflective practice	Is able to link theory to practice Demonstrates current best practice in the care provided Assesses own performance					
Practises within safety and quality assurance guidelines	Reviews against facility/organisation policy Performs hand hygiene					
Documentation and communication	Explains and communicates the activity clearly to the individual Communicates outcome and ongoing care to the individual and significant others Communicates abnormal findings to appropriate personnel Reports and documents all relevant information and any complications correctly in the healthcare record Reports any complications and/or inability to perform the procedure to the RN and/or medical officer Asks the individual to report any complications during and post procedure					

Educator/Facilitator Feedback:

Educator/Facilitator Score: Competent   Needs further development

How would you rate your overall performance while undertaking this clinical activity? (use a ✓ & initial)

Unsatisfactory   Satisfactory   Good   Excellent

Student Reflection: (discuss how you would approach your practice differently or more effectively)

EDUCATOR/FACILITATOR NAME/SIGNATURE:

STUDENT NAME/SIGNATURE: **DATE:**

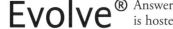 Answer guide for the Critical Thinking Exercises and Critical Thinking Questions in Case Studies is hosted on Evolve: http://evolve.elsevier.com/AU/Koutoukidis/Tabbner/

References

Australian Commission on Safety and Quality in Health Care (ACSQHC), 2021. *National Safety and Quality Health Service Standards*, 2nd ed. Available at: <https://www.safetyandquality.gov.au/sites/default/files/migrated/National-Safety-and-Quality-Health-Service-Standards-second-edition.pdf>.

Brown, D., Edwards, H., Buckley, T., et al., 2020. *Lewis's medical-surgical nursing ANZ*, 5th ed. Elsevier, Sydney.

European Pressure Ulcer Advisory Panel, National Pressure Injury Advisory Panel and Pan Pacific Pressure Injury Alliance (EPUAP/NPIAP/PPPIA), 2019. Prevention and treatment of pressure ulcers/injuries: Quick reference guide. In: Haesler, E. (ed.). EPUAP/NPIAP/PPPIA.

Department of Health, Government of Western Australia, 2014. Falls risk assessment and management plan. Available at: <https://ww2.health.wa.gov.au/Articles/F_I/Falls-Risk-Assessment-and-Management-Plan>.

Jensen, S., 2019. *Nursing health assessment: A best practice approach*, 3rd ed. Wolters Kluwer, Philadelphia.

Jensen, S., Smock, R. 2022. *Nursing health assessment: A clinical judgment approach*. Lippincott Williams & Wilkins.

Lewis, P., Foley, D., 2020. *Health assessment in nursing, Australia and New Zealand edition*, 3rd ed. Wolters Kluwer, North Ryde.

McCormack, B., McCance, T., 2017. *Person-centred practice in nursing and healthcare theory and practice*, 2nd ed. Wiley Blackwell, Chichester.

NSW Government, Ministry of Health, 2017. Nutrition care. Available at: <https://www1.health.nsw.gov.au/pds/ActivePDSDocuments/PD2017_041.pdf>.

NSW Government, Ministry of Health, 2019. Prevention of venous thromboembolism. Available at: <https://www1.health.nsw.gov.au/pds/Pages/doc.aspx?dn=PD2019_057>.

Nursing and Midwifery Board of Australia (NMBA), 2020. Decision-making framework for nursing and midwifery. Available at: <https://www.nursingmidwiferyboard.gov.au/Codes-Guidelines-Statements/Frameworks.aspx>.

VITAL SIGNS

Rachel Wassink

Overview

Vital signs involve the measurement and assessment of the body's temperature, pulse, respiration, oxygen saturation and blood pressure, and are the core component of a basic physical assessment. Vital sign measurement is an essential aspect of a nurse's role and not only forms part of the nursing process but also identifies deterioration in an individual's condition. Nurses must know the normal limits and perform repeat observations to observe for trends and determine how often to do these observations according to the individual's condition, to decrease the chance of their condition becoming critical (Crisp et al 2021).

Vital signs information is used throughout the healthcare team to inform and assist diagnosis and treatment plans and therefore accurate and timely measurements are extremely important. This information needs to be communicated effectively, both verbally and written, to ensure and support good decision-making. Vital signs are part of the assessment step of the nursing process and it is necessary to measure vital signs to detect changes in condition (even signalling life-threatening events) and gain data on treatment response (Sorrentino & Remmert 2017).

There are a variety of different situations in which vital signs are measured and collected, including:

- When an individual is admitted or discharged from a healthcare facility or department
- Before and after surgical procedures
- Before and after administration of medications that affect vital signs such as cardiovascular or respiratory medications
- Before and after invasive procedures
- If an individual's condition changes
- Before and after any interventions which may affect vital signs
- If an individual reports a non-specific symptom of physical distress; for example, 'I just don't feel right'.
- Routine monitoring, which should be determined by the individual's condition and each organisation's protocols.
  (Crisp et al 2021)

After the measurement and assessment of the individual's vital signs, the observations are documented. Observation charts usually provide for the documentation of a range of assessments including vital signs. Given the importance of these charts in identifying people at risk, the Australian Commission on Safety and Quality in Health Care (ACSQHC) has developed a range of observation charts designed to show trend data (ACSQHC 2023). It is clear on the national observation chart where assessment parameters are breached and require further urgent assessment and management (ACSQHC 2023). Any interventions provided in response to changes in vital signs must be documented, including the details of who these changes were reported to.

An abnormality or change in one vital sign can affect other vital signs; therefore, it is important to complete a full set to support critical thinking. A change in one vital sign, such as pulse, can reflect changes in other vital signs, such as blood pressure, as they are interlinked to support homeostasis (Crisp et al 2021).

When measuring vital signs in an individual, the nurse should observe the following points:
- Ensure the equipment is appropriate and functioning
- Have knowledge of the normal range of vital sign measurements
- Have knowledge of the individual's usual range of vital signs
- Know and understand the individual's medical history, therapies and medications prescribed
- Perform measurements in an appropriate environment that will have minimal effect on vital signs
- Have an organised systematic approach
- Have the knowledge to interpret the significance of vital signs and consequently make decisions about individual care
- Determine the frequency of vital sign measurement based on the individual's condition
- Have the knowledge to analyse results
- Be aware of other physical signs and symptoms of abnormal vital signs
- Verify and communicate findings and changes of an individual's condition to the relevant Registered Nurse (RN) or medical officer.

This chapter will describe the skills needed in measuring and assessing vital signs. These include assessing respirations (Clinical Skill 16.1), measuring oxygen saturation (Clinical Skill 16.2), measuring blood pressure (Clinical Skill 16.3), assessing pulse rate (Clinical Skill 16.4) and assessing body temperature (Clinical Skill 16.5).

OLDER ADULTS

Measuring vital signs in individuals with dementia may be difficult. The person may move about, strike out at the nurse and grab equipment. This is not safe for the person or the nurse. Two staff may be needed; one to use touch and a soothing voice to calm and distract the person while the other measures the vital signs.

Trying the procedure when the person is calmer may help, as may taking the respirations and pulse at one time, then taking temperature and blood pressure later.

The person should always be approached in a calm manner. The nurse should use a soothing voice and inform the person what they are about to do. Do not rush. Follow the care plan. If vital signs cannot be measured, the RN should be informed (Sorrentino & Remmert 2017).

 CASE STUDY 16.1

George Callahan, a 65-year-old male, is admitted to the cardiac ward with atrial fibrillation. This is a new presentation and George has never been admitted to hospital before. George's wife has many questions about what atrial fibrillation is and how it will affect his life. George wants to know why he finds it difficult to breathe when he is walking.

- Past history: Hypertension, high cholesterol.
- Allergies: None known.
  Observations:
- Pulse: 110 beats/min and irregular
- Blood pressure: 100/55 mmHg
- Temperature: 36.8°C
- Respiratory rate: 14 breaths/min
- Oxygen saturation: 96% on room air
  > Which observations are abnormal?
  > Why is George's pulse irregular?
  > Explain why George's blood pressure is slightly low at 100 mmHg.
  > What advice would you give to George's family about his admission?
  > Why does George become short of breath on exertion?

CRITICAL THINKING EXERCISE 16.1

1. Why are unequal bilateral breath sounds clinically significant?
2. Changes in respiratory rate can be an early indicator for clinical deterioration. Explain why.
3. When auscultating breath sounds, what difference would you expect before and after Ventolin administration?
4. Mr Lui was admitted in the medical ward with pneumonia. What would you expect Mr Lui's respiratory rate and oxygen saturations to be? Explain your rationale.

CLINICAL SKILL 16.1 Assessing respirations

Please adhere to the policy and procedures of the facility/organisation prior to undertaking the skill. Ensure this skill is in your scope of practice.

NMBA Decision-making Framework considerations (refer to NMBA Decision-making framework for nursing and midwifery 2020):	Equipment:
1. Am I educated? 2. Am I authorised? 3. Am I competent? If you answer 'no' to any of these, do not perform that activity. Seek guidance and support from your teacher/a nurse team leader/clinical facilitator/educator.	Watch Pen (blue/black) Observation chart

 PREPARE FOR THE SKILL

(Please refer to the Standard Steps on p. xii for related rationales.)
- Mentally review the steps of the skill.
- Discuss the skill with your instructor/supervisor/team leader, if required.
- Confirm correct facility/organisation policy/safe operating procedures.
- Validate the order in the individual's record.
- Identify indication and rationale for performing the activity.
- Assess for any contraindications.
- Locate and gather equipment.
- Perform hand hygiene.
- Ensure therapeutic interaction.
- Identify the individual using three individual identifiers.
- Gain the individual's consent.
- Assess for pain relief.
- Prepare the environment.
- Provide and maintain privacy.
- Assist the individual to assume an appropriate position of comfort.

Skill activity	Rationale
Check individual's previous baseline respirations.	It is important to know the individual's usual respiration rate to allow a comparison to be made.

 PERFORM THE SKILL

(Please refer to the Standard Steps on p. xii for related rationales.)
- Perform hand hygiene.
- Apply PPE: gloves, eyewear, mask and gown as appropriate.
- Ensure the individual's safety and comfort throughout skill.
- Promote independence and involvement of the individual if possible and/or appropriate.
- Assess the individual's tolerance to the skill throughout.
- Dispose of used supplies, equipment, waste and sharps appropriately.
- Remove PPE and discard or store appropriately.
- Perform hand hygiene.

Skill activity	Rationale
Ensure that the individual is resting in a position of comfort, preferably sitting or lying with the head of the bed elevated 45–60 degrees.	Exercise or discomfort alters the nature of respirations. Sitting erect promotes full ventilator movement.
Assess for signs and symptoms of respiratory alterations such as cyanotic appearance, restlessness, irritability, confusion, reduced level of consciousness, pain, difficulty breathing, production of sputum, presence of a cough.	Physical signs and symptoms may indicate alterations in respiratory status related to ventilation.

CLINICAL SKILL 16.1 Assessing respirations—cont'd

Position yourself to ensure you can see or feel the rise and fall of the chest: Place your fingers on the location of the radial pulse and watch the chest rise and fall and/or place second hand on upper back/chest to feel the rise and fall.	Feeling the rise and fall during the respiratory cycle makes it easier to count the respirations. It is important to note that if the individual is aware you are checking their respiratory rate, they become aware of their breathing which can alter the rate and depth. By placing fingers on the radial pulse, the individual will assume you are checking their pulse, potentially not altering their respiratory rate.
Once you have observed one full cycle, counting can commence. Using a watch with a second hand, with your hand on the radial pulse site, count the respirations for one minute.	Positioning yourself to appear to be checking the pulse prevents the individual from being aware that their respirations are being assessed. Inconspicuous assessment prevents individual from consciously or unintentionally altering rate and depth of breathing. The intervals between respirations may be inconsistent, and counting for a full minute enables an accurate measurement of rate.
If rhythm is regular, count number of respirations in 30 seconds and multiply by two. If rhythm is greater than 16 respirations per minute, count for a full minute.	Respiratory rate is equivalent to number of respirations per minute. Suspected irregularities require assessment for at least one minute.
While measuring the rate, also observe the rhythm (regular and irregular), depth (shallow, normal or deep) and sound of respirations.	A complete assessment of respirations is necessary.
Observe for evidence of dyspnoea (increased effort to inhale and exhale). Ask individual to describe subjective experience of shortness of breath compared with usual breathing pattern.	Individuals with chronic lung disease may experience difficulty breathing all the time and can best describe their own discomfort from shortness of breath.

NOTE: Occasional periods of apnoea are a symptom of underlying disease in an adult and must be reported to the medical officer or relevant Registered Nurse. Irregular respirations and short episodes of apnoea are normal in a newborn. Sighing is not an abnormality and should not be confused with an abnormal rhythm; it is one deep breath that opens up the small airways in the individual.

 AFTER THE SKILL

(Please refer to the Standard Steps on p. xii for related rationales.)
- Communicate outcome to the individual, any ongoing care and to report any complications.
- Restore the environment.
- Report, record and document assessment findings, details of the skill performed and the individual's response.
- Report, record and document any abnormalities and/or inability to perform the skill.
- Reassess the individual to ensure there are no adverse effects/events from the skill.

(Crisp et al 2021; Forbes & Watt 2021)

OBSERVATION CHECKLIST: ASSESSMENT OF RESPIRATIONS

STUDENT NAME: _____

CLINICAL SKILL 16.1: Assessment of respirations

DEMONSTRATION OF: The ability to effectively measure and assess respirations

If the observation checklist is being used as an assessment tool, the student will need to obtain a scale of independence for each of the performance criteria/evidence

Independent (I)
Supervised (S)
Assisted (A)
Marginal (M)
Dependent (D)

COMPETENCY ELEMENTS	PERFORMANCE CRITERIA/EVIDENCE	I	S	A	M	D
Preparation for the activity	Identifies indications and rationale for performing the activity Identifies the individual using three individual identifiers Ensures therapeutic interaction Gains the individual's consent Checks facility/organisation policy Validates the order in the individual's record Locates and gathers equipment Checks the individual's previous baseline resting respiration rate					
Performs activity informed by evidence	Ensures the individual is in a position of comfort, preferably sitting or lying with the head of the bed elevated 45–60 degrees Assesses for signs and symptoms of respiratory alterations Places individual's arm or their hand in a relaxed position across the abdomen or lower chest, directly over individual's upper abdomen Observes complete respiratory cycle Using a watch, counts the respirations for one minute If the rhythm is regular, counts number of respirations in 30 seconds and multiplies by two If rhythm is greater than 16 respirations per minute, counts for a full minute When measuring the rate, also observes rhythm, depth and sound Observes for evidence of dyspnoea Asks individual to describe subjective experience of shortness of breath					
Applies critical thinking and reflective practice	Is able to link theory to practice Demonstrates current best practice in the care provided If this is the first time respiration has been measured, if in normal range, establishes as a baseline Compares with the baseline and acceptable respiration rate range for the individual Assesses own performance					
Practises within safety and quality assurance guidelines	Reviews against facility/organisation policy Performs hand hygiene, dons appropriate PPE as per infection control protocols Cleans and disposes of equipment and waste appropriately					

COMPETENCY ELEMENTS	PERFORMANCE CRITERIA/EVIDENCE	I	S	A	M	D
Documentation and communication	Explains and communicates the activity clearly to the individual Communicates outcome and ongoing care to individual and significant others Communicates abnormal findings to appropriate personnel Reports and documents all relevant information and any complications correctly in the healthcare record Reports any complications and/or inability to perform the procedure to the RN and/or medical officer Asks the individual to report any complications during and post procedure					

Educator/Facilitator Feedback:

Educator/Facilitator Score: Competent   Needs further development

How would you rate your overall performance while undertaking this clinical activity? (use a ✓ & initial)

Unsatisfactory   Satisfactory   Good   Excellent

Student Reflection: (discuss how you would approach your practice differently or more effectively)

EDUCATOR/FACILITATOR NAME/SIGNATURE:

STUDENT NAME/SIGNATURE: **DATE:**

CLINICAL SKILL 16.2 Measuring oxygen saturation

Please adhere to the policy and procedures of the facility/organisation prior to undertaking the skill. Ensure this skill is in your scope of practice.

NMBA Decision-making Framework considerations (refer to NMBA Decision-making framework for nursing and midwifery 2020):	Equipment:
1. Am I educated? 2. Am I authorised? 3. Am I competent? If you answer 'no' to any of these, do not perform that activity. Seek guidance and support from your teacher/a nurse team leader/clinical facilitator/educator.	Pulse oximeter monitor Sensor probe and cord Pen (blue/black) Observation chart Nail polish remover if required Alcohol-based wipes

PREPARE FOR THE SKILL

(Please refer to the Standard Steps on p. xii for related rationales.)
- Mentally review the steps of the skill.
- Discuss the skill with your instructor/supervisor/team leader, if required.
- Confirm correct facility/organisation policy/safe operating procedures.
- Validate the order in the individual's record.
- Identify indication and rationale for performing the activity.
- Assess for any contraindications.
- Locate and gather equipment.
- Perform hand hygiene.
- Ensure therapeutic interaction.
- Identify the individual using three individual identifiers.
- Gain the individual's consent.
- Assess for pain relief.
- Prepare the environment.
- Provide and maintain privacy.
- Assist the individual to assume an appropriate position of comfort.

Skill activity	Rationale
Check individual's previous baseline SaO_2 measurement.	It is important to know the individual's usual SaO_2 measurement to allow for evaluation of changes.

PERFORM THE SKILL

(Please refer to the Standard Steps on p. xii for related rationales.)
- Perform hand hygiene.
- Apply PPE: gloves, eyewear, mask and gown as appropriate.
- Ensure the individual's safety and comfort throughout skill.
- Promote independence and involvement of the individual if possible and/or appropriate.
- Assess the individual's tolerance to the skill throughout.
- Dispose of used supplies, equipment, waste and sharps appropriately.
- Remove PPE and discard or store appropriately.
- Perform hand hygiene.

Skill activity	Rationale
Assess for signs and symptoms of alterations in oxygen saturation such as altered respiratory status, cyanotic appearance, restlessness, irritability, confusion, reduced level of consciousness, laboured or difficulty breathing.	Physical signs and symptoms may indicate abnormal oxygen saturation.
Assess for factors that normally influence measurement of SpO_2 including oxygen therapy, haemoglobin level and temperature.	Allows for accurate assessment of oxygen saturation variations. Peripheral vasoconstriction related to hypothermia can interfere with SpO_2 determination.
Instruct individual to breathe normally.	Prevents large fluctuations in respiration and possible error in reading.

Continued

CLINICAL SKILL 16.2 Measuring oxygen saturation—cont'd

Assess the site most appropriate for sensor probe placement. Site must have adequate local circulation and be free of moisture. If finger is to be used, remove nail polish, dirt or dried blood.	Peripheral vasoconstriction can interfere with SpO_2 determination. Opaque coatings such as nail polish decrease light transmission.
Determine capillary refill at site. If less than three seconds, select alternative site.	Cool temperature with vasoconstriction or vascular disease may decrease circulation, impede refill and prevent sensor from measuring SpO_2.
Position individual comfortably. If finger is chosen as monitoring site, support lower arm. Instruct individual to keep sensor probe site still.	Movement interferes with SpO_2 determination. Pressure of sensor probe's spring tension on finger or earlobe may be uncomfortable.
Attach sensor probe to monitoring site.	Select sensor site based on peripheral circulation and extremity temperature.
Turn on oximeter by activating power and observe pulse waveform. Correlate oximeter pulse rate with individual's radial pulse.	Enables detection of valid pulse.
Leave probe in place until oximeter readout reaches constant value and pulse display reaches full strength during each cardiac cycle. Read SpO_2 on digital display.	Pulse waveform and intensity display enables detection of valid pulse or presence of interfering signal. Reading may take from 10 to 30 seconds.
If continuous SpO_2 monitoring is planned, verify SpO_2 alarm limits, which are pre-set by the manufacturer at a low of 85% and a high of 100%. Limits for SpO_2 and pulse rate should be determined as indicated by individual's condition. Verify that alarms are on, assess skin integrity under sensor every two hours. Relocate sensor at least every four hours, and more frequently if skin integrity is altered.	Spring tension of sensor or sensitivity to disposable sensor adhesive can cause skin irritation and lead to disruption of skin integrity.
If intermittent or spot-checking SpO_2 measurements are planned, remove sensor probe and turn oximeter power off. Clean with alcohol-based wipes. Store sensor probe in appropriate location.	Sensor probes are expensive and vulnerable to damage. Maintains battery charge, reduces risk of transmission of microorganisms.

NOTE:
- Do not attach probe to finger, ear or bridge of nose if area is oedematous or skin integrity is compromised.
- Do not attach sensor to fingers that are hypothermic as vasoconstriction will alter the reading.
- Do not place sensor on same extremity as electronic blood pressure cuff. Blood flow to finger will be temporarily interrupted when cuff inflates and cause inaccurate blood pressure reading that triggers alarm.
- Do not place pulse oximeter on a limb that has an arterial or intravenous line in situ as fluid entering the arterial line may dilute the blood to alter the reading, and an intravenous line may reduce the outflow of blood from the limb so there is congestion of the venous blood, also altering the reading.
- If oximeter pulse rate, individual's radial pulse rate and apical pulse rate are different, re-evaluate oximeter sensor placement and reassess pulse rates.

 AFTER THE SKILL

(Please refer to the Standard Steps on p. xii for related rationales)
- Communicate outcome to the individual, any ongoing care and to report any complications.
- Restore the environment.
- Report, record and document assessment findings, details of the skill performed and the individual's response.
- Report, record and document any abnormalities and/or inability to perform the skill.
- Reassess the individual to ensure there are no adverse effects/events from the skill.

(Crisp et al 2021; Forbes & Watt 2021)

OBSERVATION CHECKLIST: MEASURING OXYGEN SATURATION (PULSE OXIMETRY, SpO$_2$)

STUDENT NAME: _____

CLINICAL SKILL 16.2: Measuring oxygen saturation (pulse oximetry, SpO$_2$)

DEMONSTRATION OF: The ability to effectively measure and assess oxygen saturation

If the observation checklist is being used as an assessment tool, the student will need to obtain a scale of independence for each of the performance criteria/evidence

Independent (I)

Supervised (S)

Assisted (A)

Marginal (M)

Dependent (D)

COMPETENCY ELEMENTS	PERFORMANCE CRITERIA/EVIDENCE	I	S	A	M	D
Preparation for the activity	Identifies indications and rationale for performing the activity Identifies the individual using three individual identifiers Ensures therapeutic interaction Gains the individual's consent Checks facility/organisation policy Validates the order in the individual's record Locates and gathers equipment Assesses for signs and symptoms of alterations in oxygen saturation Assesses for factors that normally influence measurement of SpO$_2$ Assesses the site most appropriate for sensory probe placement Determines capillary refill at site Checks the individual's previous baseline oxygen saturation level Assists the individual into an appropriate position					
Performs activity informed by evidence	Instructs individual to breathe normally If finger is chosen as monitoring site, supports lower arm and instructs individual to keep sensor probe still Attaches sensor probe to monitoring site Turns on oximeter by activating power and observes pulse waveform Correlates oximeter pulse rate with individual's pulse rate Leaves probe in place until oximeter readout reaches constant value and pulse display reaches full strength through each cardiac cycle Reads SpO$_2$ on digital display If continuous SpO$_2$ monitoring: • Verifies SpO$_2$ alarm limits • Verifies alarms are on • Assesses skin integrity under sensor every two hours • Relocates sensor at least every four hours If intermittent SpO$_2$: • Removes sensor probe • Turns oximeter power off • Cleans equipment and stores appropriately • Discusses findings with individual as needed					

Continued

COMPETENCY ELEMENTS	PERFORMANCE CRITERIA/EVIDENCE	I	S	A	M	D
Applies critical thinking and reflective practice	Is able to link theory to practice Demonstrates current best practice in the care provided If this is the first time oxygen saturation has been measured, if in normal range, establishes as a baseline Compares with the baseline and acceptable oxygen saturation range for the individual Assesses own performance					
Practises within safety and quality assurance guidelines	Reviews against facility/organisation policy Cleans and disposes of equipment appropriately					
Documentation and communication	Explains and communicates the activity clearly to the individual Communicates outcome and ongoing care to individual and significant others Communicates abnormal findings to appropriate personnel Reports and documents all relevant information and any complications correctly in the healthcare record Reports any complications and/or inability to perform the procedure to the RN and/or medical officer Asks the individual to report any complications during and post procedure					

Educator/Facilitator Feedback:

Educator/Facilitator Score: Competent   Needs further development

How would you rate your overall performance while undertaking this clinical activity? (use a ✓ & initial)

Unsatisfactory   Satisfactory   Good   Excellent

Student Reflection: (discuss how you would approach your practice differently or more effectively)

EDUCATOR/FACILITATOR NAME/SIGNATURE:

STUDENT NAME/SIGNATURE: **DATE:**

CLINICAL SKILL 16.3 Measuring blood pressure

Please adhere to the policy and procedures of the facility/organisation prior to undertaking the skill. Ensure this skill is in your scope of practice.

NMBA Decision-making Framework considerations (refer to NMBA Decision-making framework for nursing and midwifery 2020):	Equipment:
1. Am I educated? 2. Am I authorised? 3. Am I competent? If you answer 'no' to any of these, do not perform that activity. Seek guidance and support from your teacher/a nurse team leader/clinical facilitator/educator.	Sphygmomanometer—including manometer, an appropriate-sized cuff and bladder, and a bulb and pressure valve Stethoscope Alcohol swab Pen (blue/black) Observation chart For electronic blood pressure: • Electronic blood pressure machine • Blood pressure cuff of appropriate size as recommended by manufacturer • Source of electricity • Alcohol-based wipes

 PREPARE FOR THE SKILL

(Please refer to the Standard Steps on p. xii for related rationales.)
- Mentally review the steps of the skill.
- Discuss the skill with your instructor/supervisor/team leader, if required.
- Confirm correct facility/organisation policy/safe operating procedures.
- Validate the order in the individual's record.
- Identify indication and rationale for performing the activity.
- Assess for any contraindications.
- Locate and gather equipment.
- Perform hand hygiene.
- Ensure therapeutic interaction.
- Identify the individual using three individual identifiers.
- Gain the individual's consent.
- Assess for pain relief.
- Prepare the environment.
- Provide and maintain privacy.
- Assist the individual to assume an appropriate position of comfort.

Skill activity	Rationale
Before measuring BP, you need this information from the nurse and the care plan: • when to measure BP • what arm to use • the person's normal blood pressure range • if the person needs to be lying down, sitting or standing • what size cuff to use—regular, child-sized, extra-large, bariatric • what observations to report and record • when to report the BP measurement.	It is important to know the individual's usual blood pressure to allow for a comparison to be made.
Ensure that the individual is rested and in a position of comfort. Encourage individual to avoid exercise, caffeine and smoking for 30 minutes prior to assessment of blood pressure and have them rest at minimum 5–10 minutes before measuring. Provide privacy and reduce environmental noise.	Activity or discomfort may increase blood pressure. Allows you to hear the blood pressure sounds more accurately and puts the individual at ease.
Observe for signs and symptoms of blood pressure alterations, either high (headache, face flushing, nosebleed, fatigue) or low (dizziness, mental confusion, restlessness, pale skin, cool and mottled skin over extremities).	Physical signs and symptoms may indicate alterations in blood pressure.

CLINICAL SKILL 16.3 Measuring blood pressure—cont'd

 PERFORM THE SKILL

(Please refer to the Standard Steps on p. xii for related rationales.)
- Perform hand hygiene.
- Apply PPE: gloves, eyewear, mask and gown as appropriate.
- Ensure the individual's safety and comfort throughout skill.
- Promote independence and involvement of the individual if possible and/or appropriate.
- Assess the individual's tolerance to the skill throughout.
- Dispose of used supplies, equipment, waste and sharps appropriately.
- Remove PPE and discard or store appropriately.
- Perform hand hygiene.

Skill activity	Rationale
Determine best site for blood pressure assessment. Avoid applying cuff to extremity when: • Intravenous fluids are infusing. • An arteriovenous shunt or fistula is present. • Breast or axillary surgery has been performed on that side. • Extremity has been traumatised, is diseased or requires a cast or bulky bandage. • Cast in place. • Side affected by stroke symptoms. The lower extremities may be used when the brachial arteries are inaccessible.	Inappropriate site selection may result in poor amplification of sounds causing inaccurate readings. Application of pressure from inflated bladder temporarily impairs blood flow and can further compromise circulation in extremity that already has impaired blood flow.
Select an appropriate cuff size for person's arm. Use a larger cuff if the person is obese or has a large arm. Use a small cuff if the person has a very small arm. The person's cuff size should be listed in the care plan.	Ensure snug fit of cuff. A cuff that is too small may result in a false high reading, while a cuff that is too large may result in a false low reading. Cuff size according to age: • paediatric cuff • infant cuff • large cuff for large size arm.
Have the individual assume a sitting position if possible, with back support and feet on the ground. Ensure the individual has rested at least five minutes in this position.	Sitting is preferred to lying. Diastolic pressure measured while sitting is approximately 5 mmHg higher than when measured supine. In the older adult, a significant 20 mmHg difference between lying and sitting can occur in patients with diabetes and those with symptoms suggestive of postural hypotension, such as dizziness, syncope and falls on changing position.
Remove any constricting clothing from the individual's arm. Support the arm in an extended position with the palm facing up. Position the arm so that the brachial artery is at the level of the heart.	Tight clothing may reduce blood flow or create venous congestion in the arm. Correct arm placement enables accurate blood pressure measurement. Placement of arm above the level of the heart causes false low readings. Placement of arm lower than the level of the heart causes false high readings. For every 2.5 cm that the arm is above the level of the heart, the pressure reading will be 1 mmHg lower; similarly, if the arm is lower than the level of the heart, the reading will be too high. It may not always be possible to position the person in a seated position. If arm is extended and not supported, individual may perform isometric exercise that can increase diastolic pressure 10%. Even in the supine position a diastolic increase of as much as 3–4 mmHg can occur for each 5 cm the arm is below the level of the heart.
Clean the stethoscope earpieces and diaphragm with the wipes.	Reduces risk of transmission of microorganisms.

Continued

CLINICAL SKILL 16.3 Measuring blood pressure—cont'd

Check for air leaks in the cuff, tubing and valves of the sphygmomanometer.	Leakage of air may result in an inaccurate measurement.
Squeeze the cuff to expel any air, then tighten the valves by turning anticlockwise.	Prepares the cuff for use. Inflating bladder directly over artery ensures proper pressure is applied during inflation.
Make sure the room and the individual are quiet.	Talking, TV, music and sounds from the hallway can affect an accurate measurement.
Two-step method	
Clean the stethoscope earpieces and diaphragm with the wipes.	Reduces risk of transmission of microorganisms.
Position the sphygmomanometer on a level surface, at eye level.	If incorrectly placed, or not clearly visible by nurse, an inaccurate measurement may result. Errors in measurement can occur if the manometer is not vertical.
Palpate the radial pulse and, with the fingers on the pulse, rapidly inflate cuff to 30 mmHg above point at which pulse disappears, slowly deflate cuff and note point when pulse reappears.	This measurement provides an approximation of the systolic pressure and prevents the cuff from subsequently being overinflated.
Deflate the cuff completely and allow 30 seconds for arm to rest before reinflating the cuff.	Releases remaining air. Allows blood trapped in the veins to be returned to circulation.
Place the disc of the warmed stethoscope over the brachial artery in the antecubital fossa and hold in place with the thumb and index finger of the non-dominant hand. Reflate the cuff 30 mmHg above the palpated systolic pressure reading during the previous inflation. When placing the diaphragm of the stethoscope firmly over the brachial artery ensure entire diaphragm has full contact with the skin.	Pulse beat can be heard when the disc is placed directly over the artery, allowing for precise measurement of the systolic pressure. Warming the stethoscope with your palm will decrease discomfort for the individual.
Use the valve on the hand pump to release air, and slowly deflate the cuff at 2–3 mmHg per second—no faster than 5 mmHg per second.	If the cuff is deflated too rapidly, there will be insufficient time to assess the pressure accurately. Deflating too rapidly or too slowly gives false readings. Avoid contact of the stethoscope tubing with the clothing, cuff or tubing of the sphygmomanometer to decrease the possibility of extraneous noise.
Note the pressure reading on the manometer as soon as the pulse beat is heard through the stethoscope. The sound slowly increases in intensity.	This measurement indicates the systolic pressure.
Continue to slowly deflate the cuff. Note the pressure reading as soon as the pulse sounds muffled or disappears. Listen for 10–20 mmHg after the last sound then allow the remaining air to escape quickly.	This measurement indicates the diastolic pressure, releases remaining air and decreases individual's discomfort.
Remove the cuff and adjust the individual's clothing.	Promotes comfort.
If this is the first assessment of individual, repeat procedure on other extremity.	Comparison of blood pressure in both extremities detects circulation problems (normal difference of 5–10 mmHg exists between extremities).
One-step method	
Place stethoscope earpieces in ears and be sure sounds are clear and not muffled.	Ensures each earpiece follows angle of ear canal to facilitate hearing.

CLINICAL SKILL 16.3 Measuring blood pressure—cont'd

Locate brachial artery, and place diaphragm of stethoscope over it. Do not allow chest-piece to touch cuff or clothing.	Proper stethoscope placement ensures optimal reception.
Close valve of pressure bulb clockwise until tight.	Tightening of valve prevents air leak during inflation.
Quickly inflate cuff to 30 mmHg above individual's usual systolic pressure.	Inflation above systolic level ensures accurate measurement of systolic pressure.
Slowly release pressure bulb valve and allow manometer needle to fall at a rate of 2–3 mmHg/sec. Note point on manometer when first sound is heard. The sound will slowly increase in intensity.	Too rapid or slow a decline in pressure release causes inaccurate readings. The first Korotkoff sounds reflect systolic pressure.
Continue to deflate cuff gradually, noting point at which sound disappears in adults. Note pressure to nearest 2 mmHg. Listen for 20–30 mmHg after the last sound, and then allow remaining air to escape quickly.	Beginning of the fifth Korotkoff sound is an indicator of diastolic pressure in adults. Fourth Korotkoff sound involves distinct muffling of sounds and is an indication of diastolic pressure in children.
Remove the cuff and adjust the individual's clothing.	Promotes comfort.
Assessing blood pressure electronically	
Determine appropriateness of using electronic blood pressure measurement.	Individuals with irregular heart rate, peripheral vascular disease, seizures, tremors and shivering are not candidates for this device.
Determine best site for blood pressure assessment. Avoid applying cuff to extremity when intravenous fluids are infusing; an arteriovenous shunt or fistula is present; breast or axillary surgery has been performed on that side; extremity has been traumatised, is diseased or requires a cast or bulky bandage. The lower extremities may be used when the brachial arteries are inaccessible.	Inappropriate site selection may result in poor amplification of sounds causing inaccurate readings. Application of pressure from inflated bladder temporarily impairs blood flow and can further compromise circulation in extremity that already has impaired blood flow.
Assist individual to comfortable position, either lying or sitting. Plug in device and place near individual ensuring that connector hose reaches between cuff and machine.	Ensures individual's comfort and that equipment is prepared and in a good position to use.
Locate on/off switch and turn on machine to enable device to self-test computer systems.	Ensures it is working.
Select appropriate cuff size for individual's extremity and appropriate cuff for machine.	Ensures accurate reading. Electronic blood pressure cuff and machine are matched by manufacturer and are not interchangeable.
Expose extremity for measurement by removing constricting clothing.	To ensure proper cuff application, cuff must not be placed over clothing.
Prepare blood pressure cuff by manually squeezing the air out of the cuff and connecting cuff to connector hose.	Prepares the cuff for use.
Wrap flattened cuff snugly around extremity, verifying that only one finger fits between cuff and individual's skin. Make sure that the 'artery' arrow marked on the outside of the cuff is correctly placed.	An incorrectly placed, or loosely applied, cuff may result in an inaccurate measurement.
Verify that connector hose between cuff and machine is not kinked.	Kinking prevents proper inflation and deflation of cuff.

Continued

CLINICAL SKILL 16.3 Measuring blood pressure—cont'd

Following manufacturer's directions, set the frequency control to automatic or manual, and then press start button. The first blood pressure measurement pumps the cuff to a peak pressure of about 180 mmHg. After this pressure is reached, the machine begins a deflation sequence that determines blood pressure. The first reading determines the peak pressure inflation for additional measurements.	Following manufacturer's directions is important in obtaining an accurate measure.
When deflation is complete, digital display provides the most recent values and flashes time in minutes that have elapsed since the measurement occurred.	If the individual is having their blood pressure measured at intervals, this function can inform you of when the last measurement was.
Set frequency of blood pressure measurements and upper and lower alarm limits for systolic, diastolic and mean blood pressure readings. Intervals between blood pressure measurements are set from 1 to 90 minutes.	The nurse determines frequency and alarm limits based on individual's acceptable range of blood pressure, nursing judgment, facility/organisation's standards or healthcare provider order.
Obtain additional readings at any time by pressing the start button. Pressing the cancel button immediately deflates the cuff.	Additional readings may be needed if the individual's condition changes.
If frequent blood pressure measurements are required keep the cuff in place. Remove cuff every two hours to assess underlying skin integrity and if possible alternate blood pressure sites.	Individuals with abnormal bleeding tendencies are at risk for microvascular rupture from repeated inflations.
Compare electronic blood pressure readings with auscultated blood pressure measurements to verify accuracy of electronic blood pressure device.	Individuals with hypertension, hypotension or an arrhythmia may have inaccurate electronic blood pressure monitor readings.

 AFTER THE SKILL

(Please refer to the Standard Steps on p. xii for related rationales.)
- Communicate outcome to the individual, any ongoing care and to report any complications.
- Restore the environment.
- Report, record and document assessment findings, details of the skill performed and the individual's response.
- Report, record and document any abnormalities and/or inability to perform the skill.
- Reassess the individual to ensure there are no adverse effects/events from the skill.

(Crisp et al 2021; Forbes & Watt 2021; Scott et al 2018; Sorrentino & Remmert 2017)

OBSERVATION CHECKLIST: MEASURING BLOOD PRESSURE

STUDENT NAME: _____

CLINICAL SKILL 16.3: Measuring blood pressure

DEMONSTRATION OF: The ability to effectively measure and assess blood pressure

If the observation checklist is being used as an assessment tool, the student will need to obtain a scale of independence for each of the performance criteria/evidence

Independent (I)
Supervised (S)
Assisted (A)
Marginal (M)
Dependent (D)

COMPETENCY ELEMENTS	PERFORMANCE CRITERIA/EVIDENCE	I	S	A	M	D
Preparation for the activity	Identifies indications and rationale for performing the activity Identifies the individual using three individual identifiers Ensures therapeutic interaction Gains the individual's consent Checks facility/organisation policy Validates the order in the individual's record Locates and gathers equipment Checks the individual's previous baseline blood pressure Assists the individual into an appropriate position					
Performs activity informed by evidence	Selects appropriate cuff size Removes any constricting clothing Supports the arm in an extended position with palm facing up Positions the arm so the brachial artery is at the level of the heart Checks for air leaks in the cuff, tubing and valves of the sphygmomanometer Squeezes the cuff to expel any air and then tightens the valve Two-step method: • Palpates the brachial artery • Positions the cuff so the rubber bag is centred over brachial artery with the lower edge 2.5–5 cm above the antecubital fossa • Wraps the cuff firmly around the upper arm • Positions the sphygmomanometer on a level surface at eye level • Palpates the radial pulse and inflates cuff to 30 mmHg above where the pulse disappears • Slowly deflates cuff and notes point where pulse reappears • Deflates cuff completely • Allows arm 30 seconds to rest • Places disc of stethoscope over brachial artery • Reflates cuff to 30 mmHg above palpated systolic pressure reading • Uses the valve to deflate the cuff • Notes the pressure reading on the manometer when the pulse beat is heard • Continues to slowly deflate cuff • Notes the pressure reading when the pulse sound muffles or disappears • Allows remaining air to escape • Removes cuff and adjusts individual's clothing					

Continued

COMPETENCY ELEMENTS	PERFORMANCE CRITERIA/EVIDENCE	I	S	A	M	D
	One-step method: • Places stethoscope earpieces in ears • Relocates brachial artery and places diaphragm of stethoscope over it • Closes pressure bulb valve • Inflates cuff to 30 mmHg above individual's usual systolic pressure • Slowly releases pressure bulb valve • Notes the pressure reading on the manometer when the pulse beat is heard • Continues to slowly deflate cuff • Notes the pressure reading when the pulse sound muffles or disappears • Allows remaining air to escape • Removes cuff and adjusts individual's clothing					
	Assessing blood pressure electronically: • Determines appropriateness of using electronic blood pressure measurement • Determines best site for blood pressure assessment • Removes any constricting clothing • Selects appropriate cuff size • Manually squeezes air out of cuff and connects it to connector hose • Wraps cuff around extremity • Verifies connector hose between cuff and machine is not kinked • Turns machine on • Following manufacturer's directions, presses the start button • Compares electronic blood pressure readings with auscultated blood pressure measurements to verify accuracy					
Applies critical thinking and reflective practice	Is able to link theory to practice Demonstrates current best practice in the care provided If this is the first time blood pressure has been measured, if in normal range, establishes as a baseline Compares with the baseline and acceptable blood pressure range for the individual Assesses own performance					
Practises within safety and quality assurance guidelines	Reviews against facility/organisation policy Cleans and disposes of equipment appropriately					
Documentation and communication	Explains and communicates the activity clearly to the individual Communicates outcome and ongoing care to individual and significant others Communicates abnormal findings to appropriate personnel Reports and documents all relevant information and any complications correctly in the healthcare record Reports any complications and/or inability to perform the procedure to the RN and/or medical officer Asks the individual to report any complications during and post procedure					

Educator/Facilitator Feedback:

Educator/Facilitator Score: Competent   Needs further development

How would you rate your overall performance while undertaking this clinical activity? (use a ✓ & initial)

Unsatisfactory   Satisfactory   Good   Excellent

Student Reflection: (discuss how you would approach your practice differently or more effectively)

EDUCATOR/FACILITATOR NAME/SIGNATURE:

STUDENT NAME/SIGNATURE: **DATE:**

CLINICAL SKILL 16.4 Assessing pulse (radial)

Please adhere to the policy and procedures of the facility/organisation prior to undertaking the skill. Ensure this skill is in your scope of practice.

NMBA Decision-making Framework considerations (refer to NMBA Decision-making framework for nursing and midwifery 2020):	Equipment:
1. Am I educated? 2. Am I authorised? 3. Am I competent? If you answer 'no' to any of these, do not perform that activity. Seek guidance and support from your teacher/a nurse team leader/clinical facilitator/educator.	Watch Pen (blue/black) Observation chart

PREPARE FOR THE SKILL

(Please refer to the Standard Steps on p. xii for related rationales.)
- Mentally review the steps of the skill.
- Discuss the skill with your instructor/supervisor/team leader, if required.
- Confirm correct facility/organisation policy/safe operating procedures.
- Validate the order in the individual's record.
- Identify indication and rationale for performing the activity.
- Assess for any contraindications.
- Locate and gather equipment.
- Perform hand hygiene.
- Ensure therapeutic interaction.
- Identify the individual using three individual identifiers.
- Gain the individual's consent.
- Assess for pain relief.
- Prepare the environment.
- Provide and maintain privacy.
- Assist the individual to assume an appropriate position of comfort.

Skill activity	Rationale
Check individual's previous baseline resting pulse rate.	It is important to know the individual's usual pulse rate to compare changes with that measurement.

PERFORM THE SKILL

(Please refer to the Standard Steps on p. xii for related rationales.)
- Perform hand hygiene.
- Apply PPE: gloves, eyewear, mask and gown as appropriate.
- Ensure the individual's safety and comfort throughout skill.
- Promote independence and involvement of the individual if possible and/or appropriate.
- Assess the individual's tolerance to the skill throughout.
- Dispose of used supplies, equipment, waste and sharps appropriately.
- Remove PPE and discard or store appropriately.
- Perform hand hygiene.

Skill activity	Rationale
The radial pulse is normally assessed unless indicated. If individual is supine, place individual's forearm straight alongside or across lower chest or upper abdomen with wrist extended straight. If sitting, bend individual's elbow 90 degrees and support lower arm on chair or on nurse's arm. If not using the radial pulse, position individual so appropriate peripheral pulse point is accessible.	Radial is most common and least invasive site. Relaxed position of lower arm permits full exposure of artery to palpation.

CLINICAL SKILL 16.4 Assessing pulse (radial)—cont'd

Place the index and middle fingers over the site and press gently until pulsation can be felt. Obliterate pulse initially and then relax pressure so pulse becomes easily palpable. Slightly extend the wrist with palm down until you note the strongest pulse.	The assessor's thumb is not used since it has a strong pulse and may be felt instead of the individual's pulse. Pressure that is too light will fail to detect the pulse, and firm pressure may obliterate the pulse.
Determine: Strength of the pulse, noting whether it is bounding, strong, weak or thready.	Strength reflects volume of blood ejected against arterial wall with each heart contraction. Accurate description of strength improves communication among nurses and other healthcare professionals and allows better assessment of the individual's blood circulation status.
There are two ways of measuring pulse rate: 1. Using a watch with a second hand, count the pulse for one minute. While the rate is being counted, the rhythm and volume are also assessed. 2. If pulse is regular, count rate for 30 seconds and multiply total by two. If pulse is irregular, count rate for 60 seconds. Assess frequency and pattern of irregularity and compare radial pulses bilaterally.	Allows sufficient time to detect the rate and any abnormalities. It requires 30 seconds to determine if the pulse is regular in rhythm. Inefficient contraction of heart fails to transmit pulse wave, interfering with cardiac output, resulting in irregular pulse. Longer time period ensures more accurate count. A marked difference between radial pulses may indicate that arterial flow is compromised in one extremity and action should be taken immediately.
When pulse is irregular, compare radial pulses bilaterally and consider cardiac monitoring.	A marked inequality indicates compromised arterial flow to one extremity, and action needs to be taken.

NOTE: If pulse is irregular, assess for a pulse deficit. Count apical pulse while colleague counts radial pulse. Begin apical pulse, initiating counting by a signal to simultaneously assess pulses for a full minute. If pulse count differs by more than 2 beats/min, a pulse deficit exists, which may indicate alteration in cardiac output.

 ## AFTER THE SKILL

(Please refer to the Standard Steps on p. xii for related rationales.)
- Communicate outcome to the individual, any ongoing care and to report any complications.
- Restore the environment.
- Report, record and document assessment findings, details of the skill performed and the individual's response.
- Report, record and document any abnormalities and/or inability to perform the skill.
- Reassess the individual to ensure there are no adverse effects/events from the skill.

(Crisp et al 2021; Forbes & Watt 2021; Scott et al 2018; Sorrentino & Remmert 2017)

OBSERVATION CHECKLIST: ASSESSING PULSE (RADIAL)

STUDENT NAME: _____

CLINICAL SKILL 16.4: Assessing pulse (radial)

DEMONSTRATION OF: The ability to effectively measure and assess a radial pulse

If the observation checklist is being used as an assessment tool, the student will need to obtain a scale of independence for each of the performance criteria/evidence.

Independent (I)
Supervised (S)
Assisted (A)
Marginal (M)
Dependent (D)

COMPETENCY ELEMENTS	PERFORMANCE CRITERIA/EVIDENCE	I	S	A	M	D
Preparation for the activity	Identifies indications and rationale for performing the activity Identifies the individual using three individual identifiers Ensures therapeutic interaction Gains the individual's consent Checks facility/organisation policy Validates the order in the individual's record Locates and gathers equipment Determines appropriate site to assess pulse Checks the individual's previous baseline resting pulse rate Assists the individual into an appropriate position					
Performs activity informed by evidence	Assessing radial pulse: • If the individual is supine, places their forearm across their lower chest or upper abdomen with wrist extended straight • If sitting, bends the individual's elbow at 90 degrees and supports lower arm on chair or nurse's arm • Places the index and middle fingers over the site and presses gently until pulsation can be felt • Obliterates pulse initially and then relaxes pressure so pulse becomes easily palpable • Slightly extends the wrist with palm down until the strongest pulse is noted • Determines the strength of the pulse (bounding, strong, weak or thready) • Using a watch counts the pulse for one minute • If the pulse is regular, counts rate for 30 seconds and multiplies by two • If pulse is irregular, counts rate for 60 seconds • Assesses frequency and pattern of irregularity and compares radial pulses bilaterally • Discusses findings with individual as needed					
Applies critical thinking and reflective practice	Is able to link theory to practice Demonstrates current best practice in the care provided If this is the first time pulse has been measured, if in normal range, establishes as a baseline Compares with the baseline and acceptable heart rate range for the individual Assesses own performance					

COMPETENCY ELEMENTS	PERFORMANCE CRITERIA/EVIDENCE	I	S	A	M	D
Practises within safety and quality assurance guidelines	Reviews against facility/organisation policy Performs hand hygiene					
Documentation and communication	Explains and communicates the activity clearly to the individual Communicates outcome and ongoing care to individual and significant others Communicates abnormal findings to appropriate personnel Reports and documents all relevant information and any complications correctly in the healthcare record Reports any complications and/or inability to perform the procedure to the RN and/or medical officer Asks the individual to report any complications during and post procedure					

Educator/Facilitator Feedback:

Educator/Facilitator Score: Competent   Needs further development

How would you rate your overall performance while undertaking this clinical activity? (use a ✓ & initial)

Unsatisfactory   Satisfactory   Good   Excellent

Student Reflection: (discuss how you would approach your practice differently or more effectively)

EDUCATOR/FACILITATOR NAME/SIGNATURE:

STUDENT NAME/SIGNATURE: **DATE:**

CLINICAL SKILL 16.5 Assessing body temperature

Please adhere to the policy and procedures of the facility/organisation prior to undertaking the skill. Ensure this skill is in your scope of practice.

NMBA Decision-making Framework considerations (refer to NMBA Decision-making framework for nursing and midwifery 2020):	Equipment:
1. Am I educated? 2. Am I authorised? 3. Am I competent? If you answer 'no' to any of these, do not perform that activity. Seek guidance and support from your teacher/a nurse team leader/clinical facilitator/educator.	Appropriate thermometer Disposable probe cover or sleeve Pen (blue/black) Observation Adult Deterioration Detection System (ADDS) chart ABHR handwash Alcohol-based wipes

 PREPARE FOR THE SKILL

(Please refer to the Standard Steps on p. xii for related rationales.)
- Mentally review the steps of the skill.
- Discuss the skill with your instructor/supervisor/team leader, if required.
- Confirm correct facility/organisation policy/safe operating procedures.
- Validate the order in the individual's record.
- Identify indication and rationale for performing the activity.
- Assess for any contraindications.
- Locate and gather equipment.
- Perform hand hygiene.
- Ensure therapeutic interaction.
- Identify the individual using three individual identifiers.
- Gain the individual's consent.
- Assess for pain relief.
- Prepare the environment.
- Provide and maintain privacy.
- Assist the individual to assume an appropriate position of comfort.

Skill activity	Rationale

Before taking temperatures, you need this information from the nurse and the care plan:
- what site to use for each person—oral, rectal, axillary, tympanic membrane or temporal artery
- what thermometer to use for each person
- when to take temperatures
- which persons are at risk for a fever
- what observations to report and record
- when to report observations
- what concerns to report when:
  > a temperature is changed from a past measurement
  > a temperature is above or below the normal range for the site used.	

 PERFORM THE SKILL

(Please refer to the Standard Steps on p. xii for related rationales.)
- Perform hand hygiene.
- Apply PPE: gloves, eyewear, mask and gown as appropriate.
- Ensure the individual's safety and comfort throughout skill.
- Promote independence and involvement of the individual if possible and/or appropriate.
- Assess the individual's tolerance to the skill throughout.
- Dispose of used supplies, equipment, waste and sharps appropriately.
- Remove PPE and discard or store appropriately.
- Perform hand hygiene.

Continued

CLINICAL SKILL 16.5 Assessing body temperature—cont'd

Skill activity	Rationale
Assess the individual for temperature alterations and anything that may interfere with the accuracy of temperature measurement. Wait 15–20 minutes if the individual has smoked or ingested hot or cold foods or fluids. Remove hearing aid if required.	Physical signs and symptoms of temperature alterations may be present such as the individual being flushed or shivering. Respiratory rate greater than 18 breaths/min can influence measurement. If using an oral thermometer, intake of some foods can cause inaccurate readings. If using a tympanic thermometer, hearing aids can increase temperature readings.
Assess appropriate temperature site and temperature device for the individual.	Different individuals will have different requirements due to their health conditions. The oral site is not used for infants and children younger than four to five years. Use other routes as directed by the nurse and the care plan. Rectal temperatures are dangerous for persons with heart disease. The thermometer can stimulate the vagus nerve and slow the heart rate to dangerous levels. Tympanic membrane and temporal artery thermometers are used for persons who are confused and resist care. A standard electronic thermometer can injure the mouth and teeth if the person bites down on it. It also can cause injury if the person moves quickly and without warning.

Assessing body temperature with a tympanic membrane electronic thermometer

Skill activity	Rationale
Assist the individual in assuming a comfortable position, with head turned away from the nurse.	Ensures comfort and exposes auditory canal for accurate temperature measurement. Ensures individual's safety and comfort. Do not use side that was on pillow.
Observe for ear wax (cerumen) in individual's ear canal.	Lens cover of speculum must not be impeded by ear wax (will not obtain an accurate measurement). Switch to other ear or select an alternative measurement site.
Remove thermometer from charging base and slide disposable speculum cover over otoscope-like tip until it locks into place, being careful not to touch lens cover.	Base provides battery power. Soft plastic probe cover prevents transmission of microorganisms.
If holding hand-held unit with right hand, obtain temperature from individual's right ear; left-handed persons should obtain temperature from individual's left ear.	The less acute the angle of approach the better the probe will seal inside the auditory canal.
Insert speculum into ear canal, following manufacturer's instructions for tympanic probe positioning. Pull pinna backwards, up and out for an adult, move thermometer in a figure-eight pattern, fit probe snugly in canal and do not move, point towards the nose.	Correct positioning of probe will ensure accurate readings as there will be maximum exposure of tympanic membrane.
As soon as probe is in place, depress scan button. Leave thermometer probe in place until an audible signal is given and individual's temperature appears on the digital display (usually in 1–3 seconds).	Depression of scan button causes infrared energy to be detected. Otoscope tip must stay in situ until signal occurs to ensure accurate measurement.
Carefully remove speculum from auditory meatus. Push ejection button on unit to discard plastic probe cover into an appropriate receptacle. Wipe down speculum with alcohol-based wipes.	Reduces transmission of microorganisms.
Return hand-held unit to charging base.	Protects sensor tip from damage and keeps unit charged ready for next use. The electronic tympanic thermometer is a shared device; a nurse should notify before removing it for use and return it to charging area in a timely manner.

CLINICAL SKILL 16.5 Assessing body temperature—cont'd

If this is the first time temperature has been measured, if in normal range establish as baseline.	Used to compare future readings.
If this is not the first time, compare with baseline and acceptable temperature range for individual's age group.	Normal body temperature fluctuates within normal range; comparison of readings can reveal presence of abnormality.

Measurement of body temperature with electronic thermometer

Oral temperature

Remove thermometer from charging unit. Slide disposable plastic probe cover over thermometer probe until cover locks in place.	Charging provides battery power. Soft plastic cover prevents transmission of microorganisms. Usually oral/axilla site electronic thermometer is blue in colour (and red for rectal).
Ask the individual to open their mouth then gently place thermometer probe under the tongue in posterior sublingual pocket lateral to centre of jaw.	Heat from superficial blood vessels in sublingual pocket produces temperature reading.
Ask individual to hold thermometer probe with lips closed.	Maintains proper position of thermometer during recording.
Leave thermometer probe in place until audible signal occurs and individual's temperature appears on digital display.	To ensure accurate reading, probe must stay in place until signal occurs.
Remove thermometer probe from under individual's tongue, push ejection button and discard plastic probe cover into an appropriate receptacle. Wipe down speculum with alcohol-based wipes.	Reduces risk of transmission of microorganisms.
Return thermometer to storage position of thermometer unit and return to charger.	Maintains battery charge.
If this is the first time temperature has been measured, if in normal range establish as baseline.	Used to compare future readings.
If this is not the first time, compare with baseline and acceptable temperature range for individual's age group.	Normal body temperature fluctuates within normal range; comparison of readings can reveal presence of abnormality.

Measurement of axillary temperature

Remove thermometer from charging unit. Slide disposable plastic probe cover over thermometer probe until cover locks in place.	Charging provides battery power. Soft plastic cover prevents transmission of microorganisms. Usually oral/axilla site electronic thermometer is blue in colour (and red for rectal).
Raise individual's arm away from torso and make sure the axilla is dry.	Moisture may interfere with accurate reading and give a false low reading.
Place thermometer into centre of axilla, lower arm over probe and place arm across individual's chest.	Maintains position of thermometer against blood vessels in axilla.
Hold thermometer in place until audible signal occurs and individual's temperature appears on digital display; remove probe from axilla.	Ensures an accurate reading.
Push ejection button on thermometer probe stem to discard plastic probe cover into an appropriate receptacle. Wipe down speculum with alcohol-based wipes.	Reduces risk of transmission of microorganisms.
Return thermometer to storage position of thermometer unit and return to charger.	Maintains battery charge.

Continued

CLINICAL SKILL 16.5 Assessing body temperature—cont'd

If this is the first time temperature has been measured, if in normal range establish as baseline.	Used to compare future readings.
If this is not the first time, compare with baseline and acceptable temperature range for individual's age group.	Normal body temperature fluctuates within normal range; comparison of readings can reveal presence of abnormality.
Measuring temporal artery temperature	
Ensure the forehead is dry.	Moisture may interfere with accurate readings.
Place sensor flush on individual's forehead.	Ensures accurate measurement.
Press red scan button with your thumb. Then slowly slide the thermometer straight across the forehead while keeping the sensor flush with the skin.	Scanning for the highest temperature continues until you release the scan button.
Keeping the scan button pressed, lift the sensor from the forehead and touch the sensor to the skin on the neck just below the earlobe. Peak temperature occurs when the clicking sound during scanning stops. Then release scan button.	Sensor confirms highest temperature behind the ear lobe (usually 3–4 seconds).
Clean sensor with alcohol-based wipes.	Prevents transmission of microorganisms.
If this is the first time temperature has been measured, if in normal range establish as baseline.	Used to compare future readings.
If this is not the first time, compare with baseline and acceptable temperature range for individual's age group.	Normal body temperature fluctuates within normal range; comparison of readings can reveal presence of abnormality.

NOTE:
- In an infant or young child, it may be necessary to hold the arm against the child's side when using axillary method. If infant is in a side-lying position, the lower axilla will record the higher temperature.
- Do not use axilla if skin lesions are present because local temperature may be altered and area may be painful to touch.

 AFTER THE SKILL

(Please refer to the Standard Steps on p. xii for related rationales.)
- Communicate outcome to the individual, any ongoing care and to report any complications.
- Restore the environment.
- Report, record and document assessment findings, details of the skill performed and the individual's response.
- Report, record and document any abnormalities and/or inability to perform the skill.
- Reassess the individual to ensure there are no adverse effects/events from the skill.

(Crisp et al 2021; Forbes & Watt 2021; Scott et al 2018; Sorrentino & Remmert 2017)

OBSERVATION CHECKLIST: ASSESSING BODY TEMPERATURE

STUDENT NAME: _____

CLINICAL SKILL 16.5: Assessing body temperature

DEMONSTRATION OF: The ability to effectively measure and assess body temperature

If the observation checklist is being used as an assessment tool, the student will need to obtain a scale of independence for each of the performance criteria/evidence.

Independent (I)

Supervised (S)

Assisted (A)

Marginal (M)

Dependent (D)

COMPETENCY ELEMENTS	PERFORMANCE CRITERIA/EVIDENCE	I	S	A	M	D
Preparation for the activity	Identifies indications and rationale for performing the activity Identifies the individual using three individual identifiers Ensures therapeutic interaction Gains the individual's consent Checks facility/organisation policy Validates the order in the individual's record Locates and gathers equipment Assesses the individual for temperature alterations Determines appropriate temperature site Assists the individual into an appropriate position					
Performs activity informed by evidence	Assessing body temperature with a tympanic membrane electronic thermometer: • Ensures individual's head is turned away from nurse • Observes for cerumen • Removes thermometer from charging base • Slides the cover into place • Inserts speculum into ear canal • Depresses scan button and leaves thermometer probe in place until audible signal is heard and temperature appears on digital screen • Removes speculum from auditory meatus • Ejects plastic probe cover • Returns hand-held unit to charging base					
	Assessing body temperature with electronic thermometer—oral temperature: • Removes thermometer from charging unit • Slides cover into place • Asks the individual to open their mouth and gently places thermometer probe under tongue in posterior sublingual pocket lateral to centre of jaw • Asks the individual to hold thermometer in place with lips closed • Leaves the thermometer probe in place until audible signal occurs and temperature appears on digital screen • Removes thermometer probe from under individual's tongue • Pushes ejection button and discards plastic probe cover • Returns thermometer to charger					

Continued

COMPETENCY ELEMENTS	PERFORMANCE CRITERIA/EVIDENCE	I	S	A	M	D
	Assessing body temperature with electronic thermometer—axillary temperature: • Positions the individual—either supine or sitting • Removes clothing from shoulder and arm • Removes thermometer from charging unit • Slides disposable plastic probe cover over thermometer • Raises individual's arm away from torso and ensures axilla is dry • Places thermometer into centre of axilla, lowers arm over probe and places arm across individual's chest • Holds thermometer in place until audible signal occurs and temperature appears on digital screen • Removes probe from axilla • Pushes ejection button on thermometer and discards plastic probe cover • Returns thermometer to charger					
	Assessing temporal artery temperature: • Ensures forehead is dry • Places sensor flush on individual's forehead • Presses scan button with thumb • Slowly slides the thermometer straight across the forehead, keeping sensor flush with the skin • Keeping the scan button pressed, lifts the sensor from the forehead and touches it to the skin on the neck just below the earlobe • When clicking sound stops releases the scan button • Cleans sensor • Restores the individual's environment					
Applies critical thinking and reflective practice	Is able to link theory to practice Demonstrates current best practice in the care provided If this is the first time temperature has been measured, and it is in normal range, establishes as a baseline Compares with the baseline and acceptable temperature range for the individual Assesses own performance					
Practises within safety and quality assurance guidelines	Reviews against facility/organisation policy Performs hand hygiene, dons appropriate PPE as per infection control protocols Cleans and disposes of equipment appropriately					

COMPETENCY ELEMENTS	PERFORMANCE CRITERIA/EVIDENCE	I	S	A	M	D
Documentation and communication	Explains and communicates the activity clearly to the individual Communicates outcome and ongoing care to individual and significant others Communicates abnormal findings to appropriate personnel Reports and documents all relevant information and any complications correctly in the healthcare record Reports any complications and/or inability to perform the procedure to the RN and/or medical officer Asks the individual to report any complications during and post procedure					

Educator/Facilitator Feedback:

Educator/Facilitator Score: Competent   Needs further development

How would you rate your overall performance while undertaking this clinical activity? (use a ✓ & initial)

Unsatisfactory   Satisfactory   Good   Excellent

Student Reflection: (discuss how you would approach your practice differently or more effectively)

EDUCATOR/FACILITATOR NAME/SIGNATURE:

STUDENT NAME/SIGNATURE: **DATE:**

Evolve® Answer guide for the Critical Thinking Exercises and Critical Thinking Questions in Case Studies is hosted on Evolve: http://evolve.elsevier.com/AU/Koutoukidis/Tabbner/

References

Australian Commission on Safety and Quality in Health Care (ACSQHC), 2023. Action 8.04 Recognising acute deterioration. Available at: <https://www.safetyandquality.gov.au/standards/nsqhs-standards/recognising-and-responding-acute-deterioration-standard/detecting-and-recognising-acute-deterioration-and-escalating-care/action-804>.

Nursing and Midwifery Board of Australia (NMBA), 2020. Decision-making framework summary for nursing and midwifery. Available at: <https://www.nursingmidwiferyboard.gov.au/Codes-Guidelines-Statements/Frameworks.aspx>.

Crisp, J., Douglas, C., Rebeiro, G., et al., 2021. *Potter & Perry's fundamentals of nursing*, 6th ed. Elsevier, Sydney.

Forbes, H., Watt, E., 2021. *Jarvis's physical examination and health assessment*, 3rd ed. Elsevier, Australia.

Scott, K., Webb, M., Kostelnick, C., 2018. Health assessment. In: *Long-term caring*, 4th ed. Elsevier, Australia, Ch 11, pp. 236–252.

Sorrentino, S., Remmert, L., 2017. Oxygen needs. In: *Mosby's textbook for nursing assistants*, 9th ed. Elsevier, St Louis, Ch 39, pp. 642–657.

ADMISSION, TRANSFER AND DISCHARGE

Janine Bothe, Gabrielle Koutoukidis

Overview

When an individual is admitted into hospital or transferred to a ward or care facility, an individual health history and nursing assessment is completed. This generally consists of the individual's biographical data, reason for admission, a brief medical and surgical history, allergies, current medications, the individual's own perceptions about their health status and a review of their health risk factors. During this process a physical assessment of the individual is also completed (Crisp et al 2020; Lippincott et al 2022). Therefore, the nursing admission contains a collection of both subjective data from the individual and objective data from the completion of a physical assessment (Perry et al 2019). It is also important during admission to gain an understanding on the individual's perspective of their health condition to ensure the care provided to the individual is person-centred (Perry et al 2019).

Healthcare facilities individually have policies regarding the admission and discharge process for elective and emergency admissions. In most cases, individuals presenting for elective procedures will report to an admitting department on a prearranged date and time for the purpose of commencing the admission process. Prior to reporting for their procedure, the individual should have received some written material with information regarding their diet prior to admission (e.g. fasting for surgery), whether to cease taking particular prescription or over-the-counter medications, what items to bring (e.g. toiletries, clothing) and information regarding visiting hours, the provision of telephones and televisions and location of the cafeteria. An efficient admission process can reduce waiting times for both admitted and discharged persons as well as reducing the stress factors related to admission to hospital (Reynolds et al 2023; ANZCA 2023).

The approach to the admission process, transferring and discharge process will need to be adapted and modified depending on the individual, for example, children, adolescents and adults. The nurse's role is integral to ensuring these processes cause minimal disruption and maintain each individual's safety.

The admission interview is an important component of nursing care. It is an opportunity to establish rapport with the individual, begin any necessary health teaching processes and to commence discharge planning (Tollefson et al 2021). Often when an individual is admitted into a healthcare facility, they will experience many negative emotions, including being anxious, stressed, nervous and fearful; therefore, it is important for the nurse to assist in alleviating this state of stress by reassuring and collaborating with the individual in their care (Burton et al 2018). Effective communication throughout the admission process can help to alleviate the individual's fears and establish a positive relationship between the nurse and the individual (Tollefson et al 2021). The admission forms contain routine questions and require the collection of all data; therefore, it is important to adjust questioning and interview techniques to suit the individual, their needs and current health status (Tollefson et al 2021). For example, if the individual is fatigued and in pain, the admission process may be completed in two or three sessions. Family/carers can also be utilised to assist with gathering further information regarding the individual; however, consideration must be demonstrated to ensure the individual's privacy and confidentiality are maintained and, where possible and applicable, consent has been gained.

Once the admission data has been collected, it can be used by the healthcare team to identify, plan, implement and evaluate individualised care for that person. Accurate assessment data will be collected by each member of the multidisciplinary team; this will then provide an overview of the individual's current, previous and expected health status and enable the team to provide holistic care to the individual (Crisp et al 2020). It is important that the admission process is appropriate and effective for the individual—disruptive admissions that the individual feels are careless or impersonal can result in reduced cooperation and increased anxiety and can even aggravate symptoms such as pain (Lippincott et al 2022).

Discharge planning also begins at the individual's admission and is often incorporated into the admission process. This ensures that the individual's needs are met and continuity of care is provided throughout their admission. The individual's family/carer, community and individual self-care actions may also be incorporated (Tollefson et al 2021). The discharge plan can always be revised and updated as the individual's condition changes. The general process for discharge planning involves first assessing the individual and their family/carer, then interpreting this data to identify any discharge needs and planning to meet those needs when the individual leaves the facility. If the individual does not have any significant others, their need for assistance and support systems in place at home should also be assessed. The nurse then begins to psychologically prepare the individual and their family/carer for discharge while also implementing and evaluating the discharge plan. Often discharge planning involves the nurse providing information to the individual and teaching them health practices such as information about their illness and how it may impact on their life, medication administration, specific treatments needed such as blood glucose testing or dressing changes, and also teaching different methods for adapting back into their home environment (Burton et al 2018).

Discharge planning occurs at different times in the individual's admission to hospital. It is an ongoing process that is discussed between team members and involves the individual to ensure individual preferences are included in the planning process (Tollefson et al 2021). In order to ensure effective discharge planning there needs to be an interdisciplinary approach, including collaboration with the individual, effective communication and early assessment of interventions needed at home. These need to be achieved with every discharge and ensure a smooth transition for the individual from care to home, nursing home, respite, palliation, rehabilitation setting or family/carer member's home. It has been found that an individual's outcomes improve when the discharge process is commenced early, includes the individual, incorporates their wishes into planning and appropriate follow-up at home is provided, either in the form of a telephone call or postoperative counselling.

On discharge, individuals and their families/carers need to be informed of a variety of health management issues. These include any potential post-discharge complications, the provision of ongoing health management practices, follow-up appointments, medication management and emergency numbers (Crisp et al 2020). The individual will be given a discharge summary that will be completed by members of the multidisciplinary team and is used by the individual as a tool for their ongoing management of their health. Copies can also be provided to their general practitioner, home healthcare agency, rehabilitation or long-term care agency (Crisp et al 2020).

CASE STUDY 17.2

You are caring for John, a 45-year-old man, who is day 1 post cardiac angiogram and insertion of three stents. While you are taking his morning observations, he states that he wants to go out for a cigarette. You discuss his care plan with him as documented by the cardiologist. You explain that it would be unsafe for him to go outside, especially to smoke and the reasons why. He becomes angry and starts yelling at you, stating that it is none of your business if he goes out for a cigarette. You as the nurse reiterate in an objective manner that while he is on cardiac monitoring you are legally not permitted to disconnect him. You state you need a medical officer's order to disconnect the telemetry. John yells at you to contact the medical officer and tell him he will be going out for a cigarette no matter what he says. You contact the medical officer and advise him of the situation. The medical officer refuses to give the order to disconnect the monitoring equipment. The medical officer orders nicotine patches for John and asks you to tell John that he will be in later to discuss his treatment plan. You advise John of the medical officer's orders. He refuses the nicotine patches and starts to take the monitor leads off. You contact the charge nurse who attempts to change John's mind about leaving. John remains adamant that he is leaving and asks for the paper to sign since he was leaving against medical advice.

1. Discuss the ramifications of self-discharge from hospital.
2. What are the legal requirements a nurse must complete in this situation?

CRITICAL THINKING EXERCISE 17.4

What would you say to make an anxious person and their family more relaxed during admission?

CLINICAL SKILL 17.1 Admission and discharge process

Please adhere to the policy and procedures of the facility/organisation prior to undertaking the skill. Ensure this skill is in your scope of practice.

NMBA Decision-making Framework considerations (refer to NMBA Decision-making framework for nursing and midwifery 2020):

1. Am I educated?
2. Am I authorised?
3. Am I competent?

If you answer 'no' to any of these, do not perform that activity. Seek guidance and support from your teacher/a nurse team leader/clinical facilitator/educator.

Equipment:

For admission:
Thermometer
Vital sign monitor (or sphygmomanometer, digital watch or pulse oximeter)
Stethoscope
Penlight torch
Scales
Tape measure
Computer on wheels (or facility/organisation admission forms and charts)
ID bands
Relevant information brochures
Pen (blue/black)
For discharge:
Relevant information brochures
Discharge medications and instructions for administration
Appointment cards and referral letters
X-rays and relevant scans and reports
Any further discharge supplies (e.g. mobility aids, appliances)

 PREPARE FOR THE SKILL

(Please refer to the Standard Steps on p. xii for related rationales.)
Mentally review the steps of the skill.
Discuss the skill with your instructor/supervisor/team leader, if required.
Confirm correct facility/organisation policy/safe operating procedures.
Validate the order in the individual's record.
Identify indication and rationale for performing the activity.
Assess for any contraindications.
Locate and gather equipment.
Perform hand hygiene.
Ensure therapeutic interaction.
Identify the individual using three individual identifiers.
Gain the individual's consent.
Assess for pain relief.
Prepare the environment.
Provide and maintain privacy.
Assist the individual to assume an appropriate position of comfort.

 PERFORM THE SKILL

(Please refer to the Standard Steps on p. xii for related rationales.)
Perform hand hygiene.
Apply PPE: gloves, eyewear, mask and gown as appropriate.
Ensure the individual's safety and comfort throughout skill.
Promote independence and involvement of the individual if possible and/or appropriate.
Assess the individual's tolerance to the skill throughout.
Dispose of used supplies, equipment, waste and sharps appropriately.
Remove PPE and discard or store appropriately.
Perform hand hygiene.

CLINICAL SKILL 17.1 Admission and discharge process—cont'd

Skill activity	Rationale
Admission	
Ensure room is clean and welcoming and that the room and environment is ready for the individual. Bed may need to be adapted for the individual, check the oxygen and suction equipment. Extra items such as intravenous poles and pumps may need to be placed in room if required.	Ensures the individual's needs will be met and they will be comfortable when entering the room.
Confirm the individual's identity and place identification band on individual's wrist and ankle as per facility/organisation policy. Ensure identify is verified by using at least two patient identifiers.	Safety precaution to ensure individual's identity.
Introduce self, other staff and their roles to the individual. Inform the individual about mealtimes, visiting hours, ward/hospital facilities, smoking rules and use of mobile phones. Familiarise the individual with the call bell, bathroom, space for their belongings, TV, how to adjust the bed and introduce them to other people in the room. Inform the person of their rights while in the hospital.	Allows individual to feel comfortable in the environment. Also gives individuals a sense of security and belonging, therefore decreasing stress and anxiety.
Check if the individual has brought in any valuables and if they need to be stored and recorded as per facility/organisation policy. An inventory may be made of the individual's personal belongings and any prostheses such as dentures, hearing aids or glasses, as per facility/organisation protocol.	Decreases the risk of theft and loss of personal belongings while in the facility/organisation.
Obtain a complete set of vital signs and document findings, reporting on any abnormalities.	Acts as baseline individual data and also gives information regarding their current physiological status.
If indicated, perform a pain assessment on the individual using a pain assessment tool.	Adds to baseline data regarding the individual.
Complete weight and height of individual and document.	Some medications and treatments are height and weight dependent. This will also act as a baseline for the individual.
Complete a urinalysis on the individual, if indicated, according to facility/organisation policy.	For a baseline assessment.
Identify any allergies. If individual has allergies, place a medical alert band around their wrist and document in the patient notes and in the allergy section of the medical record or medication chart.	Alerts staff that the individual has an allergy and decreases the possibility of potentially adverse events occurring.
Obtain a complete nursing history, including data about the individual's social and cultural background, surgical and medical history, history of the current illness and reason for admission. Assess any cultural/language barriers. Ask if the person has an advance health directive and, if so, obtain a copy for their medical record.	Gains a broader understanding of the individual's health history and ensures accurate and effective treatment is provided to the individual. It can also be used to identify any potential knowledge deficits the individual has regarding their health.
Throughout the assessment, note the individual's verbal and non-verbal behaviours, determine their conscious state and orientation by observing and talking to the individual.	Behaviours may reflect specific physical abnormalities. Note timing of medications, especially analgesics and sedatives, which may cause the individual to be groggy or less responsive.
Note the individual's affect and mood, whether they are demonstrating appropriate emotional responses.	Reflects the individual's mental and emotional status, consciousness and feelings.

Continued

CLINICAL SKILL 17.1 Admission and discharge process—cont'd

Note individual's ability to communicate and understand English; also, their speech and ability to speak clearly.	Alterations reflect neurological impairment, injury or impairment of mouth, improperly fitting dentures or differences in dialect and language.
If uncertain whether the individual has understood a question, rephrase or ask a similar question.	Inappropriate response from an individual may be caused by language barriers, deterioration of mental status, preoccupation with illness or decrease in hearing acuity.
During the admission process, observe how the individual interacts with family/carer. Be alert for any indications of fear, hesitancy to report health status or willingness to let caregiver control interview. Also observe for any signs of abuse and note if the individual has any obvious physical injuries.	Suspect abuse in individuals who have suffered obvious physical injury or neglect, show signs of malnutrition or have bruises on the extremities or trunk. Report as per facility/organisation protocol.
Identify next of kin, contact details and who to contact when the individual is ready for discharge.	In case of an emergency and for any notifications needed to be provided to the next of kin.
List all medications currently being taken by the individual; this should include both prescription and non-prescription. Any medications present should be locked in a medication drawer or ward cupboard as per facility/ organisation policy and returned to the individual on discharge.	Administration and storage of medications is completed as per the hospital policy. Medications taken prior to admission need to be listed so they can be reviewed by a medical officer and/or a pharmacist to determine their effectiveness, side effects and contraindications with other medications or treatments.
Note the presence of any additional treatments and invasive tubes on or with the individual (e.g. catheters, intravenous cannulas or drain tubes). Check each device and note the following: device and location, patency and position, correct fluid/medication infusing, any presence of redness, swelling or tenderness, drainage rate or infusion rate and date of last tubing change.	Ensures continuity of care to the individual. Any invasive tubes present need careful and accurate monitoring and consequently documentation. Any medical orders regarding additional treatments and invasive tubes need to be recognised and documented.
Review the individual's fluid intake and output. Ask about their appetite, bowel function, bladder function and oral intake. Commence a fluid balance chart if indicated.	Important for fluid and electrolyte balance, especially if the individual is at risk for imbalance due to electrolyte losses associated with vomiting, diarrhoea, gastrointestinal drainage or wounds such as burns.
Note the individual's general physical appearance (weight, age, sex, height, body build) and their personal hygiene and any body odour.	Grooming may reflect activity level before examination, resources available to purchase grooming supplies, individual's mood and self-care practices. Can also reflect their culture, lifestyle and personal preferences. Body odour can result from, for example, physical exercise or deficient hygiene.
Inspect skin integrity, ensure that it is a normal colour for race with no areas of skin colour variation, neither dry nor moist, normal temperature, smooth, elastic, no lesions. Ask the individual if they have noticed any changes in their skin condition including pruritus, oozing, bleeding, changes in moles. While doing this, identify any wounds present and their management. Complete a wound care chart. Inspect pressure points observing for signs of any pressure injury.	Changes in colour can indicate pathological alterations. Changes in moles can indicate cancer. Itching could be a result from dry skin, oozing could indicate infection and bleeding may indicate a blood disorder.
Complete a pressure injury risk assessment (Braden, Waterlow or Norton).	Most facilities/organisations will complete a pressure injury risk assessment on admission to determine if an individual is at risk of developing a pressure injury. If they are at high risk this allows strategies to be implemented immediately to decrease this risk.
Assess hair, taking note of quality, texture, distribution and cleanliness.	Changes in hair can reflect hormone changes, ageing changes, poor nutrition or use of certain hair care products.

CLINICAL SKILL 17.1 Admission and discharge process—cont'd

Monitor nails for any deviations from normal (both hands and feet).	Changes in condition of nails can indicate inadequate nutrition or grooming practices, nervous habits or systemic diseases.
Note visual acuity and if need for any visual aids. Assess pupils for size, shape and equality. Assess eyes, inspect the position of eyes, colour and condition of conjunctivae and movement.	If the individual has vision acuity loss, they may need to make adjustments to support self-caring measures. Normal pupils are round, clear and equal in size. If eyes are asymmetrical in position, this can reflect trauma or tumour growth. Changes in colour of conjunctivae can be due to local infection or symptomatic of another abnormality.
Assess ears for cleanliness and discharge, assess hearing acuity. Note any hearing aids in situ.	Hearing impairment can be caused by impacted cerumen, external otitis or swelling; therefore, the ear structure needs to be inspected.
Assess mouth, look at lips, mucosa, gums, teeth and tongue, noting any abnormalities.	Ill-fitting dentures can cause lesions in the mouth. Inadequate oral hygiene or unhealthy teeth may cause bad breath.
Assess thorax and lungs, listen to breath sounds and note shape of chest, assess respiratory status, determine rate and rhythm of breathing.	Abnormal airflow into the lungs can indicate airway obstruction or mucus. A 'barrel chest' (ribs become more horizontal) can be present in chronic lung disease. Individuals with breathing problems can also assume positions that improve ventilation.
Assess abdomen, listen to bowel sounds if indicated, ask the individual about their current bowel and bladder function.	Changes in symmetry or contour of abdomen can reveal underlying masses, fluid collection or gaseous distension. Normal bowel sounds occur in irregular sequence every 5–15 seconds. If absent, can indicate cessation of gastric motility. Hyperactive bowel sounds not related to hunger or recent meal can indicate diarrhoea or early intestinal obstruction. Hypoactive bowel sounds can indicate paralytic ileus or peritonitis.
Note level of consciousness and orientation. If individual's responses are inappropriate, ask them short, direct questions regarding information they should know (e.g. 'What is your name?', 'What is the name of this place?', 'Where do you live?', 'What day is it today?', 'What month is it?').	Measures individual's orientation to person, place and time. Document this as oriented $\times$ 3. If disoriented in any way, include subjective and objective data rather than documenting 'disoriented'.
If indicated, perform a focused neurological assessment. This will include using the Glasgow Coma Scale, pupil size and reaction and limb assessment. A mental state examination may be performed if indicated.	Gives further focused baseline data regarding the individual and their condition.
Note gait and posture and if the individual is able to sit, stand and walk normally. Assess their body movements: are they purposeful? Do they display tremors? Are movements coordinated or uncoordinated? When assessing posture, note the alignment of the shoulders and hips, observe if they appear slumped, erect or bent.	Reveals musculoskeletal problems, mood and presence of pain or difficulty breathing in certain positions. Can also indicate neurological or muscular problems.
Note degree of mobility, level of independence and range of motion (ROM).	Assessment of individual's normal range of motion provides baseline for assessing changes. It also identifies muscle strength and detects limited ROM.
Note use of prostheses or aids.	May affect discharge home and indicates other devices that may be required. It can also indicate any current health deficits.

Continued

CLINICAL SKILL 17.1 Admission and discharge process—cont'd

Complete a falls risk assessment if indicated.	Most hospitals will complete a falls risk assessment on admission to determine if an individual is a falls risk and, if they are, to implement strategies immediately to decrease the risk of falling.
Ask the individual if there is any information about physical conditions or their health that have not been discussed with them.	Allows individuals to discuss any health concerns they have. This is important since they may perceive other health concerns as being more important to them than the one that they have presented with; therefore, it is important to address this for provision of person-centred care.
Identify and provide any relevant individual learning needs and provide teaching and brochures regarding these (e.g. pain management or what to expect post surgery).	It is important to ensure information is repeated when necessary and provided in written format if available. The individual may be stressed and demonstrating poor concentration and therefore may not remember the information provided to them.
Conduct a physical assessment of individual if indicated.	If the individual needs further physical assessments in any area of concern, these need to be completed.
Discuss findings with individual as needed.	Promotes participation in care and understanding of health status.
Before leaving the individual, ensure they are comfortable, that they have a water jug (if they are not fasting), that they have the call bell within reach and that they have no further questions.	If you are unable to answer any questions, it is important to refer the individual to the appropriate person who can.
Develop nursing care plan suitable for the individual. Inform the medical practitioner and any relevant allied health professionals of the individual's admission.	Allows effective and efficient nursing treatment of the individual to commence in conjunction with a medical treatment plan.
Skill activity	**Rationale**
Discharge	
Identify the following information about the individual's discharge: • location on discharge • who will pick up the individual • how they will travel to their discharge location • what time they will be picked up • if there is a need to use a facility/organisation 'transit lounge' to wait to go home (this should be organised the day before discharge).	Ensures the individual and their family/carer are prepared for discharge.
Ensure the individual is confident about performing any self-care activities that have been taught.	Ensures compliance on discharge and that the individual will be able to care for themselves on discharge, reducing the risk of readmission.
Assess the individual and family/carer needs for health education (e.g. self-care actions, use of equipment, changes to lifestyle as a result of the illness, understanding illness or changing personal behaviours that influence health, use of medications).	Allows education to be provided to the individual and their family/carer to help them cope more effectively at home and decrease the risk of deterioration and readmission.
Check all referrals to community agencies such as Commonwealth Home Support Programme (CHSP), Hospital in the Home (HITH) and physiotherapy have been completed and the individual has the relevant follow-up appointment cards.	Ensures the individual will not miss any further follow-up care and that they will have continuity of care once they leave the facility/organisation.

CLINICAL SKILL 17.1 Admission and discharge process—cont'd

Ensure the individual has in their possession any aids and equipment necessary.	Individuals will grow to rely on the facility/organisation's aids during their stay; therefore, it is important that they have aids available to them on discharge if necessary to ensure a smooth transition home.
Give the individual advice if needed on where they can obtain any long-term supplies or equipment.	If the individual is undecided about buying or hiring equipment while in the facility/organisation, it is important to give them options for when they are discharged to obtain anything they may require. Refer them to an occupational therapist to assist in this if required.
If wound care is required, identify and teach the person who will be providing that care (unless it is a community nurse) and supply materials if indicated.	Ensures wounds heal appropriately prior to and post discharge and decreases the likelihood of readmission. It is also important to identify if someone may need community nursing for wound care early in their admission process since there may be a waiting period for these services.
Ensure any intravenous cannulas, drain tubes and so on have been removed.	Once they have been removed, also educate the individual on signs of infection from the site.
Ensure individual has received discharge medications with instructions on their administration. They may need verbal instructions along with written instructions.	Medication mismanagement can have dire consequences for the individual; therefore, it is important they understand the correct administration of their medications. Provision of a Webster pack by a pharmacist may also be necessary as well as a pharmacist review.
Ensure private X-rays are returned to the individual.	These are generally the property of the individual and may be needed for follow-up care in the community.
Give any paperwork needed by the individual (e.g. medical certificates or Work Cover certificates).	Depending on the individual's circumstances, they may need a variety of different forms and certificates filled out; it is important that these are completed while in the facility/organisation (generally a few days before discharge).
Give the individual a copy of their discharge summary and explain any further details needed. Ensure individual has all details of discharge. Review all discharge advice.	Discharge forms include a summary from the multidisciplinary team and are concise and instructive. They are a good tool for the individual on discharge to assist in the ongoing management of their health.
Provide the individual with any relevant brochures (e.g. routine guidelines about postoperative care, cast care, driving etc.).	Written information is preferred over verbal since the individual may need this on discharge to clarify any doubts or concerns they have.
Ensure the individual and their family/carer understand potential complications following discharge and what to do if these occur. Also ensure they are provided with contact details in lieu of any problems.	Often this information is also provided on the discharge summary. If not, this needs to be supplied to the individual, preferably in written form.
Ensure all belongings, clothing and valuables are returned to the individual. Help the individual collect and pack all their personal belongings. Assist the individual from the area with a wheelchair if needed and assist them to transfer into the vehicle.	Ensures a safe transition for the individual.

Note:
- During the admission general health survey assessment, the nurse may need to perform more focused specific assessments as indicated by the individual's health condition.
- Discharge planning occurs at different points during the individual's admission to a facility/organisation and is an ongoing procedure. Therefore, on the individual's day of discharge the discharge process will consist of ensuring the individual understands and has all information required for their discharge. Key elements needed for effective discharge planning include collaboration with the individual, efficient communication, prompt assessment of potential interventions needed at home and an interdisciplinary approach. The goal is to assist the individual in making a smooth transition from one setting to another.

Continued

CLINICAL SKILL 17.1 Admission and discharge process—cont'd

 AFTER THE SKILL

(Please refer to the Standard Steps on p. xii for related rationales.)
Communicate outcome to the individual, any ongoing care and to report any complications.
Restore the environment.
Report, record and document assessment findings, details of the skill performed and the individual's response.
Report, record and document any abnormalities and/or inability to perform the skill.
Reassess the individual to ensure there are no adverse effects/events from the skill.

(Crisp et al 2021; Lippincott, Williams & Wilkins 2022; Perry et al 2019; Tollefson et al 2021)

OBSERVATION CHECKLIST: ADMISSION AND DISCHARGE PROCESS

STUDENT NAME: _____

CLINICAL SKILL 17.1: Admission and discharge process

DEMONSTRATION OF: The ability to effectively admit and discharge an individual from a healthcare setting

If the observation checklist is being used as an assessment tool, the student will need to obtain a scale of independence for each of the performance criteria/evidence.

Independent (I)
Supervised (S)
Assisted (A)
Marginal (M)
Dependent (D)

COMPETENCY ELEMENTS	PERFORMANCE CRITERIA/EVIDENCE	I	S	A	M	D
Preparation for the activity	Identifies the individual using three individual identifiers Ensures therapeutic interaction Gains the individual's consent Checks facility/organisation policy Locates and gathers equipment					
Performs activity informed by evidence	For admission: • Confirms individual's identity and places identification bands on individual • Informs the individual about healthcare organisation's procedures such as meal times, visiting hours, facilities and use of phones • Orientates individual to the room and shows them the call bell, bathroom, TV, how to adjust the bed and space for their belongings • Checks if individual has any valuables and stores according to healthcare organisation's policy • Completes vital signs • Performs a pain assessment • Completes record of height and weight of the individual • Completes a urinalysis on the individual • Identifies allergies and applies alert band if indicated • Obtains a complete nursing history including social and cultural background, surgical and medical history, history of current illness and reason for admission • Notes the individual's verbal and non-verbal behaviours • Determines conscious state and orientation • Determines affect and mood • Determines ability to communicate and understand English • Observes how the individual interacts with family and caregivers • Identifies next of kin • Lists all medication currently being taken by the individual • Locks any medications as per healthcare organisation's policy • Notes the presence of any additional treatments and invasive tubes					

Continued

COMPETENCY ELEMENTS	PERFORMANCE CRITERIA/EVIDENCE	I	S	A	M	D
	• Reviews the individual's fluid intake and output including bowel function • Notes the individual's general appearance including weight, age, sex, height, body build, personal hygiene and body odour • Inspects skin integrity • Completes a pressure injury risk assessment if indicated • Assesses hair • Assesses nails • Assesses visual acuity • Assesses ears • Assesses mouth • Assesses thorax and lungs • Assesses abdomen • Assesses orientation • If indicated performs a focused neurological assessment • Assesses gait and posture • Assesses degree of mobility, level of independence and range of motion • Notes any use of prostheses or aids • Completes a falls risk assessment • Asks the individual if there is anything additional the individual would like to discuss • Identifies any learning needs • Provides teaching and brochures regarding learning needs of the individual • Conducts a physical assessment of the individual if indicated • Discusses findings with the individual as needed • Ensures the individual is comfortable and has a water jug and call bell within reach • Asks individual if the individual has any questions For discharge: • Identifies where the individual is going on discharge, who will pick up the individual, how they will travel to their location, what time they will be picked up, whether they need to use a hospital transit lounge • Ensures the individual is confident about performing any self-care activities • Assesses the individual's need for any health teaching • Checks referrals to community agencies • Ensures the individual has the relevant follow-up appointments • Ensures the individual has in their possession any aids and equipment necessary for discharge • If indicated, gives advice on where the individual can obtain supplies or equipment on discharge • Ensures wound care services are in place if indicated					

COMPETENCY ELEMENTS	PERFORMANCE CRITERIA/EVIDENCE	I	S	A	M	D
	• Ensures any intravenous cannulas/tubing/drain tubes have been removed • Ensures the individual has received their discharge medications and understands administration • Ensures X-rays are returned to the individual • Gives any paperwork needed to the individual such as medical certificates • Gives the individual a copy of their discharge summary • Provides the individual with any relevant brochures • Ensures the individual and their family/carer understand potential complications on discharge and what to do if these occur • Ensures all belongings and valuables are returned to the individual • Assists the individual to their transportation					
Applies critical thinking and reflective practice	Is able to link theory to practice Demonstrates current best practice in the care provided Performs further physical assessments and focused assessments with the individual as required during the admission process Ensures discharge begins at admission Assesses own performance					
Practises within safety and quality assurance guidelines	Reviews against facility/organisation policy Performs hand hygiene, dons appropriate PPE as per infection control protocols Cleans and disposes of equipment and waste appropriately					
Documentation and communication	Explains and communicates the activity clearly to the individual Communicates outcome and ongoing care to the individual and significant others Provides education to the individual on admission and discharge as necessary Communicates abnormal findings to appropriate personnel Reports and documents all relevant information and any complications correctly in the healthcare record Reports any complications and/or inability to perform the procedure to the RN and/or medical officer					

Educator/Facilitator Feedback:

Educator/Facilitator Score: Competent   Needs further development

How would you rate your overall performance while undertaking this clinical activity? (use a ✓ & initial)

Unsatisfactory   Satisfactory   Good   Excellent

Student Reflection: (discuss how you would approach your practice differently or more effectively)

EDUCATOR/FACILITATOR NAME/SIGNATURE:

STUDENT NAME/SIGNATURE: **DATE:**

Evolve® Answer guide for the Critical Thinking Exercises and Critical Thinking Questions in Case Studies is hosted on Evolve: http://evolve.elsevier.com/AU/Koutoukidis/Tabbner/

References

Australian and New Zealand College of Anaesthetists (ANZCA), 2023. PG07(A) Guideline on pre-anesthesia consultation and patient preparation. Available at: <https://www.anzca.edu.au/getattachment/d2c8053c-7e76-410e-93ce-3f9a56ffd881/PG07(A)-Guideline-on-pre-anaesthesia-consultation-and-patient-preparation-2017>.

Burton, M., Smith, D., Ludwig, L., 2018. *Fundamentals of nursing care: Concepts, connections and skills*, 3rd ed. F.A. Davis Company, Pennsylvania.

Crisp, J., Douglas, C., Rebeiro, G., Waters, D., 2021. *Potter and Perry's fundamentals of nursing*, 6th ed. Elsevier, Chatswood.

Lippincott Williams & Wilkins, 2022. *Lippincott's nursing procedures*, 9th ed. Wolters Kluwer, Philadelphia.

Nursing and Midwifery Board of Australia (NMBA), 2020. Decision-making framework for nursing and midwifery. Available at: <https://www.nursingmidwiferyboard.gov.au/Codes-Guidelines-Statements/Frameworks.aspx>.

Perry, A., Potter, P., Ostendorf, M., 2019. *Nursing interventions and clinical skills*, 7th ed. Elsevier, St Louis.

Reynolds, L., Debona, D., Travaglia, J., 2023. *Understanding the Australian health care system*, 5th ed. Churchill Livingstone, Chatswood.

Tollefson, J., Watson, G., Jelly, E., Tambree, K., 2021. *Essential clinical skills*, 5th ed. Cengage Learning, Melbourne.

INFECTION PREVENTION AND CONTROL

Ann Bolton and Meagan Gaskett

Overview

Effective infection prevention and control is essential to providing high-quality healthcare for individuals and a safe environment for those who work in and visit healthcare settings. Infection prevention and control is everybody's business. Knowledge and understanding of the modes of transmission of infectious organisms and when to apply the basic principles of infection prevention and control is critical to the success of any evidence-based infection control program.

Infectious diseases have not disappeared and are still prevalent today: in the last 100 years there has been the outbreak of Spanish flu, H2N2 (Asian flu), HIV/AIDS and the COVID-19 pandemic. With advances in drug and medical therapy, treatments have improved life expectancy, but in some cases microorganisms have developed drug-resistant strains commonly known as 'super bugs'. It is essential that healthcare workers (HCWs) receive updates to their education and develop their knowledge about microorganisms, the infectious process and infection control principles, applying them to their daily activities to prevent the spread of microorganisms and transmission of infection. This chapter is intended to further your knowledge of infection prevention and control mechanisms, which will help to minimise the incidence of healthcare-associated infections (HAIs) and the spread of infection between individuals, as well as protecting the individual HCW and other HCWs from contact with infectious material or exposure to communicable diseases. Nurses are in a prime position to educate individuals about activities that increase personal resistance to infection, modes of transmission and prevention methods to assist in controlling the spread of infection in the home as well as in healthcare facilities and the community.

Individuals in healthcare settings are at risk of acquiring infections because of lowered resistance and increased exposure to disease-causing microorganisms, and due to assisting with invasive procedures. Sources of infection can be people or environmental objects, such as medical or nursing equipment, that has become contaminated with infective microorganisms.

This chapter outlines the more common skills associated with infection control in the healthcare setting. Hand hygiene is the single most effective measure to prevent the spread of infection and to protect individuals and staff against infection. Hand hygiene can be performed using either an alcohol-based hand rub or an antimicrobial soap and water (for most situations). Other skills look at donning and doffing personal protective equipment (PPE) and donning sterile gloves.

 CASE STUDY 18.1

Recently a person was transferred from an aged-care home into the acute medical ward. The person had a severe case of psoriasis. His skin was very itchy, and his body was covered in a raised, reddened rash, with areas of inflammation and broken skin especially in the creases of the elbows, behind the knees and in finger webbing where he had scratched so much the skin was no longer intact. The person was nursed for two weeks in the acute ward before he was diagnosed with a Norwegian scabies infestation. As soon as the diagnosis was made, transmission-based precautions (contact precautions) were implemented and the person was cared for with the appropriate medication treatment.

During the first week of his admission standard precautions should have been used at all times, particularly when applying the various lotions and creams that he was being treated with, and also when dealing with his linen. However, in the ensuing weeks, several staff members acquired the scabies infestation along with a couple of other inpatients.

Upon reflection: Transmission occurred because it was noted that on several occasions staff did not wear PPE (gloves or aprons) when in contact with his non-intact skin, staff did sit on the person's bed on many occasions and staff carried his used linen up against their bodies and uniforms before depositing the linen in the linen receptacle. This showed there was a breakdown of the minimum standard of infection prevention and control.

Outcome: What ensued was the closure of that ward, the treatment of every staff member, every person and every family member who had been in contact with the individuals in that particular ward, the steam cleaning of the carpet in that department, the removal and laundering of every individual privacy curtain as well as the laundering of every piece of clothing that the individuals had in their rooms. This was at a very large cost to the facility: a cost that was preventable if the correct infection control and prevention strategies had been used when applicable.

1. What infection prevention and control strategy should have been implemented on this person's admission?
2. What is considered best practice when handling used linen?
3. How would you describe the mode of transmission of scabies to other individuals including staff within the facility?

CRITICAL THINKING EXERCISE 18.3

Louise is a PCA working in an aged-care home. She attends to the activities of daily living of a person in a private room including taking them to the toilet, showering, dressing and taking them to the dining room for breakfast. When the person is comfortable Louise leaves the dining room to attend to another resident. When should Louise have performed hand hygiene? What PPE should Louise have utilised?

CRITICAL THINKING EXERCISE 18.4

You notice one of your colleagues wears multiple rings on each hand, bracelets and a large wrist watch, which is not removed for hand hygiene. You also note that recently your colleague has long artificial nails and is using hand moisturiser brought in from home. She wears gloves to cover her nails and jewellery. Is this considered best practice? What can you do to help your colleague understand what is best practice? How does this impact the spread of infection during COVID-19?

CLINICAL SKILL 18.1 Handwashing/hand hygiene

Please adhere to the policy and procedures of the facility/organisation prior to undertaking the skill. Ensure this skill is in your scope of practice.

NMBA Decision-making Framework considerations (refer to **NMBA Decision-making framework for nursing and midwifery 2020**):	Equipment:
1. Am I educated? 2. Am I authorised? 3. Am I competent? If you answer 'no' to any of these, do not perform that activity. Seek guidance and support from your teacher/a nurse team leader/clinical facilitator/educator.	Accessible sink with warm running water Antimicrobial/regular soap solution or alcohol-based hand rub (ABHR) Disposable or sanitised towel Waste bin/receptacle

 PREPARE FOR THE SKILL

(Please refer to the Standard Steps on p. xii for related rationales.)
Mentally review the steps of the skill.
Discuss the skill with your instructor/supervisor/team leader, if required.
Confirm correct facility/organisation policy/safe operating procedures.
Validate the order in the individual's record.
Identify indication and rationale for performing the activity.
Assess for any contraindications.
Locate and gather equipment.
Perform hand hygiene.
Ensure therapeutic interaction.
Identify the individual using three individual identifiers.
Gain the individual's consent.
Assess for pain relief.
Prepare the environment.
Provide and maintain privacy.
Assist the individual to assume an appropriate position of comfort.

Skill activity	Rationale
Inspect surface of hands for breaks or cuts in skin or cuticles. Cover lesions with a waterproof dressing before providing care.	Open cuts or wounds can harbour high concentrations of microorganisms.
Inspect hands for heavy soiling.	Soiled hands may require a lengthier handwash.
Ensure nails are short and free of nail polish and/or artificial nails.	Most microbes on hands come from beneath the fingernails. Artificial nails can harbour four times the microorganisms than non-artificial nails.
Remove all jewellery including wristwatch, rings and bracelets.	Jewellery can harbour microbes and rub against skin, causing shedding of skin cells.

 PERFORM THE SKILL

(Please refer to the Standard Steps on p. xii for related rationales.)
Perform hand hygiene.
Apply PPE: gloves, eyewear, mask and gown as appropriate.
Ensure the individual's safety and comfort throughout use of the skill.
Promote independence and involvement of the individual if possible and/or appropriate.
Assess the individual's tolerance to the skill throughout.
Dispose of used supplies, equipment, waste and sharps appropriately.
Remove PPE and discard or store appropriately.
Perform hand hygiene.

Continued

CLINICAL SKILL 18.1 Handwashing/hand hygiene—cont'd

Skill activity	Rationale
Handwash	
Wash hands when visibly soiled. Otherwise, use hand rub. Duration of entire procedure: 40–60 seconds. Stand in front of sink, keeping hands and uniform away from sink surface (if hands touch sink during handwashing, repeat).	The inside of the sink is considered a contaminated area. Reaching over the sink increases the risk of touching the edge, which is contaminated.
Turn on water, regulate flow and temperature so that the temperature is warm. Avoid splashing water against uniform.	Warm water is more comfortable and it removes less of the skin's protective oils than hot water. Microorganisms multiply in moisture and can travel elsewhere on the body.
Wet hands and wrists thoroughly under running water. Keep hands and forearms higher than elbows during washing. Apply the recommended amount of liquid soap or antimicrobial solution.	Keeping hands elevated allows water to flow from least to most contaminated areas. The amount applied should be as per the manufacturer's instructions.
Wash hands using plenty of lather and friction for at least 15 seconds. Interlace fingers and rub palms, sides and back of hands, paying attention to the tips of the fingers, thumbs and the webbing between the fingers.	Soap cleans by emulsifying fat and oils. Friction and rubbing mechanically will loosen and remove debris and transient bacteria. Interlacing the fingers and thumbs helps to ensure all surfaces are cleaned.
Rinse hands and wrists thoroughly.	Rinsing mechanically washes away debris and microorganisms. Rinse well to prevent residual soap from irritating skin.
Gently pat hands dry with paper towel. Dry from fingers to wrists and forearms.	Drying from cleanest (fingertips) to the least clean (forearms) areas avoids contamination. Gently patting hands dry helps prevent chapping and roughened skin.
Discard paper towel into the correct receptacle.	Prevents transfer of microorganisms.
Turn off water (use clean, dry paper towel if using a hand-operated tap; avoid touching handles with hands).	Minimises contamination of hands.
Alcohol-based hand rub	
Alcohol-based hand rub can be used if hands are visibly clean and dry. Duration of the entire procedure: 20–30 seconds.	Alcohol-based hand rub has been demonstrated to reduce microbial load on hand when solution is vigorously rubbed over all hands and finger surfaces.
Apply the amount recommended by the manufacturer onto dry hands (usually 15–30 mL).	Minimises wastage. Cost efficient.
Rub your hands together, ensuring that the solution comes into contact with all the surfaces of the hand. Interlace fingers and rub palms, sides and back of hands, paying attention to the tips of the fingers, thumbs and the webbing between the fingers.	Reduces microorganisms.
Continue rubbing until the solution has evaporated and the hands are dry (usually 10–15 seconds).	This is of great importance when donning gloves, because if hands are not dry, manipulation of gloves is difficult and it may cause reactive dermatitis.

CLINICAL SKILL 18.1 Handwashing/hand hygiene—cont'd

 AFTER THE SKILL

(Please refer to the Standard Steps on p. xii for related rationales.)
Communicate outcome to the individual, any ongoing care and to report any complications.
Restore the environment.
Report, record and document assessment findings, details of the skill performed and the individual's response.
Report, record and document any abnormalities and/or inability to perform the skill.
Reassess the individual to ensure there are no adverse effects/events from the skill.

Skill activity	Rationale
If hands are dry or chapped, a small amount of lotion or barrier cream can be applied.	Chapped skin becomes a reservoir for microorganisms.
Inspect hands for obvious signs of debris and contamination.	If found, indicates poor technique. Handwashing should be repeated.
Inspect hands for dermatitis or cracked skin since this may indicate complications from excessive handwashing or an allergic reaction to the antimicrobial or soap solution.	Seek advice from infection control professional. Note: Use small, single-use containers of barrier cream since large, refillable containers have been associated with nosocomial infections.

(Berman et al 2021a & b; NHMRC 2019; Rebeiro et al 2021; Tollefson & Hillman 2022; World Health Organization 2009)

OBSERVATION CHECKLIST: HANDWASHING/HAND HYGIENE

STUDENT NAME: _____

CLINICAL SKILL 18.1: Handwashing/hand hygiene

DEMONSTRATION OF: The ability to safely and correctly demonstrate handwashing techniques

If the observation checklist is being used as an assessment tool, the student will need to obtain a scale of independence for each of the performance criteria/evidence.

Independent (I)
Supervised (S)
Assisted (A)
Marginal (M)
Dependent (D)

COMPETENCY ELEMENTS	PERFORMANCE CRITERIA/EVIDENCE	I	S	A	M	D
Preparation for the activity	Identifies indications and rationale for performing the activity Checks facility/organisation policy Locates and gathers equipment					
Performs activity informed by evidence	Wets hands under running water and applies the recommended amount of liquid soap Rubs hands together for a minimum of 15 seconds Ensures solution comes into contact with all surfaces of the hand Pays attention to the tips of the fingers, the thumbs and the webbing between fingers Rinses hands thoroughly under running water Pats dry with single-use paper towel					
Applies critical thinking and reflective practice	Is able to link theory to practice Demonstrates current best practice Assesses skin integrity, removes jewellery Demonstrates or states when handwash/hand rub should be used (e.g. routine handwash for the beginning of a shift/return from breaks or gross contamination) Assesses own performance					
Practises within safety and quality assurance guidelines	Reviews against facility/organisation policy Disposes of waste appropriately Restocks equipment as required					
Documentation and communication	Reports any skin irritation/breaks to infection control professional as per facility/organisation policy					

Educator/Facilitator Feedback:

Educator/Facilitator Score: Competent   Needs further development

How would you rate your overall performance while undertaking this clinical activity? (use a ✓ & initial)

Unsatisfactory   Satisfactory   Good   Excellent

Student Reflection: (discuss how you would approach your practice differently or more effectively)

EDUCATOR/FACILITATOR NAME/SIGNATURE:

STUDENT NAME/SIGNATURE: **DATE:**

CLINICAL SKILL 18.2 Donning and doffing PPE (gloves, gown, mask, eyewear)

Please adhere to the policy and procedures of the facility/organisation prior to undertaking the skill. Ensure this skill is in your scope of practice.

NMBA Decision-making Framework considerations (refer to NMBA Decision-making framework for nursing and midwifery 2020):	**Equipment:**
1. Am I educated? 2. Am I authorised? 3. Am I competent? If you answer 'no' to any of these, do not perform that activity. Seek guidance and support from your teacher/a nurse team leader/clinical facilitator/educator.	Gown Mask Protective eyewear or face shield Disposable gloves Face shield

 PREPARE FOR THE SKILL

(Please refer to the Standard Steps on p. xii for related rationales.)
Mentally review the steps of the skill.
Discuss the skill with your instructor/supervisor/team leader, if required.
Confirm correct facility/organisation policy/safe operating procedures.
Validate the order in the individual's record.
Identify indication and rationale for performing the activity.
Assess for any contraindications.
Locate and gather equipment.
Perform hand hygiene.
Ensure therapeutic interaction.
Identify the individual using three individual identifiers.
Gain the individual's consent.
Assess for pain relief.
Prepare the environment.
Provide and maintain privacy.
Assist the individual to assume an appropriate position of comfort.

Skill activity	**Rationale**
Determine which equipment or supplies you may need to take into the room based on type of precautions in place or activity to be performed.	Ensures efficiency. Reduces contamination. Some PPE needs to be put on before entering room.

 PERFORM THE SKILL

(Please refer to the Standard Steps on p. xii for related rationales.)
Perform hand hygiene.
Apply PPE: gloves, eyewear, mask and gown as appropriate.
Ensure the individual's safety and comfort throughout use of the skill.
Promote independence and involvement of the individual if possible and/or appropriate.
Assess the individual's tolerance to the skill throughout.
Dispose of used supplies, equipment, waste and sharps appropriately.
Remove PPE and discard or store appropriately.
Perform hand hygiene.

Skill activity	**Rationale**
Donning PPE	
Gown Fully cover torso from neck to knees, arms to end of wrists, and wrap around the back. Fasten at the back of neck and waist.	Fastening the gown will keep it from falling away from the body and prevent contamination of clothing.
Mask Secure ties or elastic bands at middle of head and neck.	The mask must cover the nose and mouth to be effective as air moves in and out of both.

CLINICAL SKILL 18.2 Donning and doffing PPE (gloves, gown, mask, eyewear)—cont'd

Protective eyewear or face shield Place over face and eyes and adjust to fit.	Prevents infection. Ensures comfort.
Gloves Extend to cover wrist of isolation gown.	Maintains sterility.
Doffing/removing PPE	
Gloves Outside of gloves is contaminated. Pinch the palm of glove with opposite gloved hand; peel off. Hold removed glove in gloved hand. Slide fingers of ungloved hand under remaining glove at wrist. Peel glove off over first glove. Discard gloves in waste container.	Remove gloves first because they are the most contaminated. Reduces the risk of spreading infection. Encloses the contaminated outside area. Used gloves are contaminated with the microbes of the wearer and handled contaminants.
Perform hand hygiene.	Microorganisms multiply in dark, moist, warm conditions (e.g. on hands when gloves are worn). Gloves may contain microscopic perforations permitting the entry of microbes, which can proliferate on the wearer's hands.
Protective eyewear or face shield Outside of eye protection or face shield is contaminated. To remove, handle by head band or ear pieces. Place in designated receptacle for reprocessing or in waste container.	Reduces the risk of spreading infection.
Gown Gown front and sleeves are contaminated. Unfasten ties. Pull away from neck and shoulders, touching inside of gown only. Turn gown inside out. Fold or roll into a bundle and discard.	Reduces the risk of spreading infection.
Mask Front of mask is contaminated—DO NOT TOUCH. Grasp bottom, then top ties or elastics and remove. Discard in infectious waste container. Surgical masks can be removed at the point of care. To remove a P2 respirator, perform hand hygiene and step outside the room or into an anteroom before removing and disposing of the respirator in a closed container and performing hand hygiene again.	Reduces the risk of spreading infection.
Perform hand hygiene immediately after removing all PPE.	Gloves do not provide 100% protection Reduces the risk of developing an allergy to the latex in the gloves.

 AFTER THE SKILL

(Please refer to the Standard Steps on p. xii for related rationales.)
Communicate outcome to the individual, any ongoing care and to report any complications.
Restore the environment.
Report, record and document assessment findings, details of the skill performed and the individual's response.
Report, record and document any abnormalities and/or inability to perform the skill.
Reassess the individual to ensure there are no adverse effects/events from the skill.

(Berman et al 2021a & b; NHMRC 2019; Tollefson & Hillman 2022; World Health Organization 2009)

OBSERVATION CHECKLIST: DONNING AND DOFFING PPE (GLOVES, GOWN, MASK, EYEWEAR)

Independent (I)
Supervised (S)
Assisted (A)
Marginal (M)
Dependent (D)

STUDENT NAME: _____

CLINICAL SKILL 18.2: Donning and doffing PPE (gloves, gown, mask, eyewear)

DEMONSTRATION OF: The ability to safely and correctly don and doff PPE

If the observation checklist is being used as an assessment tool, the student will need to obtain a scale of independence for each of the performance criteria/evidence.

COMPETENCY ELEMENTS	PERFORMANCE CRITERIA/EVIDENCE	I	S	A	M	D
Preparation for the activity	Identifies indications and rationale for performing the activity Identifies the individual using three individual identifiers Ensures therapeutic interaction Gains the individual's consent Checks facility/organisation policy Validates the order in the individual's record Locates and gathers equipment					

Performs activity informed by evidence	Donning PPE:
	• Puts on the gown with the opening at the back. Ties the gown securely at neck and waist
	• Places mask over nose, mouth and chin
	• Secures ties or elastic bands around the middle of head and neck
	• Places eye protection over eyes and adjusts to fit
	• Puts on clean disposable gloves and extends the gloves to cover the cuffs of the gown
	Doffing PPE:
	• Removes the gloves
	• Performs hand hygiene
	• Removes eye protection
	• Performs hand hygiene
	• Removes gown, ensuring not to contaminate uniform
	• Disposes of gown
	• Performs hand hygiene
	• Steps outside the room and closes the door:
	  > Removes mask
	  > Disposes of mask appropriately
	  > Performs hand hygiene					

Applies critical thinking and reflective practice	Is able to link theory to practice Demonstrates current best practice Demonstrates or states when PPE should be used Assesses own performance					
Practises within safety and quality assurance guidelines	Reviews against facility/organisation policy Disposes of equipment and waste appropriately Performs hand hygiene Restocks equipment as required					
Documentation and communication	Communicates with the individual, staff and visitors the need for precautions Reports and documents all relevant information and any complications correctly in the healthcare record Reports any complications and/or inability to perform the procedure to the RN and/or medical officer					

Educator/Facilitator Feedback:

Educator/Facilitator Score: Competent   Needs further development

How would you rate your overall performance while undertaking this clinical activity? (use a ✓ & initial)

Unsatisfactory   Satisfactory   Good   Excellent

Student Reflection: (discuss how you would approach your practice differently or more effectively)

EDUCATOR/FACILITATOR NAME/SIGNATURE:

STUDENT NAME/SIGNATURE: **DATE:**

CLINICAL SKILL 18.3 Open gloving (donning and removing sterile gloves)

Please adhere to the policy and procedures of the facility/organisation prior to undertaking the skill. Ensure this skill is in your scope of practice.

NMBA Decision-making Framework considerations (refer to NMBA Decision-making framework for nursing and midwifery 2020):	Equipment:
1. Am I educated? 2. Am I authorised? 3. Am I competent? If you answer 'no' to any of these, do not perform that activity. Seek guidance and support from your teacher/a nurse team leader/clinical facilitator/educator.	Sterile gloves of appropriate size A clean work surface on which to open the gloves

 PREPARE FOR THE SKILL

(Please refer to the Standard Steps on p. xii for related rationales.)
Mentally review the steps of the skill.
Discuss the skill with your instructor/supervisor/team leader, if required.
Confirm correct facility/organisation policy/safe operating procedures.
Validate the order in the individual's record.
Identify indication and rationale for performing the activity.
Assess for any contraindications.
Locate and gather equipment.
Perform hand hygiene.
Ensure therapeutic interaction.
Identify the individual using three individual identifiers.
Gain the individual's consent.
Assess for pain relief.
Prepare the environment.
Provide and maintain privacy.
Assist the individual to assume an appropriate position of comfort.

 PERFORM THE SKILL

(Please refer to the Standard Steps on p. xii for related rationales.)
Perform hand hygiene.
Apply PPE: gloves, eyewear, mask and gown as appropriate.
Ensure the individual's safety and comfort throughout use of the skill.
Promote independence and involvement of the individual if possible and/or appropriate.
Assess the individual's tolerance to the skill throughout.
Dispose of used supplies, equipment, waste and sharps appropriately.
Remove PPE and discard or store appropriately.
Perform hand hygiene.

Skill activity	Rationale
Remove gloves from outer packaging and place gloves in the inner wrapper on a clean, dry surface above waist level.	Maintains integrity of the gloves; any moisture on the surface contaminates the gloves.
Carefully remove inner wrapper to expose sterile gloves. Keep gloves on inner surface of the inside wrapper. Position gloves with wrist opening nearest to the body.	The inner packaging must remain sterile.
Identify the right and left gloves. Prepare to glove dominant hand first.	Correct identification helps with correct gloving. Gloving the dominant hand first helps with dexterity.
Use thumb and first two fingers of non-dominant hand to pick up first glove. Lift at least 12 cm off wrapper.	Prevents accidental contamination.

CLINICAL SKILL 18.3 Open gloving (donning and removing sterile gloves)—cont'd

Grasp the folded-over part of the cuff (each glove has a cuff about 5 cm wide that is folded back to reveal inside of glove). Take care to touch only the inside surface of the glove.	The hands are not sterile, so by only touching the inside of the glove contamination is avoided.
Insert fingers of other hand into the held glove and pull the glove up over the dominant hand without touching the outer surface of the glove.	
With gloved hand, slide fingers underneath the cuff of the second glove. Ease second glove up over non-dominant hand. Be careful not to touch outside of glove or other gloved hand with bare skin. Keep thumb of dominant hand abducted back. Once hand is settled in glove, slide cuff carefully up over the wrist, being careful to touch only the sterile sides.	This helps to prevent accidental contamination.
Adjust fingers in gloves by pulling glove fingers out with the opposite hand to straighten and adjust until fitted neatly. Hands can be interlocked to help ease gloves into correct position.	Ensures a smooth fit.
Removing gloves Pinch the palm of one glove with the other gloved hand. Pull glove off, turning inside out. Hold removed glove in your gloved hand, then use the fingers of your bare hand to pull the remaining glove from the cuff over the hand. Discard in appropriate waste receptacle. Perform hand hygiene.	Minimises contamination of underlying skin. Contains contaminated gloves.

 AFTER THE SKILL

(Please refer to the Standard Steps on p. xii for related rationales.)
Communicate outcome to the individual, any ongoing care and to report any complications.
Restore the environment.
Report, record and document assessment findings, details of the skill performed and the individual's response.
Report, record and document any abnormalities and/or inability to perform the skill.
Reassess the individual to ensure there are no adverse effects/events from the skill.

(Berman et al 2021; NHMRC 2019; Tollefson & Hillman 2022; World Health Organization 2009)

OBSERVATION CHECKLIST: OPEN GLOVING (DONNING AND REMOVING STERILE GLOVES)

	Independent (I)
	Supervised (S)
	Assisted (A)
	Marginal (M)
	Dependent (D)

STUDENT NAME: _____

CLINICAL SKILL 18.3: Open gloving (donning and removing sterile gloves)

DEMONSTRATION OF: The ability to safely and correctly don and doff sterile gloves

If the observation checklist is being used as an assessment tool, the student will need to obtain a scale of independence for each of the performance criteria/evidence.

COMPETENCY ELEMENTS	PERFORMANCE CRITERIA/EVIDENCE	I	S	A	M	D
Preparation for the activity	Identifies indications and rationale for performing the activity Identifies the individual using three individual identifiers Ensures therapeutic interaction Gains the individual's consent Checks facility/organisation policy Validates the order in the individual's record Locates and gathers equipment					
Performs activity informed by evidence	Donning sterile gloves: • Opens sterile gloves, touching only the outside of the packet • Opens the inner packet by pulling each edge to the side, does not touch the inside of the inner pack • With the thumb and fingers of the non-dominant hand, grasps only the folded-back cuff area • Slides the dominant hand in. Does not touch the outside of the glove with ungloved hand • Slides the fingers of gloved hand under the cuff of second glove and slides second hand into the glove • Adjusts the finger and thumb fit of the gloves (sterile to sterile), ensuring unsterile surfaces are not touched Removing gloves: • Grasps outside of one cuff with other gloved hand, removes glove turning inside out • Uses the fingers of bare hand to pull the remaining glove from the cuff over the hand					
Applies critical thinking and reflective practice	Is able to link theory to practice Demonstrates current best practice in the care provided Assesses own performance					
Practises within safety and quality assurance guidelines	Reviews against facility/organisation policy Disposes of equipment and waste appropriately Performs hand hygiene					
Documentation and communication	Explains and communicates the activity clearly to the individual Reports and documents all relevant information and any complications correctly in the healthcare record Reports any complications and/or inability to perform the procedure to the RN and/or medical officer					

Educator/Facilitator Feedback:

Educator/Facilitator Score: Competent   Needs further development

How would you rate your overall performance while undertaking this clinical activity? (use a ✓ & initial)

Unsatisfactory   Satisfactory   Good   Excellent

Student Reflection: (discuss how you would approach your practice differently or more effectively)

EDUCATOR/FACILITATOR NAME/SIGNATURE:

STUDENT NAME/SIGNATURE: **DATE:**

Evolve® Answer guide for the Critical Thinking Exercises and Critical Thinking Questions in Case Studies is hosted on Evolve: http://evolve.elsevier.com/AU/Koutoukidis/Tabbner/

References

Berman, A., Frandsen, G., Snyder, S., Levett-Jones, T., et al., 2021a. *Kozier and Erb's fundamentals of nursing concepts, process and practice*, 5th ed. Pearson, Frenchs Forest.

Berman, A., Snyder, S., Levett-Jones, T., et al., 2021b. *Skills in clinical nursing*, 2nd ed. Pearson, Frenchs Forest.

National Health and Medical Research Council (NHMRC), 2019. Australian guidelines for the prevention and control of infection in healthcare. Available at: <https://www.nhmrc.gov.au/about-us/publications/australian-guidelines-prevention-and-control-infection-healthcare-2019>.

Nursing and Midwifery Board of Australia (NMBA), 2020. Decision-making framework for nursing and midwifery. Available at: <https://www.nursingmidwiferyboard.gov.au/Codes-Guidelines-Statements/Frameworks.aspx>.

Rebeiro, G., Wilson, D., Fuller, S., 2021. *Fundamentals of nursing: Clinical skills workbook*, 4th ed. Elsevier, Chatswood.

Tollefson, J., Hillman, E., 2022. *Clinical psychomotor skills: Assessment skills tools for nurses*, 8th edn. Cengage Learning Australia, South Melbourne.

World Health Organization (WHO), 2009. Guidelines on hand hygiene in healthcare. Available at: <https://www.who.int/publications/i/item/9789241597906>.

Online Resources and Recommended Reading

Australian Commission on Safety and Quality in Health Care (ACSQHC), 2019. National Hand Hygiene Initiative manual. ACSQHC, Sydney. Available at: <https://www.safetyandquality.gov.au/sites/default/files/2020-03/nhhi_user_manual_-_october_2019.pdf>.

Australian Commission on Safety and Quality in Health Care (ACSQHC), 2021. National safety and quality health service standards, 2nd ed. Version 2. ACSQHC, Sydney. Available at: <https://www.safetyandquality.gov.au/our-work/healthcare-associated-infection/national-infection-control-guidelines/>.

Clinical Excellence Commission: <http://www.cec.health.nsw.gov.au/keep-patients-safe/infection-prevention-and-control/healthcare-associated-infections/hand-hygiene>.

Hand Hygiene Australia: <http://www.hha.org.au>.

PERSONAL CARE AND COMFORT

Philippa Borjanov

Overview

People requiring nursing care will often need support to meet their hygiene needs and help to maintain an acceptable level of comfort. This section describes commonly performed hygiene and comfort activities in the clinical setting and provides step-by-step instructions with rationales to enable the nurse to plan and deliver effective care. Assisting the individual to perform personal hygiene activities supports a basic human need. It also allows the nurse to identify health concerns and assess the individual in order to implement nursing care to optimise the individual's health outcomes.

Providing assistance to the individual, or performing hygiene activities for them, affords both formal and informal opportunities for the nurse to collect subjective and objective data for ongoing assessment and care planning. This time also allows for the establishment and maintenance of the therapeutic relationship between the nurse and the individual, and for monitoring and evaluating the individual's response during care, identifying needs for education and planning for discharge.

Maintaining healthy intact skin and mucous membranes provides an important barrier to injury and infection and contributes to positive health outcomes for the individual. While personal hygiene activities form part of a person's daily routine and are often seen as a function of basic nursing care, this essential activity of daily living can be a valuable measure of an individual's functional independence.

Hygiene practices are personal to the individual and are normally private activities that are performed independently. Sensitivity is required when performing or assisting with some hygiene and comfort activities that involve intimate bodily contact with the individual. Informed consent should be obtained for these procedures and privacy and dignity must be maintained at all times. These activities can sometimes involve considerable movement and discomfort for the unwell or recovering individual. Appropriate assessment of pain and planning care according to the response to analgesia may be necessary to ensure maximum cooperation and participation of the individual in the activity. The nurse should be mindful that some hygiene activities involve considerable expenditure of energy for the individual as well as exposure of the skin to cold. This discomfort can be minimised by organised and efficient work practices that conserve energy and maintain warmth and comfort levels for the individual.

Regular repositioning of the individual is essential to promote comfort, allow an opportunity for the individual to advise of concerns and allow for therapeutic interaction with the nurse. Correct positioning promotes comfort and

helps to prevent complications associated with bed rest and reduced mobility. Encouraging the individual to continue with passive or active exercises is recommended for maintaining circulation and muscle tone.

Suitable preparation and time management skills are necessary to plan and deliver competent and efficient clinical care. The level of assistance provided during hygiene activities will depend on the individual's needs and will be assessed by the nurse on an ongoing basis. Interventions should be evidence based, consider the individual's preferences and be designed, where appropriate, to promote the restoration of functional independence.

 CASE STUDY 19.1

Mrs Betty Smith is a 70-year-old woman who was admitted to hospital 10 days ago following the sudden onset of left-sided arm and leg weakness. She has been diagnosed as having a right-sided stroke and has moderate weakness down her left side.

Mrs Smith says that she knows she has had a stroke but insists that she can attend to her own hygiene needs; she prefers to shower daily in the evening when she is at home.

Mrs Smith is right-handed and able to assist the nurse with washing herself, but she tends to only wash her chest and right leg; she forgets to wash the left side of her body unless prompted to do so by the nurse.

She requires supervision with ambulation since she is unsteady on her feet; the physiotherapist has provided her with a walking frame that she has reluctantly agreed to use. She says she prefers to walk unassisted because she is very independent. She needs to be reminded to walk with supervision since she has been found in the bathroom alone on several occasions attempting to get into the shower. She needs to sit down when showering in order to prevent a fall.

Mrs Smith also requires assistance with dressing due to her left-sided weakness.

1. What would the nurse need to do to ensure Mrs Smith's safety during the showering process?
2. What actions would the nurse take to allow Mrs Smith to remain as independent as possible with her hygiene care?
3. How would the nurse assist Mrs Smith to be as independent as possible with dressing?
4. Apart from the physiotherapist, which other members of the healthcare team would be involved in the care of Mrs Smith?
5. What hygiene equipment could the nurse use to assist Mrs Smith in the shower?

CRITICAL THINKING EXERCISE 19.1

Mr DeSilva, a 21-year-old Sri Lankan man, sustained a fractured tibia and fibula of his right leg as a result of a motorcycle accident. He was taken straight from the accident to the emergency department and then surgery, and has not washed since before the accident. He has arrived on the ward direct from the operating suite, with a plaster cast on the injured leg, and in a considerable amount of pain. Mr DeSilva has limited English. What needs to be done to meet his comfort and hygiene needs? What cultural aspects of care should be considered?

CLINICAL SKILL 19.1 Assisting with a shower or bath

Please adhere to the policy and procedures of the facility/organisation prior to undertaking the skill. Ensure this skill is in your scope of practice.

NMBA Decision-making Framework considerations (refer to NMBA Decision-making framework for nursing and midwifery 2020):	Equipment:
1. Am I educated? 2. Am I authorised? 3. Am I competent? If you answer 'no' to any of these, do not perform that activity. Seek guidance and support from your teacher/a nurse team leader/clinical facilitator/educator.	Personal toiletry items, including clothing Bath towels × 2 Bathmat Face washers × 2 Shower chair or commode Plastic apron and shoe protection Disposable gloves Soiled-linen container

 PREPARE FOR THE SKILL

(Please refer to the Standard Steps on p. xii for related rationales.)
Mentally review the steps of the skill.
Discuss the skill with your instructor/supervisor/team leader, if required.
Confirm correct facility/organisation policy/safe operating procedures.
Validate the order in the individual's record.
Identify indication and rationale for performing the activity.
Assess for any contraindications.
Locate and gather equipment.
Perform hand hygiene.
Ensure therapeutic interaction.
Identify the individual using three individual identifiers.
Gain the individual's consent.
Assess for pain relief.
Prepare the environment.
Provide and maintain privacy.
Assist the individual to assume an appropriate position of comfort.

Skill activity	Rationale
Review care plan and current treatment orders.	Provides information about individual's mobility, cognition, preferences and level and type of assistance required.
Assess bathroom and equipment for safety.	Maintains safe work environment.
Ensure bathroom is clean and the floor is dry.	Prevents cross-infection and promotes safety.
Provide a shower chair or commode, if needed.	Promotes safety.
Arrange required toiletry items within easy reach.	Promotes efficiency and functional independence.
Offer use of toilet facilities before activity.	Promotes comfort, reduces anxiety.

 PERFORM THE SKILL

(Please refer to the Standard Steps on p. xii for related rationales.)
Perform hand hygiene.
Apply PPE: gloves, eyewear, mask and gown as appropriate.
Ensure the individual's safety and comfort throughout skill.
Promote independence and involvement of the individual if possible and/or appropriate.
Assess the individual's tolerance to the skill throughout.
Dispose of used supplies, equipment, waste and sharps appropriately.
Remove PPE and discard or store appropriately.
Perform hand hygiene.

Continued

CLINICAL SKILL 19.1 Assisting with a shower or bath—cont'd

Skill activity	Rationale
Assist with a shower	
Assist individual to the bathroom and close the bathroom door.	Provides privacy and maintains individual dignity. Helps to maintain a comfortable room temperature.
Assist individual to undress as required. As applicable, remove clothing from unaffected side first.	Promotes functional independence.
Turn on taps, direct flow away from individual and adjust water temperature.	Maintains safety.
Allow individual to check the water temperature for suitability.	Promotes comfort and safety.
Allow individual to hold shower handle and direct water flow onto own body if able.	Promotes functional independence and cooperation. Promotes comfort and warmth.
Keep flow of warm water across individual's back during procedure.	Maintains comfort and warmth.
Supply soap product and washcloth to individual and encourage them to wash their own body as able.	Promotes self-help skills and functional independence.
Provide full assistance with washing if required. Wash the body in an efficient manner, starting with the face.	Provides support to meet hygiene needs. Promotes individual comfort.
Wash and rinse genital area from front to back.	Avoids transmission of microorganism and cross-contamination.
Dispose of the washcloth used to wash genitals immediately.	Maintains hygiene and infection control principles.
Assist as required with washing hard-to-reach areas such as lower legs, back and hair washing.	Provides support to meet hygiene needs.
Apply disposable gloves if skin to mucous membrane contact is likely.	Maintains infection control principles.
Assess individual's skin condition, especially pressure areas over bony prominences.	Identifies risks to skin integrity.
Ensure soap product is completely rinsed from the body, especially under skin folds.	Reduces irritants on the skin and helps maintain skin integrity.
Turn hot tap off first, then cold.	Promotes safety.
Place towel around individual's shoulders and another towel or bathmat under the feet.	Promotes comfort and warmth by maintaining body heat. Maintains dignity.
Drying, dressing and grooming continued below.	
Assisting with a bath	
Fill the bath with warm water to individual's hip level.	Promotes safety. A deep, hot bath may cause vasodilation.
Assist individual to the bathroom and close the bathroom door.	Provides privacy and maintains individual dignity. Helps to maintain a comfortable room temperature.
Assist individual to undress and to climb into bath.	Provides support and promotes safety.
Assess level of supervision required and, if safe, leave individual to perform activity, but remain within calling distance of bathroom.	

CLINICAL SKILL 19.1 Assisting with a shower or bath—cont'd

Supply soap and washcloth and encourage individual to participate.	Provides support, promotes self-care skills and functional independence.
Assist with washing hard-to-reach areas such as lower legs and back.	Provides support to meet hygiene needs.
Provide full assistance with washing, if required. Wash the body in an efficient manner, starting with the face.	Provides support to meet hygiene needs. Promotes individual comfort.
Dispose of washcloth used on individual's genitals.	Maintains infection control.
Assess individual's skin condition, especially pressure areas over bony prominences.	Identifies risks to skin integrity.
Ensure soap product is completely rinsed from the body, especially under skin folds.	Reduces irritants on the skin and helps maintain skin integrity.
Drain bath first, then assist individual to climb out of bath.	Promotes safety.

Assisting with drying, dressing and grooming

Sit individual on a chair covered with a towel and place a second towel around shoulders for warmth.	Provides comfort and warmth. Maintains dignity.
Ensure skin folds and hard-to-reach areas are completely dried, such as between toes.	Maintains skin integrity.
Apply prescribed creams or treatments such as anti-embolic stockings.	Follows treatment orders.
Assist with dressing as required. Dress injured or affected side first. Assist with zips, buttons or ties/laces.	Promotes functional independence.
Set up toiletry items and assist with grooming as required, brushing teeth, drying hair, applying make-up, shaving, hearing aids and glasses. As applicable, dress affected side first.	Maintains positive self-image and promotes independence.
Clean and dry floors, shower chair or bath and leave bathroom door open. Collect toiletries from bathroom and return them to individual's bedside locker.	Maintains safe environment, infection control and allows ventilation of bathroom.
Assist individual to return to bed or chair.	Promotes comfort and rest.

 AFTER THE SKILL

(Please refer to the Standard Steps on p. xii for related rationales.)
Communicate outcome to the individual, any ongoing care and to report any complications.
Restore the environment.
Report, record and document assessment findings, details of the skill performed and the individual's response.
Report, record and document any abnormalities and/or inability to perform the skill.
Reassess the individual to ensure there are no adverse effects/events from the skill.

(Australian Commission on Safety and Quality in Health Care [ACSQHC] 2021; JBI 2022a; 2022f; Rebeiro et al 2021; Wilkinson et al 2019)

OBSERVATION CHECKLIST: ASSISTING WITH A SHOWER OR BATH

STUDENT NAME: _____

CLINICAL SKILL 19.1: Assisting with a shower or bath

DEMONSTRATION OF: The ability to assist an individual with a shower or bath

If the observation checklist is being used as an assessment tool, the student will need to obtain a scale of independence for each of the performance criteria/evidence.

Independent (I)
Supervised (S)
Assisted (A)
Marginal (M)
Dependent (D)

COMPETENCY ELEMENTS	PERFORMANCE CRITERIA/EVIDENCE	I	S	A	M	D
Preparation for the activity	Identifies indications and rationale for performing the activity Identifies the individual using three individual identifiers Ensures therapeutic interaction Assesses for pain Gains the individual's consent Checks facility/organisation policy Validates the order in the individual's record Locates and gathers equipment					
Performs activity informed by evidence	Assists the individual to the bathroom Provides and maintains privacy Promotes and maintains cultural choices Adjusts water temperature if necessary Encourages the individual to participate in activity as able Promotes functional independence Provides assistance as required Washes from head to toe Ensures all body surfaces are washed and rinsed Ensures skin folds are dry Assists with drying and dressing as required Works efficiently to maintain warmth and promote comfort					
Applies critical thinking and reflective practice	Assesses mobility, skin integrity, cognition, functional independence Performs ongoing monitoring and assessment during procedure Is able to link theory to practice Demonstrates current best practice in the care provided Assesses own performance					
Practises within safety and quality assurance guidelines	Reviews against facility/organisation policy Performs hand hygiene, dons appropriate PPE as per infection control protocols Cleans and disposes of equipment and waste appropriately Ensures individual comfort and safety at completion of procedure					

COMPETENCY ELEMENTS	PERFORMANCE CRITERIA/EVIDENCE	I	S	A	M	D
Documentation and communication	Explains and communicates the activity clearly to the individual Communicates outcome and ongoing care to the individual and significant others Reports and documents all relevant information and any complications correctly in the healthcare record Reports any complications and/or inability to perform the procedure to the RN and/or medical officer Asks the individual to report any complications during and post procedure					

Educator/Facilitator Feedback:

Educator/Facilitator Score: Competent   Needs further development

How would you rate your overall performance while undertaking this clinical activity? (use a ✓ & initial)

Unsatisfactory   Satisfactory   Good   Excellent

Student Reflection: (discuss how you would approach your practice differently or more effectively)

EDUCATOR/FACILITATOR NAME/SIGNATURE:

STUDENT NAME/SIGNATURE: **DATE:**

CLINICAL SKILL 19.2 Performing a bed bath

Please adhere to the policy and procedures of the facility/organisation prior to undertaking the skill. Ensure this skill is in your scope of practice.

NMBA Decision-making Framework considerations (refer to NMBA Decision-making framework for nursing and midwifery 2020):	**Equipment:**
1. Am I educated? 2. Am I authorised? 3. Am I competent? If you answer 'no' to any of these, do not perform that activity. Seek guidance and support from your teacher/a nurse team leader/clinical facilitator/educator.	Washbasin two-thirds full with warm water Towels × 2 Disposable wipes Washcloths × 2 Disposable gloves Bed linen Personal clothing or gown Soiled-linen container *Toiletries items:* Soap product Deodorant Moisturiser, skin lotions or emollients Toothbrush and toothpaste Hair care products Shaving equipment

 PREPARE FOR THE SKILL

(Please refer to the Standard Steps on p. xii for related rationales.)
Mentally review the steps of the skill.
Discuss the skill with your instructor/supervisor/team leader, if required.
Confirm correct facility/organisation policy/safe operating procedures.
Validate the order in the individual's record.
Identify indication and rationale for performing the activity.
Assess for any contraindications.
Locate and gather equipment.
Perform hand hygiene.
Ensure therapeutic interaction.
Identify the individual using three individual identifiers.
Gain the individual's consent.
Assess for pain relief.
Prepare the environment.
Provide and maintain privacy.
Assist the individual to assume an appropriate position of comfort.

Skill activity	Rationale
Review care plan and current treatment orders.	Provides information about individual treatment, level of assistance required and equipment/supplies needed.
Offer the individual use of toilet bedpan or bottle before procedure begins.	Promotes comfort.

 PERFORM THE SKILL

(Please refer to the Standard Steps on p. xii for related rationales.)
Perform hand hygiene.
Apply PPE: gloves, eyewear, mask and gown as appropriate.
Ensure the individual's safety and comfort throughout skill.
Promote independence and involvement of the individual if possible and/or appropriate.
Assess the individual's tolerance to the skill throughout.
Dispose of used supplies, equipment, waste and sharps appropriately.
Remove PPE and discard or store appropriately.
Perform hand hygiene.

Continued

CLINICAL SKILL 19.2 Performing a bed bath—cont'd

Skill activity	Rationale
For the individual who requires full assistance Lower the head of the bed, as appropriate, so the dependent individual is lying, as flat as possible, with one pillow.	Promotes comfort.
For the individual who can partially assist Adjust the head of the bed to semi-recumbent position and place the wash basin within reach.	Promotes comfort.
Fill bowl two-thirds full with warm water.	Promotes safe work practices.
Untuck, fold and remove upper layers of bed linen and place on a clean, flat surface.	Promotes efficiency and maintains infection control.
Cover individual with a bath sheet or bed sheet and assist the individual to remove clothing.	Maintains warmth and maintains dignity.
Washing the front of the body	
Expose only the body part being washed.	Maintains warmth and dignity.
Place one towel under or across the body part and use the other towel to dry.	Protects bed linen from moisture.
Place a towel across the chest and wash the face with the washcloth without soap products. Take care around the eyes. Clean the ears and neck then dry carefully.	Maintains skin integrity.
Place towel lengthwise under the arm. Use a small amount of soap product on the washcloth to wash the arm, including the axilla.	Maintains skin integrity.
Use long and firm strokes and move joints through the normal range of motion as tolerated. Rinse and pat dry.	Promotes circulation and maintains joint health.
Wash individual's hand in the bowl of water if able. Take care to stabilise the basin on the bed and allow the individual's hand to rest in the water. Dry well.	Promotes comfort.
Repeat with other arm and hand. Apply deodorant and other creams, if required.	Promotes efficient work practices.
Uncover chest and place towel between water wash basin and individual. Wash chest, taking care to wash and dry thoroughly under women's breasts.	Protects bed linen. Maintains skin integrity and prevents excoriation.
Cover the upper body with the bath towel.	Maintains warmth and dignity.
Wash abdomen, rinse and pat dry, in particular, skin folds. Cover with the bath towel.	Promotes efficient work practices.
Check the warmth of the water and replace if cool or dirty.	Maintains comfort.
Repeat washing procedure with legs and feet taking care to dry thoroughly between toes.	Promotes efficient work practices and promotes individual comfort.
Apply gloves to wash the genitals. Rinse and pat dry thoroughly, in particular, skin folds.	Maintains infection control.
Change basin water and dispose of washcloth.	Maintains infection control.

CLINICAL SKILL 19.2 Performing a bed bath—cont'd

Washing the back and buttocks

Assist the individual to roll into a lateral position supported by the bed rail and a second person if required.	Provides comfort and maintains safety.
Keep individual covered with a bath towel and expose back and buttocks. Place towel on mattress and tuck gently against the back and buttocks.	Maintains comfort and dignity.
Wash the back starting at the neck using long firm strokes.	Promotes circulation.
Inspect the skin for signs of pressure or other injury.	Maintains skin integrity.
Pat dry thoroughly, especially the buttocks and skin folds. Apply creams as required.	Maintains skin integrity.
Cover back with towel, ensure individual is comfortable in the lateral position and well supported for the linen change procedure.	Promotes comfort and safety.
Remove wash basin and position clean bed linen and soiled-linen container within reach. Raise bed rail if moving away from the bed.	Promotes safety and efficiency.
Assist the individual into clean pyjamas or clothing of their choice.	Promotes individual comfort.

 AFTER THE SKILL

(Please refer to the Standard Steps on p. xii for related rationales.)
Communicate outcome to the individual, any ongoing care and to report any complications.
Restore the environment.
Report, record and document assessment findings, details of the skill performed and the individual's response.
Report, record and document any abnormalities and/or inability to perform the skill.
Reassess the individual to ensure there are no adverse effects/events from the skill.

(ACSQHC 2021; JBI 2022a; 2022f; Rebeiro et al 2021; Wilkinson et al 2019)

OBSERVATION CHECKLIST: PERFORMING A BED BATH

STUDENT NAME: _____

CLINICAL SKILL 19.2: Performing a bed bath

DEMONSTRATION OF: The ability to perform a bed bath

If the observation checklist is being used as an assessment tool, the student will need to obtain a scale of independence for each of the performance criteria/evidence.

Independent (I)
Supervised (S)
Assisted (A)
Marginal (M)
Dependent (D)

COMPETENCY ELEMENTS	PERFORMANCE CRITERIA/EVIDENCE	I	S	A	M	D
Preparation for the activity	Identifies indications and rationale for performing the activity Identifies the individual using three individual identifiers Ensures therapeutic interaction Assesses for pain Gains the individual's consent Checks facility/organisation policy Validates the order in the individual's record Assists the individual into an appropriate position					
Performs activity informed by evidence	Encourages the individual to participate in activity as able Promotes and maintains cultural choices Promotes functional independence Provides assistance as required Washes from head to toe Ensures all body surfaces are washed and rinsed Ensures skin folds are dry Assists with drying and dressing as required Works efficiently to maintain warmth and promote comfort					
Applies critical thinking and reflective practice	Is able to link theory to practice Assesses mobility, skin integrity, cognition, functional independence Demonstrates current best practice in the care provided Assesses own performance					
Practises within safety and quality assurance guidelines	Reviews against facility/organisation policy Performs hand hygiene, dons appropriate PPE as per infection control protocol Raises the bed to the appropriate working position based on nurse's height and lowers at completion of activity Cleans and disposes of equipment and waste appropriately					
Documentation and communication	Explains and communicates the activity clearly to the individual Communicates outcome and ongoing care to the individual and significant others Communicates abnormal findings to appropriate personnel Reports and documents all relevant information and any complications correctly in the healthcare record Reports any complications and/or inability to perform the procedure to the RN and/or medical officer Asks the individual to report any complications during and post procedure					

Educator/Facilitator Feedback:

Educator/Facilitator Score: Competent   Needs further development

How would you rate your overall performance while undertaking this clinical activity? (use a ✓ & initial)

Unsatisfactory   Satisfactory   Good   Excellent

Student Reflection: (discuss how you would approach your practice differently or more effectively)

EDUCATOR/FACILITATOR NAME/SIGNATURE:

STUDENT NAME/SIGNATURE: **DATE:**

CLINICAL SKILL 19.3 Performing an eye toilet

Please adhere to the policy and procedures of the facility/organisation prior to undertaking the skill. Ensure this skill is in your scope of practice.

NMBA Decision-making Framework considerations (refer to NMBA Decision-making framework for nursing and midwifery 2020):	Equipment:
1. Am I educated? 2. Am I authorised? 3. Am I competent? If you answer 'no' to any of these, do not perform that activity. Seek guidance and support from your teacher/a nurse team leader/clinical facilitator/educator.	Sterile dressing pack or kidney dish Pack sterile cottonwool balls/gauze Sodium chloride 0.9% × 1 sachet Kidney dish Extra sterile gauze swabs Towel Disposable waterproof sheet ('bluey') Rubbish bag Alcohol-based hand rub Disposable gloves Cleaning solution (alcohol) and wipe for trolley or work surface

PREPARE FOR THE SKILL

(Please refer to the Standard Steps on p. xii for related rationales.)
Mentally review the steps of the skill.
Discuss the skill with your instructor/supervisor/team leader, if required.
Confirm correct facility/organisation policy/safe operating procedures.
Validate the order in the individual's record.
Identify indication and rationale for performing the activity.
Assess for any contraindications.
Locate and gather equipment.
Perform hand hygiene.
Ensure therapeutic interaction.
Identify the individual using three individual identifiers.
Gain the individual's consent.
Assess for pain relief.
Prepare the environment.
Provide and maintain privacy.
Assist the individual to assume an appropriate position of comfort.

Skill activity	Rationale
Review care plan and current treatment orders.	Provides information about individual's treatment, equipment/supplies needed.

PERFORM THE SKILL

(Please refer to the Standard Steps on p. xii for related rationales.)
Perform hand hygiene.
Apply PPE: gloves, eyewear, mask and gown as appropriate.
Ensure the individual's safety and comfort throughout skill.
Promote independence and involvement of the individual if possible and/or appropriate.
Assess the individual's tolerance to the skill throughout.
Dispose of used supplies, equipment, waste and sharps appropriately.
Remove PPE and discard or store appropriately.
Perform hand hygiene.

Skill activity	Rationale
Use aseptic non-touch technique (ANTT) to open and prepare dressing pack or procedure tray.	Maintains infection control practices and principles.
Place cottonwool/gauze swabs in tray and pour normal saline over swabs.	Prepares supplies ready for use.
Ask or assist individual to lie flat if permitted.	Facilitates drainage of fluid away from the face.

CLINICAL SKILL 19.3 Performing an eye toilet—cont'd

Place towel or disposable waterproof sheet under individual's head.	Protects pillow and bedding.
Place kidney dish close to the individual's cheek.	Protects individual and bed linen.
Begin with the less affected or the cleaner of the two eyes.	Prevents transmission of microorganisms from an affected eye to an unaffected eye.
Ask or assist the individual to close the eyelid. Use a saline moistened swab to clean eyelid from inner canthus to outer canthus and discard swab in kidney dish.	Prevents fluid and debris from entering the nasolacrimal duct.
Use a new moistened swab for each action and continue to gently swab the eyelid and lashes until clean.	Prevents cross-contamination.
If the top and bottom eyelids or lashes are stuck together, gently swab across the eyelid until the eyelashes are free.	Promotes comfort.
Ask the individual to open the eye or assist individual to open eye if appropriate. Use a gauze swab in the hand to gently bring the lower eyelid down.	Allows inspection of the eyeball.
Inspect the eyeball and surrounding tissue and assess for signs of injury, inflammation, debris, foreign body or infection.	Identifies risks to individual's eye health.
Use gauze swab to absorb moisture and dry around the eye.	Promotes individual comfort.
Repeat the procedure for the other eye.	Prevents cross-infection to unaffected eye.
Dry any moisture from the individual's face, remove the towel from under the head.	Promotes individual comfort and maintains skin integrity.
Following the eye toilet, prescribed and non-prescribed drops may need to be instilled or ointments applied. Allow appropriate time in between instilling eye drops and applying ointment.	Applies individual treatment and care orders for irritation or infection. Maximises effectiveness of treatment.

 AFTER THE SKILL

(Please refer to the Standard Steps on p. xii for related rationales.)
Communicate outcome to the individual, any ongoing care and to report any complications.
Restore the environment.
Report, record and document assessment findings, details of the skill performed and the individual's response.
Report, record and document any abnormalities and/or inability to perform the skill.
Reassess the individual to ensure there are no adverse effects/events from the skill.

(ACSQHC 2021; JBI 2022d; 2022e; Rebeiro et al 2021)

OBSERVATION CHECKLIST: PERFORMING AN EYE TOILET

STUDENT NAME: _____

CLINICAL SKILL 19.3: Performing an eye toilet

DEMONSTRATION OF: The ability to performing an eye toilet

If the observation checklist is being used as an assessment tool, the student will need to obtain a scale of independence for each of the performance criteria/evidence.

Independent (I)
Supervised (S)
Assisted (A)
Marginal (M)
Dependent (D)

COMPETENCY ELEMENTS	PERFORMANCE CRITERIA/EVIDENCE	I	S	A	M	D
Preparation for the activity	Identifies indications and rationale for performing the activity Identifies the individual using three individual identifiers Ensures therapeutic interaction Assesses for pain Gains the individual's consent Checks facility/organisation policy Validates the order in the individual's record Locates and gathers equipment Assists the individual into an appropriate position					
Performs activity informed by evidence	Performs procedure using aseptic non-touch technique (ANTT) Promotes and maintains cultural choices Cleans unaffected/less affected eye first Uses new swab for each cleaning action Applies infection control principles					
Applies critical thinking and reflective practice	Performs visual inspection and assessment of the eye Is able to link theory to practice Demonstrates current best practice in the care provided Assesses own performance					
Practises within safety and quality assurance guidelines	Reviews against facility/organisation policy Performs hand hygiene, dons appropriate PPE as per infection control protocols Raises the bed to the appropriate working position based on nurse's height and lowers at completion of activity Cleans and disposes of equipment and waste appropriately					
Documentation and communication	Explains and communicates the activity clearly to the individual Communicates outcome and ongoing care to individual and significant others Communicates abnormal findings to appropriate personnel Reports and documents all relevant information and any complications correctly in the healthcare record Reports any complications and/or inability to perform the procedure to the RN and/or medical officer Asks the individual to report any complications during and post procedure					

Educator/Facilitator Feedback:

Educator/Facilitator Score: Competent   Needs further development

How would you rate your overall performance while undertaking this clinical activity? (use a ✓ & initial)

Unsatisfactory   Satisfactory   Good   Excellent

Student Reflection: (discuss how you would approach your practice differently or more effectively)

EDUCATOR/FACILITATOR NAME/SIGNATURE:

STUDENT NAME/SIGNATURE: **DATE:**

CLINICAL SKILL 19.4 Assisting with oral hygiene, cleaning teeth and dentures

Please adhere to the policy and procedures of the facility/organisation prior to undertaking the skill. Ensure this skill is in your scope of practice.

NMBA Decision-making Framework considerations (refer to NMBA Decision-making framework for nursing and midwifery 2020):	Equipment:
1. Am I educated? 2. Am I authorised? 3. Am I competent? If you answer 'no' to any of these, do not perform that activity. Seek guidance and support from your teacher/a nurse team leader/clinical facilitator/educator.	Kidney dish or small bowl Warm water for rinsing Soft toothbrush or electric toothbrush Fluoride tooth or denture paste Towel Alcohol-based hand rub Disposable gloves Eye protection

 PREPARE FOR THE SKILL

(Please refer to the Standard Steps on p. xii for related rationales.)
Mentally review the steps of the skill.
Discuss the skill with your instructor/supervisor/team leader, if required.
Confirm correct facility/organisation policy/safe operating procedures.
Validate the order in the individual's record.
Identify indication and rationale for performing the activity.
Assess for any contraindications.
Locate and gather equipment.
Perform hand hygiene.
Ensure therapeutic interaction.
Identify the individual using three individual identifiers.
Gain the individual's consent.
Assess for pain relief.
Prepare the environment.
Provide and maintain privacy.
Assist the individual to assume an appropriate position of comfort.

Skill activity	Rationale
Review care plan and current treatment orders.	Provides information about individual treatment, equipment/supplies needed.
Position individual seated at the basin or position clean over-bed table in front of individual at a suitable height for use.	Promotes functional independence.
Assist with preparation of items for use: apply toothpaste to brush, place towel over chest or within reach, fill cup with water.	Promotes efficiency and functional independence.

 PERFORM THE SKILL

(Please refer to the Standard Steps on p. xii for related rationales.)
Perform hand hygiene.
Apply PPE: gloves, eyewear, mask and gown as appropriate.
Ensure the individual's safety and comfort throughout skill.
Promote independence and involvement of the individual if possible and/or appropriate.
Assess the individual's tolerance to the skill throughout.
Dispose of used supplies, equipment, waste and sharps appropriately.
Remove PPE and discard or store appropriately.
Perform hand hygiene.

Skill activity	Rationale
Cleaning dentures	
Ask or assist individual to remove dentures into small bowl or kidney dish.	Facilitates cleaning.

CLINICAL SKILL 19.4 Assisting with oral hygiene, cleaning teeth and dentures—cont'd

Use a finger to carefully break the suction between the gum and denture at the end of the gum line.	Promotes individual comfort and maintains safe work practices.
Wet toothbrush in water and brush the inner and outer surface of dentures using firm strokes.	Ensures efficient cleaning.
Rinse each denture under running water and ensure all paste is removed from denture surfaces.	Promotes individual comfort and maintains oral health.
Offer individual a cup of clean warm to cool water to rinse and a bowl to spit waste before reinserting dentures.	Promotes individual comfort and oral hygiene.
Allow individual to replace own dentures in mouth if able.	Promotes individual comfort and independence.
Cleaning teeth	
Ask individual to open mouth and briefly inspect teeth and oral cavity for debris. Assist to rinse if necessary.	Allows inspection of teeth and oral cavity. Removes debris from mouth to facilitate cleaning.
Gently brush all teeth and gum surfaces using an up-and-down action or circular motion.	Facilitates removal of debris and maintains tooth and gum health.
Start at the upper back teeth and gently brush the outer surfaces of teeth and gum line towards the front teeth.	Removes debris from teeth and gums.
Repeat with inner top teeth and gums.	Removes debris from teeth and gums.
Repeat with bottom teeth in same manner as top teeth.	Removes debris from teeth and gums.
Offer water to rinse mouth before continuing to clean outer and inner surfaces of lower teeth and gums.	Facilitates removal of toothpaste from mouth.
Brush chewing surfaces of teeth.	Removes debris from teeth and gums.
Brush surface of tongue if necessary.	Promotes individual comfort.
Offer water to rinse toothpaste from mouth.	Promotes individual comfort and maintains oral health.
Dry around mouth and apply water-based moisturiser to lips.	Promotes individual comfort.

 AFTER THE SKILL

(Please refer to the Standard Steps on p. xii for related rationales.)
Communicate outcome to the individual, any ongoing care and to report any complications.
Restore the environment.
Report, record and document assessment findings, details of the skill performed and the individual's response.
Report, record and document any abnormalities and/or inability to perform the skill.
Reassess the individual to ensure there are no adverse effects/events from the skill.

(ACSQHC 2021; JBI 2022c; 2022g; 2023h; Rebeiro et al 2021)

OBSERVATION CHECKLIST: ASSISTING WITH ORAL HYGIENE, CLEANING TEETH AND DENTURES

STUDENT NAME: _____

CLINICAL SKILL 19.4: Assisting with oral hygiene, cleaning teeth and dentures

DEMONSTRATION OF: The ability to perform oral hygiene

If the observation checklist is being used as an assessment tool, the student will need to obtain a scale of independence for each of the performance criteria/evidence.

Independent (I)

Supervised (S)

Assisted (A)

Marginal (M)

Dependent (D)

COMPETENCY ELEMENTS	PERFORMANCE CRITERIA/EVIDENCE	I	S	A	M	D
Preparation for the activity	Identifies indications and rationale for performing the activity Identifies the individual using three individual identifiers Ensures therapeutic interaction Assesses for pain Gains the individual's consent Checks facility/organisation policy Validates the order in the individual's record Locates and gathers equipment Assists the individual into an appropriate position					
Performs activity informed by evidence	Prepares equipment for individual to facilitate self-care if possible Promotes and maintains cultural choices Provides support and assistance if required Ensures teeth and gum surfaces are clean and rinsed					
Applies critical thinking and reflective practice	Performs visual assessment of oral cavity Is able to link theory to practice Demonstrates current best practice in the care provided Assesses own performance					
Practises within safety and quality assurance guidelines	Reviews against facility/organisation policy Performs hand hygiene, dons appropriate PPE as per infection control protocols Raises the bed to the appropriate working position based on nurse's height and lowers at completion of activity Cleans and disposes of equipment and waste appropriately					
Documentation and communication	Explains and communicates the activity clearly to the individual Communicates outcome and ongoing care to the individual and significant others Communicates abnormal findings to appropriate personnel Reports and documents all relevant information and any complications correctly in the healthcare record Reports any complications and/or inability to perform the procedure to the RN and/or medical officer Asks the individual to report any complications during and post procedure					

Educator/Facilitator Feedback:

Educator/Facilitator Score:　　Competent　　　　Needs further development

How would you rate your overall performance while undertaking this clinical activity? (use a ✓ & initial)

Unsatisfactory　　　　　　　Satisfactory　　　Good　　　　　Excellent

Student Reflection: (discuss how you would approach your practice differently or more effectively)

EDUCATOR/FACILITATOR NAME/SIGNATURE:

STUDENT NAME/SIGNATURE:　　　　　　　　　　　　　　　　**DATE:**

CLINICAL SKILL 19.5 Performing special mouth care

Please adhere to the policy and procedures of the facility/organisation prior to undertaking the skill. Ensure this skill is in your scope of practice.

NMBA Decision-making Framework considerations (refer to NMBA Decision-making framework for nursing and midwifery 2020):

1. Am I educated?
2. Am I authorised?
3. Am I competent?

If you answer 'no' to any of these, do not perform that activity. Seek guidance and support from your teacher/a nurse team leader/clinical facilitator/educator.

Equipment:

Kidney dish or similar × 2
Large cotton swab sticks
Cup of warm water
Soft toothbrush or electric toothbrush
Fluoride toothpaste
Chlorhexidine mouthwash
Towel
Disposable waterproof sheet ('bluey')
Pen torch
Tongue depressor
Labelled denture container
Water-based lip moisturiser
Prescribed or non-prescribed medication
Alcohol-based hand rub
Disposable gloves
Eye protection
Cleaning solution (alcohol) and wipe for trolley or work surface
Rubbish bag
Suction equipment (with Yankauer or y-suction catheter)

 PREPARE FOR THE SKILL

(Please refer to the Standard Steps on p. xii for related rationales.)
Mentally review the steps of the skill.
Discuss the skill with your instructor/supervisor/team leader, if required.
Confirm correct facility/organisation policy/safe operating procedures.
Validate the order in the individual's record.
Identify indication and rationale for performing the activity.
Assess for any contraindications.
Locate and gather equipment.
Perform hand hygiene.
Ensure therapeutic interaction.
Identify the individual using three individual identifiers.
Gain the individual's consent.
Assess for pain relief.
Prepare the environment.
Provide and maintain privacy.
Assist the individual to assume an appropriate position of comfort.

Skill activity	Rationale
Review care plan and current treatment orders.	Provides information about individual treatment, equipment/supplies needed.
Assist individual into lateral position.	Allows secretions to be suctioned from the buccal cavity and protects airway from aspiration.
Place towel or waterproof sheet under head.	Protects pillow and bedding.

CLINICAL SKILL 19.5 Performing special mouth care—cont'd

 PERFORM THE SKILL

(Please refer to the Standard Steps on p. xii for related rationales.)
Perform hand hygiene.
Apply PPE: gloves, eyewear, mask and gown as appropriate.
Ensure the individual's safety and comfort throughout skill.
Promote independence and involvement of the individual if possible and/or appropriate.
Assess the individual's tolerance to the skill throughout.
Dispose of used supplies, equipment, waste and sharps appropriately.
Remove PPE and discard or store appropriately.
Perform hand hygiene.

Skill activity	Rationale
Ask the individual to open the mouth or use the tongue depressor to gently open the mouth. Carefully remove dentures or partial denture into kidney dish or denture container.	Allows dentures or dental plates to be safely removed.
Use torch to inspect oral cavity: teeth, gum surfaces, mucous membranes and tongue.	Allows for close inspection of oral cavity to identify injury, inflammation or infection, loose teeth and foreign objects.
Place kidney dish at individual's chin or cheek. Place a small amount of toothpaste on the toothbrush or prepare chlorhexidine mouth swabs for use.	Protects individual and bedding from secretions.
Brush or swab teeth and gums using a gentle up-and-down action, beginning with inside back teeth.	Removes debris and plaque from teeth and gums.
Offer water and straw (if not contraindicated) to rinse mouth (only if gag reflex is present) and encourage individual to spit into kidney dish if able.	Toothpaste and debris should be rinsed from teeth and gum surfaces.
If individual is unable to rinse and spit, or gag is absent, rinse toothbrush with water and use to remove toothpaste from teeth and gum surfaces. Suction secretions from buccal cavity as required.	Toothpaste should be removed from teeth and gum surfaces. Prevents aspiration of secretions into airway.
Use toothbrush or mouth swabs to remove coating from tongue if required.	Improves oral hygiene.
Apply prescribed ointments.	Completes individual treatment and care orders.
Clean dentures using toothbrush and toothpaste before rinsing and replacing in the mouth.	Promotes oral hygiene and comfort.
Apply a water-based lubricant to the lips.	Prevents soreness and cracking.
Dry moisture from the individual's mouth, remove the towel.	Promotes comfort.

 AFTER THE SKILL

(Please refer to the Standard Steps on p. xii for related rationales.)
Communicate outcome to the individual, any ongoing care and to report any complications.
Restore the environment.
Report, record and document assessment findings, details of the skill performed and the individual's response.
Report, record and document any abnormalities and/or inability to perform the skill.
Reassess the individual to ensure there are no adverse effects/events from the skill.

(ACSQHC 2021; JBI 2022g; Rebeiro et al 2021)

OBSERVATION CHECKLIST: PERFORMING SPECIAL MOUTH CARE

Independent (I)

Supervised (S)

Assisted (A)

Marginal (M)

Dependent (D)

STUDENT NAME: _____

CLINICAL SKILL 19.5: Performing special mouth care

DEMONSTRATION OF: The ability to perform special mouth care

If the observation checklist is being used as an assessment tool, the student will need to obtain a scale of independence for each of the performance criteria/evidence.

COMPETENCY ELEMENTS	PERFORMANCE CRITERIA/EVIDENCE	I	S	A	M	D
Preparation for the activity	Identifies indications and rationale for performing the activity Identifies the individual using three individual identifiers Ensures therapeutic interaction Assesses for pain Gains the individual's consent Checks facility/organisation policy Validates the order in the individual's record Locates and gathers equipment					
Performs activity informed by evidence	Assists the individual into lateral position to manage risk to airway Cleans and rinses teeth and gum surfaces Promotes and maintains cultural choices					
Applies critical thinking and reflective practice	Performs visual assessment of oral cavity Is able to link theory to practice Checks patency of airway management equipment Demonstrates current best practice in the care provided Assesses own performance					
Practises within safety and quality assurance guidelines	Reviews against facility/organisation policy Performs hand hygiene, dons appropriate PPE as per infection control protocols Checks bed brakes Raises the bed to the appropriate working position based on nurse's height and lowers at completion of activity Cleans and disposes of equipment and waste appropriately					
Documentation and communication	Explains and communicates the activity clearly to the individual Communicates outcome and ongoing care to the individual and significant others Communicates abnormal findings to appropriate personnel Reports and documents all relevant information and any complications correctly in the healthcare record Reports any complications and/or inability to perform the procedure to the RN and/or medical officer Asks the individual to report any complications during and post procedure					

Educator/Facilitator Feedback:

Educator/Facilitator Score: Competent   Needs further development

How would you rate your overall performance while undertaking this clinical activity? (use a ✓ & initial)

Unsatisfactory   Satisfactory   Good   Excellent

Student Reflection: (discuss how you would approach your practice differently or more effectively)

EDUCATOR/FACILITATOR NAME/SIGNATURE:

STUDENT NAME/SIGNATURE: **DATE:**

CLINICAL SKILL 19.6 Making an unoccupied bed

Please adhere to the policy and procedures of the facility/organisation prior to undertaking the skill. Ensure this skill is in your scope of practice.

NMBA Decision-making Framework considerations (refer to NMBA Decision-making framework for nursing and midwifery 2020):	Equipment:
1. Am I educated? 2. Am I authorised? 3. Am I competent? If you answer 'no' to any of these, do not perform that activity. Seek guidance and support from your teacher/a nurse team leader/clinical facilitator/educator.	Bottom sheet (flat or fitted) Top sheet (flat) Waterproof bedding protector (if required) Pillowcase/s Blanket Bedspread Disposable gloves Disposable apron (if required) Soiled-linen container

 PREPARE FOR THE SKILL

(Please refer to the Standard Steps on p. xii for related rationales.)
Mentally review the steps of the skill.
Discuss the skill with your instructor/supervisor/team leader, if required.
Confirm correct facility/organisation policy/safe operating procedures.
Validate the order in the individual's record.
Identify indication and rationale for performing the activity.
Assess for any contraindications.
Locate and gather equipment.
Perform hand hygiene
Ensure therapeutic interaction
Identify the individual using three individual identifiers.
Gain the individual's consent.
Assess for pain relief.
Prepare the environment.
Provide and maintain privacy.
Assist the individual to assume an appropriate position of comfort.

Skill activity	Rationale
Place clean bedlinen on a chair or clean flat surface near the bed. Place soiled-linen container near the bed.	Prevents cross-infection.
Move the bedside cabinet and over-bed table away from the bed.	Provides safe work space around bed.

 PERFORM THE SKILL

(Please refer to the Standard Steps on p. xii for related rationales.)
Perform hand hygiene.
Apply PPE: gloves, eyewear, mask and gown as appropriate.
Ensure the individual's safety and comfort throughout skill.
Promote independence and involvement of the individual if possible and/or appropriate.
Assess the individual's tolerance to the skill throughout.
Dispose of used supplies, equipment, waste and sharps appropriately.
Remove PPE and discard or store appropriately.
Perform hand hygiene.

Skill activity	Rationale
Remove pillowcases and place in soiled-linen container. Place pillows on a clean flat surface.	Prevents cross-infection.
Start at the top (head) of the bed, lift the mattress on one side of the bed and free the bottom sheet.	Promotes work efficiency.

CLINICAL SKILL 19.6 Making an unoccupied bed—cont'd

Move down to the end (foot) of the bed, lift the mattress and loosen and untuck each layer at the corner.	Facilitates ease of removal.
If working alone, complete one side of the bed before moving to loosen other side.	Promotes efficient work practices.
Inspect each layer of bed linen for signs of soiling or damage and replace as required.	Promotes skin integrity and individual hygiene and comfort.
Remove each item of upper bed linen separately, fold and place on a clean flat surface.	Folding facilitates replacement.
Take the top hem of bed linen and fold down towards the centre of the bed and repeat with bottom hem.	Promotes efficient work practices. Prevents cross-infection.
From the side of the bed, bring each piece towards the centre and fold bundle again.	Promotes efficient work practices. Prevents cross-infection.
Lift off the bed, holding bundle away from body and place on a clean flat surface.	Prevents cross-infection.
Remove soiled linen by rolling linen towards the centre of the bed.	Prevents cross-infection.
Lift linen off bed, holding bundle away from body and place into soiled-linen container.	Prevents cross-infection.
Inspect mattress for signs of damage. Clean and dry if soiled.	Prevents cross-infection.
If working alone, complete bed making on one side of the bed before moving to complete the other side.	Promotes efficient work practices.
If reusing bed linen Place folded bottom sheet in the centre of the mattress. Unfold sheet towards each side of the bed then unfold over the edge of mattress Unfold the sheet towards the top and bottom ends of the bed.	Bedclothes are easier to adjust or remove if they are replaced and tucked in separately.
If using a new sheet Place folded sheet in the centre of the mattress and unfold sheet along the length of mattress. Unfold the sheet across the mattress towards edge of the bed.	Promotes efficient work practices.
Position the sheet so it hangs equally on each side and move the sheet up towards the head of the bed to allow sufficient amount to tuck under mattress.	Allows sufficient sheet at each corner to complete triangular folds.
Complete a triangular fold Stand facing the head of the bed, tuck in the sheet at each corner over the top of the mattress and pull tightly under the mattress.	Maintains a neat appearance and holds the sheet firmly on the mattress.
At the side of the bed, pick up the edge of the sheet about 40 cm from head of the bed and lift up onto mattress.	Promotes individual comfort and maintains neat appearance.
Pull sheet tightly to make a 45-degree angle from the top corner of the mattress.	Promotes individual comfort and maintains neat appearance.
Tuck remaining sheet under the mattress at each side.	Promotes individual comfort and maintains neat appearance.

Continued

CLINICAL SKILL 19.6 Making an unoccupied bed—cont'd

Bring the triangular fold down over the side of the bed and tuck in tightly under the mattress.	Promotes individual comfort and maintains neat appearance.
Repeat at the foot or end of the bed then tuck in the remaining sheet along the long edge of the bed.	Promotes individual comfort and maintains neat appearance.
If working alone, move to opposite side of bed and begin tucking in the sheet at the head of the bed.	Promotes efficient work practices.
Ensure the sheet is smooth and tucked in tightly.	Promotes individual comfort and maintenance of skin integrity.
Position the waterproof bedding protector if required across the centre of the bed and tuck in along both sides.	Protects the individual and bottom sheet and facilitates ease of removal and replacement if soiled.
Place top sheet on bed and unfold along length of bed and position evenly over the bed.	Allows sufficient amount of sheet to complete triangular folds.
Bring the top edge of sheet to the level of the bed head.	Allows sufficient amount of sheet to fold over and protect the blanket.
Move to the end of the bed and tuck the sheet tightly under the bottom of the mattress.	Promotes individual comfort and maintains neat appearance.
Tuck the remaining sheet under the mattress using a triangular fold.	Promotes individual comfort and maintains neat appearance.
Place blanket on centre of bed and unfold, position as above and tuck in at the end of the bed using a triangular fold.	Promotes individual comfort and maintains neat appearance.
Move to the head of the bed and fold the blanket down 30 cm. Fold top sheet over to cover the blanket.	Folded sheet protects the blanket.
Place bedspread on centre of bed and unfold, ensuring it is evenly positioned on each side and covering the untucked portion of the blanket.	Promotes individual comfort and maintains neat appearance.
Bring top hem of bedspread level with the bed head then tuck in the remainder at the end of the bed using a triangular fold.	Promotes individual comfort and maintains neat appearance.
At the head of the bed, fold excess fabric under and bring neatly to the level of the sheet and blanket.	Maintains neat appearance.
Fold bedding back according to individual's need.	Allows easy access for individual to return to bed.
Replace pillows and arrange according to individual's need.	Promotes individual comfort and safety.

 AFTER THE SKILL

(Please refer to the Standard Steps on p. xii for related rationales.)
Communicate outcome to the individual, any ongoing care and to report any complications.
Restore the environment.
Report, record and document assessment findings, details of the skill performed and the individual's response.
Report, record and document any abnormalities and/or inability to perform the skill.
Reassess the individual to ensure there are no adverse effects/events from the skill.

(ACSQHC 2021; JBI 2022b; Rebeiro et al 2021)

OBSERVATION CHECKLIST: MAKING AN UNOCCUPIED BED

STUDENT NAME: _____

CLINICAL SKILL 19.6: Making an unoccupied bed

DEMONSTRATION OF: The ability to make an unoccupied bed

If the observation checklist is being used as an assessment tool, the student will need to obtain a scale of independence for each of the performance criteria/evidence.

Independent (I)

Supervised (S)

Assisted (A)

Marginal (M)

Dependent (D)

COMPETENCY ELEMENTS	PERFORMANCE CRITERIA/EVIDENCE	I	S	A	M	D
Preparation for the activity	Identifies indications and rationale for performing the activity Checks facility/organisation policy Locates and gathers equipment					
Performs activity informed by evidence	Folds and removes soiled sheets without contamination Promotes and maintains cultural choices Applies triangular fold to sheet at corners to secure to mattress Ensures bottom sheet is free from folds or creases Works efficiently to save time					
Applies critical thinking and reflective practice	Prepares bed according to the individual's comfort needs and clinical requirements Ensures bed linen is neatly and securely fitted Is able to link theory to practice Demonstrates current best practice in the care provided Assesses own performance					
Practises within safety and quality assurance guidelines	Reviews against facility/organisation policy Performs hand hygiene, dons appropriate PPE as per infection control protocols Checks bed brakes Raises the bed to the appropriate working position based on nurse's height and lowers at completion of activity Disposes of waste appropriately					
Documentation and communication	Not applicable					

Educator/Facilitator Feedback:

Educator/Facilitator Score: Competent   Needs further development

How would you rate your overall performance while undertaking this clinical activity? (use a ✓ & initial)

Unsatisfactory   Satisfactory   Good   Excellent

Student Reflection: (discuss how you would approach your practice differently or more effectively)

EDUCATOR/FACILITATOR NAME/SIGNATURE:

STUDENT NAME/SIGNATURE: **DATE:**

CLINICAL SKILL 19.7 Making a postoperative bed

Please adhere to the policy and procedures of the facility/organisation prior to undertaking the skill. Ensure this skill is in your scope of practice.

NMBA Decision-making Framework considerations (refer to NMBA Decision-making framework for nursing and midwifery 2020):	Equipment:
1. Am I educated? 2. Am I authorised? 3. Am I competent? If you answer 'no' to any of these, do not perform that activity. Seek guidance and support from your teacher/a nurse team leader/clinical facilitator/educator.	Flat sheet × 2 Waterproof bedding protector (if required) Pillowcase/s Blanket Disposable gloves Disposable apron Soiled-linen container

 PREPARE FOR THE SKILL

(Please refer to the Standard Steps on p. xii for related rationales.)
Mentally review the steps of the skill.
Discuss the skill with your instructor/supervisor/team leader, if required.
Confirm correct facility/organisation policy/safe operating procedures.
Validate the order in the individual's record.
Identify indication and rationale for performing the activity.
Assess for any contraindications.
Locate and gather equipment.
Perform hand hygiene.
Ensure therapeutic interaction.
Identify the individual using three individual identifiers.
Gain the individual's consent.
Assess for pain relief.
Prepare the environment.
Provide and maintain privacy.
Assist the individual to assume an appropriate position of comfort.

Skill activity	Rationale
Place clean bedlinen on a chair or clean flat surface near the bed. Place soiled-linen container near the bed.	Prevents cross-infection.
Move the bedside cabinet and over-bed table away from the bed.	Provides safe work space around bed.

 PERFORM THE SKILL

(Please refer to the Standard Steps on p. xii for related rationales.)
Perform hand hygiene.
Apply PPE: gloves, eyewear, mask and gown as appropriate.
Ensure the individual's safety and comfort throughout skill.
Promote independence and involvement of the individual if possible and/or appropriate.
Assess the individual's tolerance to the skill throughout.
Dispose of used supplies, equipment, waste and sharps appropriately.
Remove PPE and discard or store appropriately.
Perform hand hygiene.

Skill activity	Rationale
Remove pillowcases and place in soiled-linen container. Place pillows on a clean flat surface.	Prevents cross-infection.
Start at the top (head) of the bed, lift the mattress on one side of the bed and untuck the bottom sheet.	Promotes work efficiency.
If working alone, complete bed making on one side of bed before moving to complete the other side.	Promotes efficient work practices.

Continued

CLINICAL SKILL 19.7 Making a postoperative bed—cont'd

Place folded sheet in the centre of the mattress and unfold sheet along the length of mattress. Unfold the sheet across the mattress towards edge of the bed.	Promotes efficient work practices.
Position the sheet so it hangs equally on each side and move the sheet up towards the head of the bed to allow sufficient amount to tuck under mattress.	Allows sufficient amount of sheet to complete triangular folds at each corner.
Stand facing the head of the bed and tuck sheet over the top of the mattress and pull tightly under the mattress.	Provides a neat and secure fold for the sheet and promotes individual comfort.
At the side of the bed, pick up the edge of the sheet about 40 cm from head of the bed and lift up onto mattress.	Promotes individual comfort and maintains neat appearance.
Pull sheet tightly to make a 45-degree angle from the top corner of the mattress	Promotes individual comfort and maintains neat appearance.
Bring the triangular fold down over the side of the bed and tuck in tightly under the mattress.	Promotes individual comfort and maintains neat appearance.
Tuck remaining sheet under the mattress at each side.	Promotes individual comfort and maintains neat appearance.
Repeat at the foot or end of the bed then tuck in the remaining sheet along the long edge of the bed.	Promotes individual comfort and maintains neat appearance.
If working alone, move to opposite side of bed and begin tucking in the sheet at the head of the bed.	Promotes efficient work practices.
Ensure the sheet is smooth and tucked in tightly.	Promotes individual comfort and maintenance of skin integrity.
Position the waterproof bedding protector if required across the width of the bed according to surgical procedure. For example, place across the middle section of mattress for gynaecological and abdominal surgeries or at the top of the mattress for head and neck surgeries. Tuck under mattress on both sides.	Protects the individual and bottom sheet and facilitates ease of removal and replacement if soiled.
Place top sheet on bed and unfold along length of bed and position evenly over the bed.	Allows sufficient amount of sheet at each corner to complete a triangular fold.
Bring the top edge of sheet to the level of the bed head.	Allows sufficient amount of sheet to fold over blanket.
Allow the remaining sheet to hang over the end of the bed without tucking in.	Allows sheet to be folded into bundle.
Place blanket over sheet and bring to the level of the sheet at the top end of the bed and adjust to allow remaining blanket to overhang equally on both sides and over end of bed.	Allows blanket to be folded into bundle.
Place bedspread over blanket as above, if required.	Allows bedspread to be folded into bundle.
Fold bedspread down 30 cm from top. Fold blanket down over the bedspread and fold sheet over the blanket.	Prepares bedding for folding into bundle.
Move to end of the bed and fold the sheet, blanket and bedspread as above.	Prepares bedding for folding into bundle.
Pick up the sheet, blanket and bedspread at each corner and fold towards the middle of the bed making a 45-degree angle fold.	Folds bedding into bundle.

CLINICAL SKILL 19.7 Making a postoperative bed—cont'd

Pick up the point of the sheet, blanket and bedspread from each side of the bed and fold towards the centre of the bed.	Folds bedding into bundle.
Fold each edge of the bundle towards the centre of the bed and then fold one side of the bundle onto the other.	Folds bedding into bundle.
Fold each end of the bundle into the centre and then fold over again.	Folds bedding into bundle.
Place bed linen bundle at the end of the bed or place on a flat clean surface.	Facilitates efficient replacement of bed linen.
Replace pillowcase and place on bed.	Promotes individual comfort.

 AFTER THE SKILL

(Please refer to the Standard Steps on p. xii for related rationales.)
Communicate outcome to the individual, any ongoing care and to report any complications.
Restore the environment.
Report, record and document assessment findings, details of the skill performed and the individual's response.
Report, record and document any abnormalities and/or inability to perform the skill.
Reassess the individual to ensure there are no adverse effects/events from the skill.

(ACSQHC 2021; JBI 2022b; Rebeiro et al 2021)

OBSERVATION CHECKLIST: MAKING A POSTOPERATIVE BED

STUDENT NAME: _____

CLINICAL SKILL 19.7: Making a theatre bed

DEMONSTRATION OF: The ability to make a postoperative bed

If the observation checklist is being used as an assessment tool, the student will need to obtain a scale of independence for each of the performance criteria/evidence.

Independent (I)
Supervised (S)
Assisted (A)
Marginal (M)
Dependent (D)

COMPETENCY ELEMENTS	PERFORMANCE CRITERIA/EVIDENCE	I	S	A	M	D
Preparation for the activity	Identifies indications and rationale for performing the activity Checks facility/organisation policy Locates and gathers equipment					
Performs activity informed by evidence	Folds and removes soiled sheets without contamination Promotes and maintains cultural choices Applies triangular fold to sheet at corners to secure to mattress Ensures bottom sheet is free from folds or creases Works efficiently to save steps					
Applies critical thinking and reflective practice	Ensures bed linen is neatly and securely fitted Folds bed linen into theatre bundle to facilitate reapplication Prepares bed according to clinical requirements Is able to link theory to practice Demonstrates current best practice in the care provided Assesses own performance					
Practises within safety and quality assurance guidelines	Reviews against facility/organisation policy Performs hand hygiene, dons appropriate PPE as per infection control protocols Checks bed brakes Raises the bed to the appropriate working position based on nurse's height and lowers at completion of activity Disposes of waste appropriately					
Documentation and communication	Not applicable					

Educator/Facilitator Feedback:

Educator/Facilitator Score: Competent   Needs further development

How would you rate your overall performance while undertaking this clinical activity? (use a ✓ & initial)

Unsatisfactory   Satisfactory   Good   Excellent

Student Reflection: (discuss how you would approach your practice differently or more effectively)

EDUCATOR/FACILITATOR NAME/SIGNATURE:

STUDENT NAME/SIGNATURE: **DATE:**

CLINICAL SKILL 19.8 Making an occupied bed

Please adhere to the policy and procedures of the facility/organisation prior to undertaking the skill. Ensure this skill is in your scope of practice.

NMBA Decision-making Framework considerations (refer to NMBA Decision-making framework for nursing and midwifery 2020):	Equipment:
1. Am I educated? 2. Am I authorised? 3. Am I competent? If you answer 'no' to any of these, do not perform that activity. Seek guidance and support from your teacher/a nurse team leader/clinical facilitator/educator.	Flat sheet × 2 Waterproof bedding protector (if required) Pillowcase/s Blanket Bedspread Disposable gloves Disposable apron Soiled-linen container

 PREPARE FOR THE SKILL

(Please refer to the Standard Steps on p. xii for related rationales.)
Mentally review the steps of the skill.
Discuss the skill with your instructor/supervisor/team leader, if required.
Confirm correct facility/organisation policy/safe operating procedures.
Validate the order in the individual's record.
Identify indication and rationale for performing the activity.
Assess for any contraindications.
Locate and gather equipment
Perform hand hygiene.
Ensure therapeutic interaction.
Identify the individual using three individual identifiers.
Gain the individual's consent.
Assess for pain relief.
Prepare the environment.
Provide and maintain privacy.
Assist the individual to assume an appropriate position of comfort.

Skill activity	Rationale
Place clean bedlinen on a chair or clean flat surface near the bed. Place soiled-linen container near the bed.	Prevents cross-infection.
Move the bedside cabinet and over-bed table away from the bed.	Provides safe work space around bed.
Assist the individual to roll into a lateral position supported by the bed rail and a second person if required.	Provides comfort and maintains safety.

 PERFORM THE SKILL

(Please refer to the Standard Steps on p. xii for related rationales.)
Perform hand hygiene.
Apply PPE: gloves, eyewear, mask and gown as appropriate.
Ensure the individual's safety and comfort throughout skill.
Promote independence and involvement of the individual if possible and/or appropriate.
Assess the individual's tolerance to the skill throughout.
Dispose of used supplies, equipment, waste and sharps appropriately.
Remove PPE and discard or store appropriately.
Perform hand hygiene.

Skill activity	Rationale
Start at the top (head) of the bed, lift the mattress on one side of the bed and free the bottom sheet.	Promotes work efficiency.

CLINICAL SKILL 19.8 Making an occupied bed—cont'd

Move down to the end (foot) of the bed, lift the mattress and loosen and untuck each layer at the corner.	Facilitates ease of removal.
Fan fold or tightly roll sheet towards the centre of the bed and tuck under individual's back and buttocks.	Facilitates ease of retrieval by assistant from under the individual.
Inspect the mattress surface and smooth creases and remove debris.	Maintains skin integrity.
Place clean folded sheet in the centre of the bed. Unfold towards the top and bottom end of the bed.	Promotes efficient work practices.
Unfold half of the length of the sheet towards the edge of the mattress and position to allow a drop of 30 cm at the top, bottom and side edge of sheet.	Ensures sheet is evenly positioned on mattress and allows sufficient amount of sheet to complete fold.
Tuck in sheet at top and bottom using a triangular fold. Tuck in sheet along side of bed. Roll or fan fold excess sheet towards individual's back and tuck under as able. Position the waterproof bedding protector if required across the centre of the bed and unfold half of the length towards the edge of the mattress.	Ensures sheet remains in place and promotes individual's comfort. Maintains neat appearance.
Inform the individual about the need to move over the linen roll and assist as necessary. Support with the side rail as needed.	Encourages participation. Promotes comfort and safety.
Remove sheet from under individual and place carefully in soiled-linen container.	Ensures sheet remains in place and promotes individual comfort. Maintains neat appearance
Inspect mattress; clean if needed and dry thoroughly.	Maintains skin integrity. Prevents cross-contamination.
Bring the clean sheet through from under the individual and pull tightly before tucking in at the top and bottom ends and along the side of the bed.	Ensures sheet remains in place and promotes individual comfort. Maintains neat appearance.
Pull waterproof bedding protector through from under individual and tuck in firmly under mattress. Ensure the surface is free of creases or folds.	Protects bottom sheet and mattress. Maintains individual comfort and skin integrity.
Support individual to roll back to centre of the bed and assist into clean pyjamas or hospital gown.	Promotes comfort and individual wellbeing.
Replace top sheet, blanket and bedspread.	Provides warmth and individual comfort.
Unfold top sheet towards the top and bottom of the bed and fold over the top sheet at the level of the individual's chin to allow at least 30 cm to cover the chest.	Promotes efficient work practices.
Tuck in sheet at end of bed using a triangular fold. Ensure the individual has sufficient room to move feet and toes.	Promotes individual comfort and maintains neat appearance. Promotes skin integrity.
Unfold blanket as above and tuck in using triangular fold at end of bed.	Promotes individual comfort and maintains neat appearance.
Fold blanket 30 cm from top then fold sheet over blanket.	Folded sheet protects blanket from soiling. Promotes individual comfort.
Replace bedspread and tuck in using triangular fold at end of bed.	Promotes individual comfort and maintains neat appearance.
Fold under the top 30 cm of bedspread at the level of the sheet and blanket.	Promotes individual comfort and maintains neat appearance.

Continued

CLINICAL SKILL 19.8 Making an occupied bed—cont'd

Adjust the bedspread along each side of bed to cover the untucked sheet and blanket.	Promotes neat appearance.

 AFTER THE SKILL

(Please refer to the Standard Steps on p. xii for related rationales.)
Communicate outcome to the individual, any ongoing care and to report any complications.
Restore the environment.
Report, record and document assessment findings, details of the skill performed and the individual's response.
Report, record and document any abnormalities and/or inability to perform the skill.
Reassess the individual to ensure there are no adverse effects/events from the skill.

(ACSQHC 2021; JBI 2022b; Rebeiro et al 2021)

OBSERVATION CHECKLIST: MAKING THE OCCUPIED BED

STUDENT NAME: _____

CLINICAL SKILL 19.8: Making the occupied bed

DEMONSTRATION OF: The ability to make an occupied bed

If the observation checklist is being used as an assessment tool, the student will need to obtain a scale of independence for each of the performance criteria/evidence.

Independent (I)

Supervised (S)

Assisted (A)

Marginal (M)

Dependent (D)

COMPETENCY ELEMENTS	PERFORMANCE CRITERIA/EVIDENCE	I	S	A	M	D
Preparation for the activity	Identifies indications and rationale for performing the activity Identifies the individual using three individual identifiers Ensures therapeutic interaction Gains the individual's consent Checks facility/organisation policy Validates the order in the individual's record Locates and gathers equipment Assists the individual into an appropriate position					
Performs activity informed by evidence	Encourages the individual to participate in activity as able Promotes and maintains cultural choices Works efficiently to maintain warmth and promote comfort Folds and removes soiled sheets without contamination Applies triangular fold to sheet at corners to secure to mattress Ensures bottom sheet is free from folds or creases					
Applies critical thinking and reflective practice	Assists the individual during the procedure according to response Is able to link theory to practice Demonstrates current best practice in the care provided Assesses own performance					
Practises within safety and quality assurance guidelines	Reviews against facility/organisation policy Performs hand hygiene, dons appropriate PPE as per infection control protocols Checks bed brakes Raises the bed to the appropriate working position based on nurse's height and lowers at completion of activity Disposes of waste appropriately					
Documentation and communication	Explains and communicates the activity clearly to the individual Reports any complications and/or inability to perform the procedure to the RN Asks the individual to report any complications during and post procedure					

Educator/Facilitator Feedback:

Educator/Facilitator Score: Competent   Needs further development

How would you rate your overall performance while undertaking this clinical activity? (use a ✓ & initial)

Unsatisfactory   Satisfactory   Good   Excellent

Student Reflection: (discuss how you would approach your practice differently or more effectively)

EDUCATOR/FACILITATOR NAME/SIGNATURE:

STUDENT NAME/SIGNATURE: **DATE:**

Evolve®

Answer guide for the Critical Thinking Exercises and Critical Thinking Questions in Case Studies is hosted on Evolve: http://evolve.elsevier.com/AU/Koutoukidis/Tabbner/

References

Australian Commission on Safety and Quality in Health Care (ACSQHC), 2021. National safety and quality health service standards, 2nd ed. Available at: <https://www.safetyandquality.gov.au/sites/default/files/2021-05/national_safety_and_quality_health_service_nsqhs_standards_second_edition_-_updated_may_2021.pdf>.

Joanna Briggs Institute, 2022a. Bathing and showering techniques. (JBI13750.) Available at: <https://jbi.global/ebp>.

Joanna Briggs Institute, 2022b. Bed making. (JBI2299.) Available at: <https://jbi.global/ebp>.

Joanna Briggs Institute, 2022c. Dementia: Oral hygiene care. (JBI681.) Available at: <https://jbi.global/ebp>.

Joanna Briggs Institute, 2022d. Eye cleansing. (JBI1022.) Available at: <https://jbi.global/ebp>.

Joanna Briggs Institute, 2022e. Eye toilet: Older person. (JBI2133.) Available at: <https://jbi.global/ebp>.

Joanna Briggs Institute, 2022f. Hygiene management. (JBI2021.) Available at: <https://jbi.global/ebp>.

Joanna Briggs Institute. 2022g. Oral hygiene in adults: General principles. (JBI23021.) Available at: <https://jbi.global/ebp>.

Joanna Briggs Institute, 2023h. Stroke: Oral hygiene. (JBI20454.) Available at: <https://jbi.global/ebp>.

Nursing and Midwifery Board of Australia (NMBA), 2020. Decision-making framework for nursing and midwifery. Available at: <https://www.nursingmidwiferyboard.gov.au/Codes-Guidelines-Statements/Frameworks.aspx>.

Rebeiro, G., Wilson, D., Fuller, S., 2021. *Fundamentals of nursing: Clinical skills workbook*, 4th ed. Elsevier, Chatswood.

Wilkinson, J., Treas, L., Barnett, K., et al., 2019. *Fundamentals of nursing. Vol 2: Thinking, doing and caring*, 4th ed. F.A. Davis Company, Philadelphia.

ADMINISTRATION AND MONITORING OF MEDICATIONS AND INTRAVENOUS THERAPY

Heather Redmond

Overview

Medication administration is a routine nursing task, requiring the nurse to possess the necessary skills and knowledge to competently and safely administer medications and monitor individuals for therapeutic effects and adverse reactions. When used appropriately medications contribute to significant improvements in an individual's health (Australian Commission on Safety and Quality in Health Care [ACSQHC] 2021). However, medications can also be associated with harm and adverse outcomes for the individual. Adverse medication events can affect an individual in a variety of ways from mild adverse reactions to allergic reactions or death (ACSQHC 2023).

The safety of individuals in the healthcare setting is a global concern (World Health Organization 2019) and nurses have an integral role to play in ensuring their safety, particularly in the medication administration process. In 2012, the ACSQHC developed a medication safety action guide that aims to reduce harm to people from medications through safe and effective medication management.

It is important that all health professionals follow organisational policy and procedural guidelines, and understand and follow the national recommendations for terminology, abbreviations and symbols to be used in medicines documentation (ACSQHC 2016), labelling of injectable medicines, fluids and lines (ACSQHC 2016) and the National Safety and Quality Health Care Medication Standards (ACSQHC 2021) to reduce the likelihood of an individual experiencing an adverse medication event. It is not only nurses who are involved in the process of medication administration and management for individuals in the healthcare setting. Medical officers primarily are responsible for prescribing medication based on the individual's health needs; however, Nurse Practitioners or eligible midwives can also prescribe specific to their area of clinical practice, within state and/or territory legislation (Frotjold & Bloomfield 2021). The pharmacist has many roles including preparing and dispensing medicines, mixing up compounds or specific IV solutions, correct labelling, ensuring the medication is correct for the individual, and education (Frotjold & Bloomfield 2021). It is the nurse's responsibility to ensure prior to medication administration that medications are prescribed and administered accurately.

A medication error is a result of a failure to follow medication processes of the '11 rights' and can occur at any time during prescribing, dispensing, administration or ingestion of the medication. The nurse administers the medication so it is the nurse's responsibility to ensure the individual is administered medication according to the '11 rights'. The nurse is also the healthcare professional who spends the most time with individuals in the healthcare setting and is therefore most likely to observe any adverse reactions (ADRs) an individual may experience to a medication. In addition, the nurse also observes the individual for the therapeutic effectiveness of the medication treatment and can provide information to the medical officer and registered nurse of patient outcomes and provide education to the individual regarding their medication management.

To ensure that medications are administered correctly and safely, the nurse must observe the 11 rights of medication administration:

1. The right prescription
2. The right medication
3. The right dose
4. The right expiration date
5. The right route
6. The right time
7. The right form
8. The right person
9. The right documentation
10. The right to refuse
11. The right response.

Before any medication is administered, the individual's medication chart must be checked thoroughly and systematically to determine the accuracy of the prescription and medication supplied including dose and expiration date, as well as the identity of the individual receiving the medication, the route and form to be administered, and the date and time for administration of the medication prescribed. The nurse must also complete the medication documentation, assess for a therapeutic response and identify any contraindications to medication administration. If the individual refuses medication administration this should also be documented and reported to the medical officer.

The administration of an injection is an invasive procedure that must be performed using the standard aseptic non-touch technique (ANTT) as there is a risk of infection when a needle pierces the skin. The potential for infection is prevented by ANTT, ensuring all key sites are not contaminated (ANTT nd), and this is achieved through hand hygiene, ANTT when preparing the solution and in administration of the injection, and in preparing the skin prior to the injection. Principles of ANTT (see Ch 18 in *Tabbner's Nursing Care: Theory and Practice*, 9th ed) are used when preparing for and administering parenteral medications.

 CASE STUDY 20.1

Medication interactions

David had recently been prescribed two new medications by his GP for hypertension and depression. David was diligent about taking his medications as prescribed. David started experiencing dizziness and feeling faint and generally unwell and, since the symptoms continued to worsen over the next few days, he decided to make an appointment to go back and see his GP. In the meantime, he researches using the internet since he was sure the medications were making him unwell. He found that the combination of the blood pressure medication and the antidepressant were interacting with each other as well as the grapefruit juice he was drinking. David noted he was not supposed to drink grapefruit juice with the prescribed antihypertensive. David considered that he ate healthily and drank grapefruit juice every morning because it was rich in antioxidants. On return to the GP, David's blood pressure was 95/45 mmHg and his heart rate was 110 beats per minute. The GP said that blood pressure medication had caused his blood pressure to drop, which was making him feel dizzy and faint.

David's doctor immediately adjusted his medication regimen, taking him off the antidepressant and switching him to a different blood pressure medication that wouldn't interact with the one he was already taking. It took a few days for the new medication to take effect.

1. What is the role of the doctor and the pharmacist in ensuring safe medication administration for David?
2. What questions could David have asked his GP about the newly prescribed medications?

CRITICAL THINKING EXERCISE 20.3

Medication administration safety

You are working on the medical ward, and it is an extremely busy shift. You complete your medication round prior to breakfast, and notice your colleague is looking flustered. She tells you that she must attend to one of her patients that has been incontinent, and she has just drawn up Mr Park's insulin in the medication room. She asks for you to get the insulin, check this with another nurse and give it to Mr Park for her. She mentions the medication chart is in the medication room. What are the safety issues in giving a medication that you have not drawn up, or seen drawn up yourself? What is your response?

CRITICAL THINKING EXERCISE 20.4

Mr Thompson has had Crohn's disease for 10 years and went to theatre for an ileocecal resection and formation of a temporary ileostomy due to scarring and ongoing inflammation. Postoperatively, his serum potassium levels were 3 mmol/L and he was given 10 mmol/L of potassium chloride in 100 mL IV. After the potassium was administered, the medical officer ordered for Mr Thompson a 1000 mL of 0.9% normal saline with 30 mmol/L of potassium chloride to be given over eight hours IV. You complete a set of vital signs and Mr Thompson's BP is 90/58 mmHg, HR 110 beats/minute, RR 20 breaths/minute & SpO_2 96%. You inform the RN and the medical officer who instructs you to give Mr Thompson a 250 mL IV fluid bolus. What is your responsibility in giving the fluid bolus given Mr Thompson's current IV therapy?

CLINICAL SKILL 20.1 Administering oral medications

Please adhere to the policy and procedures of the facility/organisation prior to undertaking the skill. Ensure this skill is in your scope of practice.

NMBA Decision-making Framework considerations (refer to NMBA Decision-making framework for nursing and midwifery 2020):	Equipment:
1. Am I educated? 2. Am I authorised? 3. Am I competent? If you answer 'no' to any of these, do not perform that activity. Seek guidance and support from your teacher/a nurse team leader/clinical facilitator/educator.	NIMC/EMM system medication order Prescribed medication Disposable medication cups Glass of water, juice or preferred liquid Straw (if required) Medication cutting device (if required) Clean pill crusher (if required) Liquid measure or oral/enteral syringe Resource material (e.g. MIMS, *Don't Rush to Crush*)

 PREPARE FOR THE SKILL

(Please refer to the Standard Steps on p. xii for related rationales.)
Mentally review the steps of the skill.
Discuss the skill with your instructor/supervisor/team leader, if required.
Confirm correct facility/organisation policy/safe operating procedures.
Validate the order in the individual's record.
Identify indication and rationale for performing the activity.
Assess for any contraindications.
Locate and gather equipment.
Perform hand hygiene.
Ensure therapeutic interaction.
Identify the individual using three individual identifiers.
Gain the individual's consent.
Assess for pain relief.
Prepare the environment.
Provide and maintain privacy.
Assist the individual to assume an appropriate position of comfort.

Skill activity	Rationale
Ensure correct medication is given by following the '11 rights' throughout preparation and administration.	Identifies issues, which can be addressed prior to administration. Prevents medication errors from occurring and promotes correct and safe administration of medication/s.
Ensure medication orders are correctly prescribed and written. Verify indication for the medication on the NIMC/EMM system. Review name of medication on the NIMC/EMM system, dose, route, time of last administration and frequency of administration. Assess for any medication contraindications; check allergy status on the medication chart and with the individual; compare with the medication ordered; check for medication interactions. Review all necessary information about the medication, including action, purpose, normal dose, side effects, any special administration information.	Ensures correct medication administration is about to take place. Ensures the nurse understands why the individual is receiving the medication and is able to ask for a review by the medical officer if the individual's health status changes. Ensures that the right medication is being given at the right frequency and time, via the correct route and prevents medication errors from occurring. Ensures all medication allergies are recorded and determines if a medication should be given. Reduces risk of allergic reactions occurring. Promotes correct and safe administration of the medication and enables the nurse to monitor the therapeutic effects of the medication.
Assess individual's ability to receive the medication in the prescribed form via the prescribed route.	If the individual is nauseous, and is not able to tolerate medication given via the oral route, a review will need to occur to reassess the ordered route.

CLINICAL SKILL 20.1 Administering oral medications—cont'd

Check medication chart for the individual's identifiers, including asking the individual to state their full name, date of birth (DOB) and then check these as well as the UR number with the ID band and NIMC/EMM system.	Confirms the individual's identity.
Perform any necessary assessments related to the medication such as blood pressure (BP), pulse, respiratory rate (RR).	Apical pulse should be performed before administering digoxin; RR checked before opioid (narcotic) analgesics; BP checked before antihypertensives. If any abnormalities are found, the nurse should not administer medication and should contact nurse in charge and medical officer.

 PERFORM THE SKILL

(Please refer to the Standard Steps on p. xii for related rationales.)
Perform hand hygiene.
Apply PPE: gloves, eyewear, mask and gown as appropriate.
Ensure the individual's safety and comfort throughout skill.
Promote independence and involvement of the individual if possible and/or appropriate.
Assess the individual's tolerance to the skill throughout.
Dispose of used supplies, equipment, waste and sharps appropriately.
Remove PPE and discard or store appropriately.
Perform hand hygiene.

Skill activity	Rationale
Prepare medications as per administration guidelines and calculate the correct dose Review *Don't Rush to Crush* handbook if medication needs to be crushed. Ensure the right medication is being administered by comparing the label of the medication and expiry date with the name on the NIMC/EMM system three times: • First check: Before removing from the trolley or cupboard • Second check: Before removing from the container • Third check: Before returning to the trolley or cupboard, or discarding.	Following administration guidelines ensures the medication's effectiveness and the correct dosage of medication is being administered. Some individuals may require their medication to be crushed. Ensures medication order is the same as the medication supplied. Ensures the correct medication is being administered. Prevents preparation and administration errors.
Solid dose forms	
Tip the required number of tablets or capsules into the lid of the container and transfer into the medicine cup. Do not touch the medication with your bare hands.	Maintains cleanliness of medications and prevents cross-infection.
Some individuals may require their medication to be crushed. Crush medication/s using a clean pill crusher if required after reviewing the *Don't Rush to Crush* resource.	Some medications cannot be crushed. Crushing these medications can alter their effectiveness. Clean pill crusher ensures that medications are not being mixed from previous individual's medications.
Liquid dose forms	
Follow manufacturer's instructions—shake bottle thoroughly unless contraindicated.	Promotes mixing of the contents and a uniform distribution of the medication in the liquid.
Hold the bottle with the label against the palm of the hand and remove bottle cap and place it upside down.	Mixture will be poured away from the label, to avoid smearing of the label. Prevents contamination of the inside of the cap.
Place the medicine cup on a flat surface and at eye level, pour the liquid medication to the correct level on the medicine cup, ensuring the prescribed dose is poured or withdraw the required dose from the container using an approved oral/enteral syringe.	Ensures accuracy of measurement. Note that parenteral syringes should not be used for administration or administration of doses.

Continued

CLINICAL SKILL 20.1 Administering oral medications—cont'd

Administration

Assist the individual into a sitting (preferred) or side-lying position when possible.	Prevents aspiration during swallowing.
Administer the oral medication. Individual may self-administer or assist as required. Offer a glass of water, unless contraindicated. Advise individual to take a few sips of water before placing medication in the mouth.	Solid forms of medication are swallowed more easily in a moistened mouth and by swallowing with liquids.
Remain with the individual until the medication is swallowed. Never leave medication unattended at the bedside or on the medication trolley.	The nurse assumes responsibility for ensuring that the individual receives the prescribed medication. Other individuals may access the medications if left at the bedside.

 AFTER THE SKILL

(Please refer to the Standard Steps on p. xii for related rationales.)
Communicate outcome to the individual, any ongoing care and to report any complications.
Restore the environment.
Report, record and document assessment findings, details of the skill performed and the individual's response.
Report, record and document any abnormalities and/or inability to perform the skill.
Reassess the individual to ensure there are no adverse effects/events from the skill.

Skill activity	Rationale
As indicated, advise to remain sitting upright for 30 minutes after ingestion.	Prevents side effects such as oesophageal ulceration.
Record and sign for each medication administered on the NIMC/EMM system.	Prompt documentation prevents medication errors.
Safe medication management guidelines, outlined in Clinical Interest Box 20.3, should be incorporated into relevant aspects of this skill.	

(ACSQHC 2012; 2019; Frotjold & Bloomfield 2021; JBI 2022c; Rebeiro et al 2021; The Society of Hospital Pharmacists of Australia [SHPA] 2022; Tollefson et al 2022)

OBSERVATION CHECKLIST: ADMINISTERING ORAL MEDICATIONS

STUDENT NAME: _____

CLINICAL SKILL 20.1: Administering oral medications

DEMONSTRATION OF: The ability to safely and correctly administer oral medications

If the observation checklist is being used as an assessment tool, the student will need to obtain a scale of independence for each of the performance criteria/evidence.

Independent (I)

Supervised (S)

Assisted (A)

Marginal (M)

Dependent (D)

COMPETENCY ELEMENTS	PERFORMANCE CRITERIA/EVIDENCE	I	S	A	M	D
Preparation for the activity	Identifies indications and rationale for performing medication administration Identifies the individual using three individual identifiers: full name, DOB and UR number Ensures therapeutic interaction Gains the individual's consent Checks facility/organisation policy, resource material Validates the order on the individual's NIMC/EMM system Follows the 11 rights Locates and gathers appropriate equipment Prepares the work environment					
Performs activity informed by evidence	Reviews name of medication, dose, route, time of last administration and frequency of administration with NIMC/EMM system Verifies indication for medication Considers any medication administration requirements such as whether the medication must be given with food, contraindications, timing for administration, and the right form Performs any necessary assessments related to the specific medication such as blood pressure (BP), pulse rate and respiratory rate (RR) Compares the medication and expiry date with the name of medication on the NIMC/EMM system three times Positions individual as required: sitting or side-lying if unable to sit Offers fluid to assist swallowing medication					
Applies critical thinking and reflective practice	Is able to link theory to practice Demonstrates current best practice in the care provided Assesses individual's knowledge regarding medication action and provides medication education as required Assesses individual's ability to receive medication or self-administer orally Monitors individual for medication effectiveness (if applicable) Monitors individual for any ADRs to the medication Assesses own performance					

Continued

COMPETENCY ELEMENTS	PERFORMANCE CRITERIA/EVIDENCE	I	S	A	M	D
Practises within safety and quality assurance guidelines	Reviews against facility/organisation policy and NSQHS Medication Standard Performs hand hygiene, dons appropriate PPE and uses ANTT principles Checks the expiry dates and performs calculations, as required Checks individual's allergies Remains with individual until all medications are swallowed Cleans and disposes of equipment and waste appropriately					
Documentation and communication	Explains and communicates the medication delivery clearly to the individual Communicates outcome and ongoing care to individual and significant others Reports any complications and/or any reason for non-administration of medication on the NIMC/EMM system, and to RN and/or medical officer Documents all relevant information and any complications correctly in the healthcare record: • Documents and signs for medication • Records reasons for withholding any medication • Documents in accordance with state legislation for drug of dependency Provides any special instructions Asks the individual to report any complications during and post procedure					

Educator/Facilitator Feedback:

Educator/Facilitator Score: Competent   Needs further development

How would you rate your overall performance while undertaking this clinical activity? (use a ✓ & initial)

Unsatisfactory   Satisfactory   Good   Excellent

Student Reflection: (discuss how you would approach your practice differently or more effectively)

EDUCATOR/FACILITATOR NAME/SIGNATURE:

STUDENT NAME/SIGNATURE: **DATE:**

CLINICAL SKILL 20.2 Administering medications via enteral routes (nasogastric tube, percutaneous endoscopic gastrostomy tube, percutaneous endoscopic gastrojejunostomy tube)

Please adhere to the policy and procedures of the facility/organisation prior to undertaking the skill. Ensure this skill is in your scope of practice.

NMBA Decision-making Framework considerations (refer to NMBA Decision-making framework for nursing and midwifery 2020):

1. Am I educated?
2. Am I authorised?
3. Am I competent?

If you answer 'no' to any of these, do not perform that activity. Seek guidance and support from your teacher/a nurse team leader/clinical facilitator/educator.

Equipment:
NIMC/EMM system medication order
Prescribed medication
Disposable medication cups
Oral/enteral syringe for measuring and administering liquid medication forms
Clean pill crusher (if required)
Water
50 mL enteral tip syringe
Disposable gloves
pH indicator paper/strips (if nasogastric tube in use)
Resource material (e.g. MIMS, *Don't Rush to Crush*)

 PREPARE FOR THE SKILL

(Please refer to the Standard Steps on p. xii for related rationales.)
Mentally review the steps of the skill.
Discuss the skill with your instructor/supervisor/team leader, if required.
Confirm correct facility/organisation policy/safe operating procedures.
Validate the order in the individual's record.
Identify indication and rationale for performing the activity.
Assess for any contraindications.
Locate and gather equipment.
Perform hand hygiene.
Ensure therapeutic interaction.
Identify the individual using three individual identifiers.
Gain the individual's consent.
Assess for pain relief.
Prepare the environment.
Provide and maintain privacy.
Assist the individual to assume an appropriate position of comfort.

Skill activity	Rationale
Ensure correct medication is given by following the '11 rights' throughout preparation and administration. Ensure medication orders are correctly prescribed and written. Verify indication for the medication on the NIMC/EMM system. Review name of medication on the NIMC/EMM system, dose, route, time of last administration and frequency of administration. Assess for any medication contraindications; check allergy status on the medication chart and with the individual; compare with the medication ordered; check for medication interactions. Review all necessary information about the medication, including action, purpose, normal dose, side effects, any special administration information.	Identifies issues, which can be addressed prior to administration. Prevents medication errors from occurring and promotes correct and safe administration of medication/s. Ensures correct medication administration is about to take place. Ensures the nurse understands why the individual is receiving the medication and is able to ask for a review by the medical officer if the individual's health status changes. Ensures that the right medication is being given at the right frequency and time, via the correct route and prevents medication errors from occurring. Ensures all medication allergies are recorded and determines if a medication should be given. Reduces risk of allergic reactions occurring. Promotes correct and safe administration of the medication and enables the nurse to monitor the therapeutic effects of the medication.

CLINICAL SKILL 20.2 Administering medications via enteral routes (nasogastric tube, percutaneous endoscopic gastrostomy tube, percutaneous endoscopic gastrojejunostomy tube)—cont'd

Assess individual's ability to receive the medication in the prescribed form via the prescribed route.	If medication needs to be administered on an empty stomach, the nurse will need to ensure the tube feed is modified around the medication delivery times (e.g. ceasing the enteral tube feed for a certain time so medications can be administered).
Check medication chart for the individual's identifiers, including asking the individual to state their full name, date of birth (DOB) and then check these as well as the UR number with the ID band and NIMC/EMM system.	Confirms the individual's identity.
Perform any necessary assessments related to the specific medication such as blood pressure (BP), pulse rate, and respiratory rate (RR).	Apical pulse should be performed before administering digoxin; RR checked before opioid (narcotic) analgesics; BP checked before antihypertensives. If any abnormalities are found, the nurse should not administer medication and report to the nurse in charge and medical officer.

 PERFORM THE SKILL

(Please refer to the Standard Steps on p. xii for related rationales.)
Perform hand hygiene.
Apply PPE: gloves, eyewear, mask and gown as appropriate.
Ensure the individual's safety and comfort throughout skill.
Promote independence and involvement of the individual if possible and/or appropriate.
Assess the individual's tolerance to the skill throughout.
Dispose of used supplies, equipment, waste and sharps appropriately.
Remove PPE and discard or store appropriately.
Perform hand hygiene.

Skill activity	Rationale
Prepare medications as per administration guidelines and calculate the correct dose. Review *Don't Rush to Crush* handbook if medication needs to be crushed. Ensure the right medication is being administered by comparing the label of the medication and expiry date with the name on the NIMC/EMM system three times: • First check: Before removing from the trolley or cupboard • Second check: Before removing from the container • Third check: Before returning to the trolley or cupboard, or discarding.	Following administration guidelines ensures the medication's effectiveness and the correct dosage of medication is being administered. Medications should be given in liquid form if available. Other medications may require crushing as per the *Don't Rush to Crush* handbook. Ensures medication order is the same as the medication supplied. Ensures the correct medication is being administered. Prevents preparation and administration errors.
Follow steps for preparation of solid dose forms or liquid dose forms in Clinical Skill 20.1. Mix each individual crushed medication with a small amount of water. Check the fluid balance status of the individual for any fluid restrictions.	Following administration guidelines ensures medications are administered correctly. Checking to see if there is a fluid restriction may determine the amount of fluid used to flush the line before and after medication administration.
Position in semi-Fowler's position unless contraindicated.	Reduces the risk of regurgitation and aspiration.
Stop the flow of any feed solutions in progress prior to administering medications through the feeding tube.	Recommendation is not to administer feed solutions with medications. Some medications may also require the feed solution to be stopped for a set length of time to allow for effective absorption. Again, check with the pharmacist or dietitian if you are unsure.

Continued

CLINICAL SKILL 20.2 Administering medications via enteral routes (nasogastric tube, percutaneous endoscopic gastrostomy tube, percutaneous endoscopic gastrojejunostomy tube)—cont'd

Prior to administration of medications into tube check for position and patency. Determine placement of nasogastric tube (NGT) (if this route used) by aspirating stomach contents and testing the pH indicator strips. The pH should be <6. Connect the appropriate type of syringe to the tube (no less than a 30 mL syringe). Flush the tube with 30 mL of water with the plunger or remove the plunger of the oral/enteral syringe, and pour the water into the barrel and hold the barrel of the syringe above the stomach.	Ensures NGT tubing is in the stomach and prevents inadvertent delivery of medication into the lungs. The smaller the syringe, the greater the pressure, which could rupture the tubing. Flushing ensures patency of the tube. Holding the barrel of the syringe above the level of the stomach assists with gravity delivery of the medication directly into the stomach via the tube.
If more than one medication is to be given, they must be given separately. Draw up each medication separately into the oral/enteral syringe and administer into the tube. Flush with 10 mL of water between each medication.	Flushing prevents occlusion of the tube. Administering medications separately prevents clogging of the tube.
When the last medication is administered, flush the tube with at least 30 mL of water. Remove the syringe barrel and replace tube cap if enteral feed is not being administered. If the individual is receiving continuous feeding, check the facility/organisation policy on when to recommence.	Ensures patency of tube. Reduces incidence of occlusion.

 AFTER THE SKILL

(Please refer to the Standard Steps on p. xii for related rationales.)
Communicate outcome to the individual, any ongoing care and to report any complications.
Restore the environment.
Report, record and document assessment findings, details of the skill performed and the individual's response.
Report, record and document any abnormalities and/or inability to perform the skill.
Reassess the individual to ensure there are no adverse effects/events from the skill.

Skill activity	Rationale
Advise to remain in semi-Fowler's position for 30 minutes.	Reduces risk of regurgitation and aspiration. Keeps individual informed and creates an opportunity to initiate medication education. Monitors for adverse effects and ensures that complications can be prevented or addressed early.
Record and sign for each medication administered on the NIMC/EMM system.	Prompt documentation prevents medication errors.
Safe medication management guidelines, outlined in Clinical Interest Box 20.3, should be incorporated into relevant aspects of this skill.	

(ACSQHC 2012; 2019; JBI 2022b; Williams 2022; The Agency for Clinical Innovation and the Gastroenterological Nurses College of Australia 2015; The SPHA 2022; Tollefson et al 2022)

OBSERVATION CHECKLIST: ADMINISTERING MEDICATIONS VIA ENTERAL ROUTES (NASOGASTRIC TUBE, PERCUTANE-OUS ENDOSCOPIC GASTROSTOMY TUBE, PERCUTANEOUS ENDOSCOPIC GASTROJEJUNOSTOMY TUBE)

Independent (I)

Supervised (S)

Assisted (A)

Marginal (M)

Dependent (D)

STUDENT NAME: _____

CLINICAL SKILL 20.2: Administering medications via enteral routes

DEMONSTRATION OF: The ability to administer medication via enteral routes (nasogastric tube, percutaneous endoscopic gastrostomy tube, percutaneous endoscopic gastrojejunostomy tube)

If the observation checklist is being used as an assessment tool, the student will need to obtain a scale of independence for each of the performance criteria/evidence.

COMPETENCY ELEMENTS	PERFORMANCE CRITERIA/EVIDENCE	I	S	A	M	D
Preparation for the activity	Identifies indications and rationale for performing the medication administration Identifies the individual using three individual identifiers: full name, DOB and UR number Ensures therapeutic interaction Gains the individual's consent Checks facility/organisation policy, resource material Follows the 11 rights Validates the order in the individual's NIMC/EMM system Locates and gathers equipment Prepares the work environment					
Performs activity informed by evidence	Reviews name of medication, dose, route, time of last administration and frequency of administration with NIMC/EMM system Verifies indication for medication Considers any medication administration requirements such as whether the medication must be given with food, contraindications, timing for administration and the right form Verifies that medication can be crushed Performs any necessary assessments related to the medication such as BP, pulse rate and RR Compares the medication and expiry date with the name of medication on the NIMC/EMM system three times Positions individual appropriately Checks placement of tube, disconnects tube from feeding line (if in use) Flushes tube pre and post each medication Advises individual to remain sitting upright for 30 minutes post medication administration					

Continued

COMPETENCY ELEMENTS	PERFORMANCE CRITERIA/EVIDENCE	I	S	A	M	D
Applies critical thinking and reflective practice	Is able to link theory to practice Demonstrates current best practice in the care provided Assesses individual's knowledge regarding medication action and provides medication education as required Monitors individual for therapeutic effect of medication (if applicable) Monitors individual for any ADRs to the medication Assesses own performance					
Practises within safety and quality assurance guidelines	Reviews against facility/organisation policy and NSQHS Medication Standard Performs hand hygiene, dons appropriate PPE and uses ANTT principles Checks the expiry dates and performs calculations, as required Checks individual's allergies Cleans and disposes of equipment and waste appropriately					
Documentation and communication	Explains and communicates the medication administration process clearly to the individual Communicates outcome and ongoing care to individual and significant others Reports any complications and/or any reason of non-administration of the medication on the NIMC/EMM system, and to RN and/or medical officer Documents all relevant information and any complications correctly in the healthcare record: • Documents and signs for medication • Records reasons for withholding any medication • Documents in accordance with state legislation for drug of dependency Provides any special instructions Asks the individual to report any complications during and post procedure					

Educator/Facilitator Feedback:

Educator/Facilitator Score: Competent   Needs further development

How would you rate your overall performance while undertaking this clinical activity? (use a ✓ & initial)

Unsatisfactory   Satisfactory   Good   Excellent

Student Reflection: (discuss how you would approach your practice differently or more effectively)

EDUCATOR/FACILITATOR NAME/SIGNATURE:

STUDENT NAME/SIGNATURE: **DATE:**

CLINICAL SKILL 20.3 Inserting a rectal suppository or disposable enema

Please adhere to the policy and procedures of the facility/organisation prior to undertaking the skill. Ensure this skill is in your scope of practice.

NMBA Decision-making Framework considerations (refer to NMBA Decision-making framework for nursing and midwifery 2020):	**Equipment:**
1. Am I educated? 2. Am I authorised? 3. Am I competent? If you answer 'no' to any of these, do not perform that activity. Seek guidance and support from your teacher/a nurse team leader/clinical facilitator/educator.	NIMC/EMM system medication order Enema/suppository Lubricant Waterproof sheet Disposable gloves Resource material (e.g. MIMS)

 PREPARE FOR THE SKILL

(Please refer to the Standard Steps on p. xii for related rationales.)
Mentally review the steps of the skill.
Discuss the skill with your instructor/supervisor/team leader, if required.
Confirm correct facility/organisation policy/safe operating procedures.
Validate the order in the individual's record.
Identify indication and rationale for performing the activity.
Assess for any contraindications.
Locate and gather equipment.
Perform hand hygiene.
Ensure therapeutic interaction.
Identify the individual using three individual identifiers.
Gain the individual's consent.
Assess for pain relief.
Prepare the environment.
Provide and maintain privacy.
Assist the individual to assume an appropriate position of comfort.

Skill activity	Rationale
Ensure correct medication is given by following the '11 rights' throughout preparation and administration.	Identifies issues, which can be addressed prior to administration. Prevents medication errors from occurring and promotes correct and safe administration of medication/s.
Ensure medication orders are correctly prescribed and written. Verify indication for the medication on the NIMC/EMM system. Review name of medication on the NIMC/EMM system, dose, route, time of last administration and frequency of administration. Assess for any medication contraindications; check allergy status on the medication chart and with the individual; compare with the medication ordered; check for medication interactions. Review all necessary information about the medication, including action, purpose, normal dose, side effects, any special administration information.	Ensures correct medication administration is about to take place. Ensures the nurse understands why the individual is receiving the medication and is able to ask for a review by the medical officer if the individual's health status changes. Ensures that the right medication is being given at the right frequency and time, via the correct route and prevents medication errors from occurring. Ensures all medication allergies are recorded and determines if a medication should be given. Reduces risk of allergic reactions occurring. Promotes correct and safe administration of the medication and enables the nurse to monitor the therapeutic effects of the medication.
Assess individual's ability to receive the medication in the prescribed form via the prescribed route.	If the individual is not able to receive the medication given via the rectal route (e.g. haemorrhoids, rectal bleeding or diarrhoea), a review will need to occur to reassess the ordered route.
Check medication chart for the individual's identifiers, including asking the individual to state their full name, date of birth (DOB) and then check these as well as the UR number with the ID band and NIMC/EMM system.	Confirms the individual's identity.

CLINICAL SKILL 20.3 Inserting a rectal suppository or disposable enema—cont'd

Perform any necessary assessments related to the medication such as pain assessment or bowel chart.	If any abnormalities are found, the nurse should not administer medication and should contact nurse in charge and medical officer.

PERFORM THE SKILL

(Please refer to the Standard Steps on p. xii for related rationales.)
Perform hand hygiene.
Apply PPE: gloves, eyewear, mask and gown as appropriate.
Ensure the individual's safety and comfort throughout skill.
Promote independence and involvement of the individual if possible and/or appropriate.
Assess the individual's tolerance to the skill throughout.
Dispose of used supplies, equipment, waste and sharps appropriately.
Remove PPE and discard or store appropriately.
Perform hand hygiene.

Skill activity	Rationale
Prepare medication as per administration guidelines and calculate the correct dose. Ensure the right medication is being administered by comparing the label of the medication and expiry date with the name on the NIMC/EMM system three times: • First check: Before removing from the trolley or cupboard • Second check: Before removing from the container • Third check: Before returning to the trolley or cupboard, or discarding.	Following administration guidelines ensures the medication's effectiveness and the correct dosage of medication is being administered. Ensures medication order is the same as the medication supplied. Ensures the correct medication is being administered. Prevents preparation and administration errors.
Place individual in a left lateral position with the right leg flexed.	Anatomical site of the lower colon means that this position is the most effective for the introduction and retention of suppositories.
Ensure individual is adequately covered, with only the buttocks exposed. Place protective sheet under buttocks.	Promotes warmth and comfort. Provides absorption pad for any leakages and respects dignity.
Lubricate finger of glove and end of suppository/enema nozzle.	Facilitates smooth insertion of suppository/enema.
Gently insert the suppository by directing it with the finger, through the anus, about 2.5 cm into the rectum. Insert enema tip approximately 10 cm into the rectum and squeeze contents into the rectum.	Suppository/enema must pass the internal anal sphincter and come in contact with rectal mucosa. Ensures that the medication is delivered into the rectum.
During insertion, encourage the individual to take deep breaths through the mouth.	Helps to relax the anal sphincters.

AFTER THE SKILL

(Please refer to the Standard Steps on p. xii for related rationales.)
Communicate outcome to the individual, any ongoing care and to report any complications.
Restore the environment.
Report, record and document assessment findings, details of the skill performed and the individual's response.
Report, record and document any abnormalities and/or inability to perform the skill.
Reassess the individual to ensure there are no adverse effects/events from the skill.

Continued

CLINICAL SKILL 20.3 Inserting a rectal suppository or disposable enema—cont'd

Skill activity	Rationale
Advise individual to remain on their side or supine for at least five minutes and to retain the suppository/enema for the correct length of time for medication administered.	Individual must be aware whether the suppository/enema is to be retained to allow any medication to be dissipated, or whether to expect a bowel action. Suppositories/enemas to promote a bowel action should be retained for at least 20 minutes. An enema should be held for the time stated on the manufacturer's instructions. Keeps individual informed and creates an opportunity to initiate medication education.
Record and sign for each medication administered on the NIMC/EMM system.	Prompt documentation prevents medication errors.
Ensure individual has easy access to toilet facilities and a nurse call bell within reach.	Reduces anxiety related to accidental expulsion of the suppository or faeces. Can communicate with the nurse in a timely manner.
Observe faeces for odour, colour, texture and amount. Document results.	Assists to assess the effectiveness of the treatment and detects any abnormalities.
Attend to individual's personal hygiene and reposition.	Helps promote dignity and comfort.

Safe medication management guidelines, outlined in Clinical Interest Box 20.3, should be incorporated into relevant aspects of this skill.

(ACSQHC 2012; 2019; JBI 2022a; Rebeiro et al 2021; Tollefson et al 2022)

OBSERVATION CHECKLIST: INSERTING A RECTAL SUPPOSITORY OR DISPOSABLE ENEMA

STUDENT NAME: _____	Independent (I) Supervised (S) Assisted (A) Marginal (M) Dependent (D)

CLINICAL SKILL 20.3: Inserting a rectal suppository or disposable enema

DEMONSTRATION OF: The ability to safely and correctly administer a rectal suppository or enema

If the observation checklist is being used as an assessment tool, the student will need to obtain a scale of independence for each of the performance criteria/evidence.

COMPETENCY ELEMENTS	PERFORMANCE CRITERIA/EVIDENCE	I	S	A	M	D
Preparation for the activity	Identifies indications and rationale for performing medication administration Identifies the individual using three individual identifiers: full name, DOB and UR number Ensures therapeutic interaction Gains the individual's consent Checks facility/organisation policy, resource material Validates the order on the individual's NIMC/EMM system Follows the 11 rights Locates and gathers equipment Prepares the work environment					
Performs activity informed by evidence	Reviews name of medication, dose, route, time of last administration and frequency of administration with NIMC/EMM system Verifies indication for medication Considers any medication administration requirements, contraindications Compares the medication and expiry date with the name of medication on the NIMC/EMM system three times Advises individual to lie in the left lateral position for medication administration and puts in place an absorbent, protective pad Lubricates finger of glove and suppository/enema nozzle Correctly administers the rectal suppository or enema Asks the individual to remain on their side or supine for at least 15 minutes Ensures the individual has easy access to toilet facilities and nurse call bell					
Applies critical thinking and reflective practice	Is able to link theory to practice Demonstrates current best practice in the care provided Assesses individual's knowledge regarding medication action and provides medication education as required Monitors individual for medication effectiveness (if applicable) Monitors individual for any ADRs to the medication Assesses own performance					

Continued

COMPETENCY ELEMENTS	PERFORMANCE CRITERIA/EVIDENCE	I	S	A	M	D
Practises within safety and quality assurance guidelines	Reviews against facility/organisation policy and NSQHS Medication Standard Performs hand hygiene, dons appropriate PPE and uses ANTT principles Checks the expiry dates and performs calculations, as required Checks individual's allergies Cleans and disposes of equipment and waste appropriately					
Documentation and communication	Explains and communicates the medication administration clearly to the individual Communicates outcome and ongoing care to individual and significant others Reports any complications and/or any reason for non-administration of the medication on the NIMC/EMM system, and to RN and/or medical officer Documents all relevant information and any complications correctly in the healthcare record: • Documents and signs for medication • Records reasons for withholding any medication Provides any special instructions Asks the individual to report any complications during and after the procedure					

Educator/Facilitator Feedback:

Educator/Facilitator Score: Competent   Needs further development

How would you rate your overall performance while undertaking this clinical activity? (use a ✓ & initial)

Unsatisfactory   Satisfactory   Good   Excellent

Student Reflection: (discuss how you would approach your practice differently or more effectively)

EDUCATOR/FACILITATOR NAME/SIGNATURE:

STUDENT NAME/SIGNATURE: **DATE:**

CLINICAL SKILL 20.4 Administering subcutaneous and intramuscular injections

Please adhere to the policy and procedures of the facility/organisation prior to undertaking the skill. Ensure this skill is in your scope of practice.

NMBA Decision-making Framework considerations (refer to NMBA Decision-making framework for nursing and midwifery 2020):	Equipment:
1. Am I educated? 2. Am I authorised? 3. Am I competent? If you answer 'no' to any of these, do not perform that activity. Seek guidance and support from your teacher/a nurse team leader/clinical facilitator/educator.	NIMC/EMM system medication order Prescribed medication Diluent (if required) Syringe 23G needle (for IM injections) 25G needle (for subcut injections) 18G needle or 18G blunt needle Antiseptic swab (if required) Sterile gauze Injection tray Sharps container Disposable gloves (if required) Resource material (e.g. MIMS, *Australian Injectable Drugs Handbook*, APINCHS list)

 PREPARE FOR THE SKILL

(Please refer to the Standard Steps on p. xii for related rationales.)
Mentally review the steps of the skill.
Discuss the skill with your instructor/supervisor/team leader, if required.
Confirm correct facility/organisation policy/safe operating procedures.
Validate the order in the individual's record.
Identify indication and rationale for performing the activity.
Assess for any contraindications.
Locate and gather equipment.
Perform hand hygiene.
Ensure therapeutic interaction.
Identify the individual using three individual identifiers.
Gain the individual's consent.
Assess for pain relief.
Prepare the environment.
Provide and maintain privacy.
Assist the individual to assume an appropriate position of comfort.

Skill activity	Rationale
Ensure correct medication is given by following the '11 rights' throughout preparation and administration.	Identifies issues, which can be addressed prior to administration. Prevents medication errors from occurring and promotes correct and safe administration of medication/s.

CLINICAL SKILL 20.4 Administering subcutaneous and intramuscular injections—cont'd

Ensure medication orders are correctly prescribed and written. Verify indication for the medication on the NIMC/EMM system. Review name of medication on the NIMC/EMM system, dose, route, time of last administration and frequency of administration. Assess for any medication contraindications; check allergy status on the medication chart and with the individual; compare with the medication ordered; check for medication interactions. Review all necessary information about the medication, including action, purpose, normal dose, side effects, any special administration information. Review high-risk medicines on facility/organisation APINCHS list.	Ensures correct medication administration is about to take place. Ensures the nurse understands why the individual is receiving the medication and is able to ask for a review by the medical officer if the individual's health status changes. Ensures that the right medication is being given at the right frequency and time, via the correct route and prevents medication errors from occurring. Ensures all medication allergies are recorded and determines if a medication should be given. Reduces risk of allergic reactions occurring. Promotes correct and safe administration of the medication and enables the nurse to monitor the therapeutic effects of the medication. Review of APINCHS list alerts the nurse to checking procedures before, during and after high-risk medication delivery, decreasing the risk of toxic or adverse events from occurring.
Assess individual's ability to receive the medication in the prescribed form via the prescribed route.	Ensures the correct anatomical location is chosen and any abnormalities such as areas of infection, cellulitis, dermatitis, and scarring or bruising from previous injection sites are avoided.
Gain assistance of another nurse if the individual is a child, or an adult who is restless or irrational or may need assistance with positioning.	Promotes safety during administration.
Check medication chart for the individual's identifiers, including asking the individual to state their full name, date of birth (DOB) and then check these as well as the UR number with the ID band and NIMC/EMM system.	Confirms the individual's identity.
Perform any necessary assessments related to the specific medication being administered (e.g. vital signs, blood glucose level, pain levels).	Ensures safety of the individual during the administration of the medication.

 PERFORM THE SKILL

(Please refer to the Standard Steps on p. xii for related rationales.)
Perform hand hygiene.
Apply PPE: gloves, eyewear, mask and gown as appropriate.
Ensure the individual's safety and comfort throughout skill.
Promote independence and involvement of the individual if possible and/or appropriate.
Assess the individual's tolerance to the skill throughout.
Dispose of used supplies, equipment, waste and sharps appropriately.
Remove PPE and discard or store appropriately.
Perform hand hygiene.

Continued

CLINICAL SKILL 20.4 Administering subcutaneous and intramuscular injections—cont'd

Skill activity	Rationale
Calculate correct dose and prepare medication according to Table 20.4 Preparation of medications from ampoules and vials and as per the *Australian Injectable Drugs Handbook*. Check label and expiry date. Have two nurses check (one must be an RN) according to safe administration guidelines and the facility/organisation policy. Ensure the right medication is being administered by comparing the label of the medication vial/ampoule and expiry date with the name on the NIMC/EMM system three times: • First check: Before removing from the impress/DD cupboard • Second check: Before removing from the vial/ampoule • Third check: Before discarding the vial/ampoule.	Promotes safety during administration. Ensures medications are being prepared as per the recommended process. Ensures medication order is the same as the medication supplied. Ensures the correct medication is being administered. Prevents preparation and administration errors.
Select an appropriate injection site for correct volume to be administered and assist the individual into a comfortable position. Select an injection site that has not been used frequently. If possible, ask the individual the site of the last injection.	Appropriate site selection aids absorption and reduces likelihood of injury and discomfort. Rotating sites minimises tissue damage. Sites should be rotated for long-term therapy such as insulin, as repeatedly using the same site leads to thickening of skin and tissue atrophy. Comfort promotes relaxation and helps to reduce anxiety.
Locate the injection site using anatomical landmarks. Check site for any masses, lumps, signs of infection, scars or skin lesions.	Insertion of medication into the correct site avoids injury to underlying structures. Masses, scars etc., will interfere with medication absorption.
If required, cleanse the site with an antiseptic swab and allow area to dry for 30 seconds.	Removes microorganisms from the skin.
Remove the needle cap and hold the syringe in the dominant hand. Hold the individual's skin between the thumb and forefinger and either pull the skin taut (IM injection) or pinch up skin (IM or subcutaneous injection).	In an IM injection, a needle penetrates tight skin more easily than loose skin. Pinching the skin up may be necessary when a subcutaneous injection is given to an obese individual, or when an IM injection is given to an individual with small muscle mass.
Insert the needle quickly and firmly, at a 45-degree or 90-degree angle for subcutaneous injection, and at a 90-degree angle for IM injection.	Quick, firm insertion technique minimises anxiety and discomfort. 45-degree angle may need to be used in a subcutaneous injection where there is minimal subcutaneous tissue, to prevent insertion into a muscle.
For an IM injection, slowly pull back on the plunger to aspirate as per policy and procedure guidelines. If blood appears in the syringe, the needle is withdrawn, and the injection repeated at another site, using a fresh dose, syringe and needle. (**Note:** Needle aspiration does not need to be performed for a subcut injection.)	Muscles are more vascular than subcutaneous tissue. Checks whether needle has penetrated a blood vessel as insertion will be intravenous and not intramuscular.
Inject the medication slowly depressing the syringe plunger 1 mL every 10 seconds. Once injected pause for at least five seconds before withdrawing the needle.	Slow injection reduces tissue trauma and pain. Pausing permits dispersal of the medication.
Withdraw needle at same angle of insertion while applying gauze gently over the injection site. Apply pressure with sterile gauze if bleeding occurs. Do not massage.	Support of tissues minimises discomfort as the needle is withdrawn. Use of alcohol swab may cause discomfort. Massage may cause bleeding/bruising, increase the absorption rate, damage underlying tissue.

CLINICAL SKILL 20.4 Administering subcutaneous and intramuscular injections—cont'd

Activate the needle safety guard (if used) or dispose of syringe without recapping into proper receptacle (kidney dish) or straight into an appropriately labelled rigid-walled sharps container.	Recapping used needles increases the risk of a needlestick injury. Proper disposal prevents sharps injury to personnel or visitors.

 AFTER THE SKILL

(Please refer to the Standard Steps on p. xii for related rationales.)
Communicate outcome to the individual, any ongoing care and to report any complications.
Restore the environment.
Report, record and document assessment findings, details of the skill performed and the individual's response.
Report, record and document any abnormalities and/or inability to perform the skill.
Reassess the individual to ensure there are no adverse effects/events from the skill.

Skill activity	Rationale
Record and sign for each medication administered on the NIMC/EMM system.	Prompt documentation prevents medication errors.

Safe medication management guidelines, outlined in Clinical Interest Box 20.3, should be incorporated into relevant aspects of this skill.

(ACSQHC 2012; 2019; 2023a; JBI 2021d; 2022f; Rebeiro et al 2021; The SPHA 2023; Tollefson et al 2022)

OBSERVATION CHECKLIST: ADMINISTERING SUBCUTANEOUS AND INTRAMUSCULAR INJECTIONS

STUDENT NAME: _____

CLINICAL SKILL 20.4: Administering subcutaneous and intramuscular injections

DEMONSTRATION OF: The ability to safely and correctly administer subcutaneous and intramuscular injections

If the observation checklist is being used as an assessment tool, the student will need to obtain a scale of independence for each of the performance criteria/evidence.

Independent (I)
Supervised (S)
Assisted (A)
Marginal (M)
Dependent (D)

COMPETENCY ELEMENTS	PERFORMANCE CRITERIA/EVIDENCE	I	S	A	M	D
Preparation for the activity	Identifies indications and rationale for performing medication administration Identifies the individual using three individual identifiers: full name, DOB and UR number Ensures therapeutic interaction Gains the individual's consent Checks facility/organisation policy, resource material Validates the order on the individual's NIMC/EMM system Follows the 11 rights Locates and gathers equipment Prepares the work environment					
Performs activity informed by evidence	Reviews name of medication, dose, route, time of last administration and frequency of administration with NIMC/EMM system Verifies indication for medication Considers any medication administration requirements, contraindications Performs any necessary assessments related to the specific medication being administered (e.g. vital signs, blood glucose level, pain levels) Compares the medication and expiry date with the name of medication on the NIMC/EMM system three times Positions individual appropriately Selects and prepares the appropriate site for the subcut injection Safely administers injection to minimise discomfort and maximise absorption. Inserts the needle quickly and firmly, at a 45-degree or 90-degree angle for subcutaneous injection, and at a 90-degree angle for intramuscular injection Aspirates plunger of syringe for IM injection Assesses individual for correct angle for subcutaneous injection Aspirates to ensure that medication is not being delivered into a blood vessel when performing an intramuscular injection Administers the medication by depressing the plunger I mL every 10 seconds Waits five seconds and withdraws needle					

COMPETENCY ELEMENTS	PERFORMANCE CRITERIA/EVIDENCE	I	S	A	M	D
Applies critical thinking and reflective practice	Is able to link theory to practice Demonstrates current best practice in the care provided Assesses individual's knowledge regarding medication action and provides medication education as required Monitors individual for medication effectiveness (if applicable) Monitors individual for any ADRs to the medication Assesses own performance					
Practises within safety and quality assurance guidelines	Reviews against facility/organisation policy and NSQHS Medication Standard Performs hand hygiene, dons appropriate PPE and uses ANTT principles Checks the expiry dates and performs calculations, as required Checks individual's allergies Checks individual's identification requirements with second nurse (RN) at the bedside Cleans and disposes of equipment and waste appropriately					
Documentation and communication	Explains and communicates the medication administration clearly to the individual Communicates outcome and ongoing care to individual and significant others Reports any complications and/or reason for non-administration of the medication on the NIMC/EMM system, and to the RN and/or medical officer Documents all relevant information and any complications correctly in the healthcare record: • Documents and signs for medication • Records reasons for withholding any medication • Documents in accordance with state legislation for drug of dependency Provides any special instructions Asks the individual to report any complications during and post procedure					

Educator/Facilitator Feedback:

Educator/Facilitator Score: Competent   Needs further development

How would you rate your overall performance while undertaking this clinical activity? (use a ✓ & initial)

Unsatisfactory   Satisfactory   Good   Excellent

Student Reflection: (discuss how you would approach your practice differently or more effectively)

EDUCATOR/FACILITATOR NAME/SIGNATURE:

STUDENT NAME/SIGNATURE: **DATE:**

CLINICAL SKILL 20.5 Establishing intravenous (IV) therapy (assisting)

Please adhere to the policy and procedures of the facility/organisation prior to undertaking the skill. Ensure this skill is in your scope of practice.

NMBA Decision-making Framework considerations (refer to NMBA Decision-making framework for nursing and midwifery 2020):	Equipment:
1. Am I educated? 2. Am I authorised? 3. Am I competent? If you answer 'no' to any of these, do not perform that activity. Seek guidance and support from your teacher/a nurse team leader/clinical facilitator/educator.	Intravenous fluid order chart/EMM system fluid order Fluid balance chart (FBC) IV fluid IV infusion set Burette (if applicable) 10 mL syringe 10 mL normal saline 0.9% IV cannula IV cap/bung Dressing pack Antiseptic skin prep (chlorhexidine 70% solution) Disposable gloves Tourniquet Tape Occlusive dressing IV pump stand IV volumetric pump IV line label IV cannula care plan

 PREPARE FOR THE SKILL

(Please refer to the Standard Steps on p. xii for related rationales.)
Mentally review the steps of the skill.
Discuss the skill with your instructor/supervisor/team leader, if required.
Confirm correct facility/organisation policy/safe operating procedures.
Validate the order in the individual's record.
Identify indication and rationale for performing the activity.
Assess for any contraindications.
Locate and gather equipment.
Perform hand hygiene.
Ensure therapeutic interaction.
Identify the individual using three individual identifiers.
Gain the individual's consent.
Assess for pain relief.
Prepare the environment.
Provide and maintain privacy.
Assist the individual to assume an appropriate position of comfort.

Skill activity	Rationale
Ensure correct IV fluid is given by following the '11 rights' throughout preparation and administration.	Identifies issues, which can be addressed prior to administration. Prevents medication errors from occurring and promotes correct and safe administration of medication/s.
Ensure IV fluid orders are correctly prescribed and written. Verify indication for the IV fluid on the IV fluid order chart/EMM system fluid order. Review name of fluid on the IV fluid order chart/EMM system fluid order, dose, route, time of last administration and frequency of administration. Assess for any contraindications: Check allergy status on the medication/fluid order chart and with the individual; compare with the intravenous fluid ordered. Review all necessary information about the IV fluid, including action, purpose, normal dose, side effects, any special administration information.	Ensures correct IV fluid administration is about to take place. Ensures the nurse understands why the individual is receiving the IV fluid and is able to ask for a review by the medical officer if the individual's health status changes. Ensures correct IV fluid is administered. Promotes correct and safe administration of the IV fluid and prevents medication errors from occurring. Ensures all medication allergies are recorded. Promotes correct and safe administration of the IV fluid and enables the nurse to monitor the therapeutic effects of IV fluid.

Continued

CLINICAL SKILL 20.5 Establishing intravenous (IV) therapy (assisting)—cont'd

Assess individual's ability to receive the IV fluid. Review FBC for fluid volume status. Perform any necessary assessments related to the medication such as blood pressure (BP), pulse, respiratory rate (RR), SpO$_2$.	Identifies if individual has contraindications such as heart failure or kidney failure. Prevents circulatory overload. If any abnormalities are found, the nurse should not administer medication and should contact nurse in charge and medical officer.
Check IV fluid order chart/EMM system fluid order for the individual's identifiers, including asking the individual to state their full name, date of birth (DOB) and then check these as well as the UR number with the ID band and (IV) fluid order chart/EMM system fluid order.	Confirms the individual's identity.

 PERFORM THE SKILL

(Please refer to the Standard Steps on p. xii for related rationales.)
Perform hand hygiene.
Apply PPE: gloves, eyewear, mask and gown as appropriate.
Ensure the individual's safety and comfort throughout skill.
Promote independence and involvement of the individual if possible and/or appropriate.
Assess the individual's tolerance to the skill throughout.
Dispose of used supplies, equipment, waste and sharps appropriately.
Remove PPE and discard or store appropriately.
Perform hand hygiene.

Skill activity	Rationale
Prepare IV fluid as per administration guidelines and calculate the correct rate. Ensure the right IV fluid is being administered by comparing the label and expiry date with the name of the IV fluid on the intravenous fluid order chart/EMM system fluid order three times: • First check: Before removing from the storage room • Second check: Before removing IV fluid flask from the packaging • Third check: Before spiking the IV fluid flask with the IV line spike and programming the volumetric pump.	Following administration guidelines ensures the IV fluid's effectiveness and rate. Ensures IV fluid ordered is the same as the IV fluid supplied. Ensures the correct IV fluid is being administered. Abides by the legal and ethical frameworks regarding safe administration and checking procedures. Prevents preparation and administration errors.
Prepare giving set by closing the roller clamp, spiking the IV fluid bag using ANTT. Squeeze the drip chamber to allow fluid to enter and then open the roll clamp and prime the line. Continue priming with IV fluid until all of the air in the giving set has been expelled.	Ensures safe administration and ensures the tubing is filled with solution and free of air to prevent air embolus.
Assist medical officer or RN with cannulating the individual in order to establish IV access. Support the individual and help to anchor the proposed site for cannulation.	Relieves anxiety and allows for easier cannulation and securement of the IV without complications.
Vigorously rub injection port with alcohol swab for 30 seconds and allow to dry for 30 seconds.	Prevents contamination.
Connect primed line onto needleless port and secure Luer lock. Program ordered volumetric pump flow rate according to the IV fluid order chart/EMM system fluid order.	Ensures the safe administration of IV fluid.

CLINICAL SKILL 20.5 Establishing intravenous (IV) therapy (assisting)—cont'd

AFTER THE SKILL

(Please refer to the Standard Steps on p. xii for related rationales.)
Communicate outcome to the individual, any ongoing care and to report any complications.
Restore the environment.
Report, record and document assessment findings, details of the skill performed and the individual's response.
Report, record and document any abnormalities and/or inability to perform the skill.
Reassess the individual to ensure there are no adverse effects/events from the skill.

Skill activity	Rationale
Ask individual to report pain/discomfort around the cannula site or any swelling.	Monitors for adverse effects such as phlebitis and ensures that complications can be prevented or addressed early.
Ensure that the person who inserted the cannula documents the insertion and gauge of the IV cannula on appropriate form. • The commencement of the IV fluid on the IV fluid order chart/EMM system fluid order • Complete/commence a FBC as per facility/organisation policy • Date and attach a change of line label to IV tubing Handover to nursing staff on next shift: type of fluid, flow rate, condition of PIVC infusion site, any adverse drug reactions.	Alerts staff of IV cannula presence and fluid administration (if in progress). Any adverse effects can be managed promptly. Identifies potential for a fluid balance overload or deficit. Prevents fluid imbalance. Identifies when IV line is required to be changed. Provides individual's healthcare data to the healthcare team. Allows for the planning and implementation of care.
Safe medication management guidelines, outlined in Clinical Interest Box 20.3, should be incorporated into relevant aspects of this skill.	

(ACSQHC 2012; 2015; Gorski 2023; Queensland Health 2018; Rebeiro et al 2021; Tollefson et al 2022)

OBSERVATION CHECKLIST: ESTABLISHING INTRAVENOUS (IV) THERAPY (ASSISTING)

Independent (I)	
Supervised (S)	
Assisted (A)	
Marginal (M)	
Dependent (D)	

STUDENT NAME: _____

CLINICAL SKILL 20.5: Establishing intravenous (IV) therapy (assisting)

DOMAIN(S): Professional and collaborative practice; provision of care; reflective and analytical practice

If the observation checklist is being used as an assessment tool, the student will need to obtain a scale of independence for each of the performance criteria/evidence.

COMPETENCY ELEMENTS	PERFORMANCE CRITERIA/EVIDENCE	I	S	A	M	D
Preparation for the activity	Identifies indications and rationale for performing establishment of an IV line Identifies the individual using three individual identifiers: full name, DOB and UR number Ensures therapeutic interaction Gains the individual's consent Checks facility/organisation policy, resource material Validates the order on the individual's IV fluid order chart/EMM system fluid order Follows the 11 rights Locates and gathers equipment Prepares the work environment					
Performs activity informed by evidence	Assists with insertion of the peripheral intravenous catheter (PIVC) where appropriate Performs the necessary assessments prior to establishing the IV Compares the label of the IV fluid and expiry date with the name of IV fluid on the IV fluid order chart/EMM system fluid order three times Prepares the giving set by closing the roller clamp, spiking the IV fluid bag using aseptic non-touch technique (ANTT) and then filling the drip chamber with fluid Primes the line by releasing the roller clamp slowly and allowing fluid to enter the giving set line Continues priming with fluid until all of the air in the giving set has been expelled Connects primed line onto cannula hub or needleless system Programs the volumetric pump using the medication library and setting the flow rate as per the IV fluid order with an RN and/or as per facility/organisation policy Checks the PIVC site for any complications including checking for patency Ensures PIVC and IV line secured correctly, IV line is labelled and that the insertion site is visible Assesses the PIVC site and the individual for any complications using the Visual Infusion Phlebitis Score (VIPS) Stabilises limb as required					

COMPETENCY ELEMENTS	PERFORMANCE CRITERIA/EVIDENCE	I	S	A	M	D
Applies critical thinking and reflective practice	Is able to link theory to practice Demonstrates current best practice in the care provided Assesses individual's knowledge regarding medication action and provides medication education as required Monitors individual for therapeutic effect of medication (if applicable) Monitors individual for any ADRs to the medication Assesses own performance					
Practises within safety and quality assurance guidelines	Reviews against facility/organisation policy and NSQHS Medication Standard Performs hand hygiene, dons appropriate PPE and uses ANTT principles Checks the expiry dates and performs calculations, as required Checks individual's allergies Cleans and disposes of equipment and waste appropriately					
Documentation and communication	Explains and communicates the IV medication/fluid administration clearly to the individual Communicates outcome and ongoing care to individual and significant others Reports any complications and/or reasons for no administration of the IV medication/fluid to the RN and/or medical officer Documents all relevant information and any complications correctly in the healthcare record: • Documents accurately on IV fluid order chart/ EMM system fluid order, fluid balance chart and in progress notes • The PIVC site must be inspected and VIPS assessed as per facility/organisational policy Provides any special instructions Asks the individual to report any complications post procedure and throughout the IV being used					

Educator/Facilitator Feedback:

Educator/Facilitator Score: Competent   Needs further development

How would you rate your overall performance while undertaking this clinical activity? (use a ✓ & initial)

Unsatisfactory   Satisfactory   Good   Excellent

Student Reflection: (discuss how you would approach your practice differently or more effectively)

EDUCATOR/FACILITATOR NAME/SIGNATURE:

STUDENT NAME/SIGNATURE: DATE:

CLINICAL SKILL 20.6 Intravenous management

Please adhere to the policy and procedures of the facility/organisation prior to undertaking the skill. Ensure this skill is in your scope of practice.

NMBA Decision-making Framework considerations (refer to NMBA Decision-making framework for nursing and midwifery 2020):	Equipment:
1. Am I educated? 2. Am I authorised? 3. Am I competent? If you answer 'no' to any of these, do not perform that activity. Seek guidance and support from your teacher/a nurse team leader/clinical facilitator/educator.	Intravenous (IV) fluid order chart/EMM system fluid order IV fluid IV volumetric pump Fluid balance chart (FBC) IV line label IV cannula care plan

 PREPARE FOR THE SKILL

(Please refer to the Standard Steps on p. xii for related rationales.)
Mentally review the steps of the skill.
Discuss the skill with your instructor/supervisor/team leader, if required.
Confirm correct facility/organisation policy/safe operating procedures.
Validate the order in the individual's record.
Identify indication and rationale for performing the activity.
Assess for any contraindications.
Locate and gather equipment.
Perform hand hygiene.
Ensure therapeutic interaction.
Identify the individual using three individual identifiers.
Gain the individual's consent.
Assess for pain relief.
Prepare the environment.
Provide and maintain privacy.
Assist the individual to assume an appropriate position of comfort.

Skill activity	Rationale
Check the IV fluid order chart/EMM system fluid order for the individual's identifiers when changing an IV fluid flask or re-programming the rate, including asking the individual to state their full name, date of birth (DOB) and then check these as well as the UR number with the ID band and (IV) fluid order chart/EMM system fluid order.	Confirms the individual's identity prior to any changes in IV fluid administration or management.

 PERFORM THE SKILL

(Please refer to the Standard Steps on p. xii for related rationales.)
Perform hand hygiene.
Apply PPE: gloves, eyewear, mask and gown as appropriate.
Ensure the individual's safety and comfort throughout skill.
Promote independence and involvement of the individual if possible and/or appropriate.
Assess the individual's tolerance to the skill throughout.
Dispose of used supplies, equipment, waste and sharps appropriately.
Remove PPE and discard or store appropriately.
Perform hand hygiene.

Continued

CLINICAL SKILL 20.6 Intravenous management—cont'd

Skill activity	Rationale
Assess individual's ability to continue to receive the IV fluid. Perform any necessary assessments related to identifying local and systemic complications: Local signs: Assess IV insertion site using the VIPS for any signs of redness/pallor, temperature (hot or cold), pain/discomfort, swelling (infiltration or extravasation) or bleeding. Systemic signs: Assess vital signs such as blood pressure (BP), pulse, respiratory rate (RR), SpO$_2$. Review FBC for fluid volume status and assess for signs of circulatory overload or fluid volume deficit, assess for signs of infection/septicaemia or pulmonary air embolism. Check the patency of the IV cannula and IV line and IV line label.	Identifies if individual has contraindications such as heart failure or kidney failure. Prevents circulatory overload. If any abnormalities are found, the nurse should not administer medication and should contact nurse in charge and medical officer. Assessing early for local or systemic complications will mitigate the risk of developing more severe issues. Local signs and symptoms may be an early sign of phlebitis. Prevents circulatory overload. Ensures the PIVC is patent and prevents PIVC from occluding. Identifies key sites are secure along the IV line. Identifies when the IV line needs changing.
Assist individual with IV therapy with changing clothing, ambulating and personal hygiene, ensure the IV line remains intact and is not disconnected from the PIVC during these activities. Explain rationale for care to the individual when performing any of the above in order to maintain IV access.	Educates individual about importance of maintaining IV access and the risks associated with poor management. Ensures safety with IV management. Prevents a break in the continuity of the IV line and therefore preventing contamination. Prevents complications.
Change IV fluid as ordered ensuring that correct checking procedures are followed as per Clinical Skill 20.5. Program the new flow rate as per the IV fluid order. Check the IV fluid bag for expiry date, colour and leakage.	Ensures safe administration of IV fluid. Ensures IV fluid order is the same as the IV fluid supplied. Ensures the correct IV fluid is being administered. Prevents preparation and administration errors.
Monitor IV infusion every hour as per facility/organisation policy. Assess PIVC patency using VIPS, and rate of flow. Assess individual's response to treatment.	Prevents complications related to delivery of IV fluid and early detection of inflammation or tissue damage.

 ## AFTER THE SKILL

(Please refer to the Standard Steps on p. xii for related rationales.)
Communicate outcome to the individual, any ongoing care and to report any complications.
Restore the environment.
Report, record and document assessment findings, details of the skill performed and the individual's response.
Report, record and document any abnormalities and/or inability to perform the skill.
Reassess the individual to ensure there are no adverse effects/events from the skill.

Skill activity	Rationale
Ask individual to report: • Pain or discomfort • Coolness over PIVC site • Swelling of feet and hands • Shortness of breath.	Assists in identifying early signs of local or systemic complications.
Sign IV fluid order chart/EMM system fluid order, record date and time infusion commenced: • Complete and attach change of IV line label to IV tubing. • Document review of PIVC each shift and note any complications such as infection, injury or loss of patency. • Complete FBC as per facility/organisation policy. Handover to nursing staff on next shift: type of fluid, flow rate, condition of PIVC infusion site, any adverse drug reactions.	Maintains IV access and maintenance. Ensures individual is receiving recommended therapy as ordered. Prevents complications and monitors status. Provides individual's healthcare data to the healthcare team. Allows for the planning and implementation of care.

CLINICAL SKILL 20.6 Intravenous management—cont'd

Discontinue IV therapy and remove IV cannula when: • There is a medical order (verbal or written) • PIVC has been in situ for three days or has not been used for more than 24 hours • Complications have arisen (as mentioned above) and these have been discussed with an RN or medical officer (see Clinical Skill 20.8). Document date and time of removal, condition of site at time of removal and whether cannula and tip is complete and intact (see Clinical Skill 20.8).	IV cannulas are inserted to administer medications and/or fluids. The goal is to remove the PIVC if it is no longer required, reducing the risk of infection. Loss of patency or complications will mean that a PIVC will need to be removed and re-sited.

Safe medication management guidelines, outlined in Clinical Interest Box 20.3, should be incorporated into relevant aspects of this skill.

(ACSQHC 2012; 2015; Gorski 2023; Queensland Health 2018; Rebeiro et al 2021; Tollefson et al 2022; SESLHD 2019)

OBSERVATION CHECKLIST: INTRAVENOUS MANAGEMENT

STUDENT NAME: _____

CLINICAL SKILL 20.6: Intravenous management

DEMONSTRATION OF: The ability to safely and correctly manage IV therapy

If the observation checklist is being used as an assessment tool, the student will need to obtain a scale of independence for each of the performance criteria/evidence.

Independent (I)
Supervised (S)
Assisted (A)
Marginal (M)
Dependent (D)

COMPETENCY ELEMENTS	PERFORMANCE CRITERIA/EVIDENCE	I	S	A	M	D
Preparation for the activity	Identifies indications and rationale for safely and correctly managing IV therapy Identifies the individual using three individual identifiers: full name, DOB and UR number Ensures therapeutic interaction Gains the individual's consent Checks facility/organisation policy, resource material Validates the order in the individual's IV fluid order chart/EMM system fluid order Verifies name of IV fluid, volume, dose, fluid of previous order and frequency with the IV fluid order chart/EMM system fluid order Follows the 11 rights Locates and gathers equipment Prepares the work environment					
Performs activity informed by evidence	Calculates IV flow rate Checks the IV fluid order/EMM system fluid order and IV pump rate Calculates drops per minute for gravity feed Assesses the PIVC site and individual for any complications Uses VIPS to score PIVC site Reviews FBC and fluid volume status Checks patency Ensures IV pump programmed and working correctly and troubleshoots issues Ensures the IV line is labelled Ensures PIVC and IV line secured correctly, and that the insertion site is visible Stabilises limb as required Follows medical officer's orders regarding discontinuation of the IV and/or removal of the PIVC					
Applies critical thinking and reflective practice	Is able to link theory to practice Demonstrates current best practice in the care provided Assesses individual's knowledge regarding IV fluid action and provides education as required Assesses the individual's ability to cooperate with the procedure Assesses own performance Is able to link theory to practice Demonstrates current best practice in the care provided Assesses individual's knowledge regarding medication action and provides medication education as required Monitors individual for therapeutic effect of medication (if applicable) Monitors individual for any ADRs to the medication Assesses own performance					

COMPETENCY ELEMENTS	PERFORMANCE CRITERIA/EVIDENCE	I	S	A	M	D
Practises within safety and quality assurance guidelines	Reviews against facility/organisation policy and NSQHS Medication Standard Performs hand hygiene, dons appropriate PPE and uses ANTT principles Checks the expiry dates and performs calculations, as required Checks individual's allergies Cleans and disposes of equipment and waste appropriately					
Documentation and communication	Explains and communicates the IV fluid administration procedure clearly to the individual Communicates outcome and ongoing care to individual and significant others Reports any complications and/or any reason for non-administration of IV fluid to the RN and/or medical officer Documents all relevant information and any complications correctly in the healthcare record: • Documents accurately on IV fluid order chart/EMM system fluid order, FBC and in progress notes • The PIVC site must be inspected and VIPS assessed as per facility/organisational policy Provides any special instructions Asks the individual to report any complications throughout the IV therapy					

Educator/Facilitator Feedback:

Educator/Facilitator Score: Competent   Needs further development

How would you rate your overall performance while undertaking this clinical activity? (use a ✓ & initial)

Unsatisfactory   Satisfactory   Good   Excellent

Student Reflection: (discuss how you would approach your practice differently or more effectively)

EDUCATOR/FACILITATOR NAME/SIGNATURE:

STUDENT NAME/SIGNATURE: **DATE:**

CLINICAL SKILL 20.7 Administration of intravenous (IV) medications: Infusion and bolus

Please adhere to the policy and procedures of the facility/organisation prior to undertaking the skill. Ensure this skill is in your scope of practice.

NMBA Decision-making Framework considerations (refer to NMBA Decision-making framework for nursing and midwifery 2020):	Equipment:
1. Am I educated? 2. Am I authorised? 3. Am I competent? If you answer 'no' to any of these, do not perform that activity. Seek guidance and support from your teacher/a nurse team leader/clinical facilitator/educator.	(IV) fluid order chart NIMC/EMM system IV/medication orders IV fluid flask/medication vial/ampoule Diluent IV infusion set Burette Secondary bag Syringes and needleless device for administration and medication vial access (if applicable) IV additive label IV line label Alcohol or antiseptic swabs Disposable gloves IV volumetric pump Fluid balance chart (FBC) Injection tray Resource material (e.g. MIMS, *Australian Injectable Drugs Handbook*, APINCHS list)

 PREPARE FOR THE SKILL

(Please refer to the Standard Steps on p. xii for related rationales.)
Mentally review the steps of the skill.
Discuss the skill with your instructor/supervisor/team leader, if required.
Confirm correct facility/organisation policy/safe operating procedures.
Validate the order in the individual's record.
Identify indication and rationale for performing the activity.
Assess for any contraindications.
Locate and gather equipment.
Perform hand hygiene.
Ensure therapeutic interaction.
Identify the individual using three individual identifiers.
Gain the individual's consent.
Assess for pain relief.
Prepare the environment.
Provide and maintain privacy.
Assist the individual to assume an appropriate position of comfort.

Continued

CLINICAL SKILL 20.7 Administration of intravenous (IV) medications: Infusion and bolus—cont'd

Skill activity	Rationale
General procedures for administration of all IV medications	
Ensure correct IV fluid/medication is given by following the '11 rights' throughout preparation and administration.	Identifies issues, which can be addressed prior to administration. Prevents medication errors from occurring and promotes correct and safe administration of medication/s.
Ensure IV fluid/medication orders are correctly prescribed and written. Verify indication for the medication on the NIMC/EMM system. Review name of medication on the NIMC/EMM system, dose, route, time of last administration and frequency of administration. Assess for any contraindications; check allergy status on the medication chart and with the individual; compare with the medication ordered; check for medication interactions with concurrent IV therapy. Review all necessary information about the medication, including action, purpose, normal dose, side effects, any special administration information. Review high-risk medicines on facility/organisation APINCHS list.	Ensures correct medication administration is about to take place. Ensures the nurse understands why the individual is receiving the medication and is able to ask for a review by the medical officer if the individual's health status changes. Ensures that the right medication is being given at the right frequency and time, via the correct route and prevents medication errors from occurring. Ensures all medication allergies are recorded and determines if a medication should be given. Reduces risk of allergic reactions occurring. Promotes correct and safe administration of the medication and enables the nurse to monitor the therapeutic effects of the medication. Review of APINCHS list alerts the nurse to checking procedures before, during and after high-risk medication delivery, decreasing the risk of toxic or adverse events from occurring.
Assess individual's ability to receive the IV fluid/medication bolus.	Allows nurse to monitor individual's response to IV medication given that onset of action is quicker than any other route.
Check IV fluid order chart, NIMC/EMM system orders for the individual's identifiers, including asking the individual to state their full name, date of birth (DOB) and then check these as well as the UR number with the ID band and (IV) fluid order chart or NIMC/EMM system order.	Confirms the individual's identity.
Perform any necessary assessments related to the medication being administered (e.g. vital signs, chest auscultation, potassium levels, pain levels before, during and after infusion of medication as recommended and/or as per facility/organisation policy).	Ensures safety of the individual during the administration of the medication.

 PERFORM THE SKILL

(Please refer to the Standard Steps on p. xii for related rationales.)
Perform hand hygiene.
Apply PPE: gloves, eyewear, mask and gown as appropriate.
Ensure the individual's safety and comfort throughout skill.
Promote independence and involvement of the individual if possible and/or appropriate.
Assess the individual's tolerance to the skill throughout.
Dispose of used supplies, equipment, waste and sharps appropriately.
Remove PPE and discard or store appropriately.
Perform hand hygiene.

CLINICAL SKILL 20.7 Administration of intravenous (IV) medications: Infusion and bolus—cont'd

Skill activity	Rationale
Prepare medications as per administration guidelines and calculate the correct dose. Ensure the right IV medication is being administered by comparing the label and expiry date with the name on the NIMC/EMM system three times: • First check: Before removing from the storage room • Second check: Before preparing IV medication • Third check: Before adding to IV fluid or administering as a bolus through the PIVC.	Ensures medication order is the same as the medication supplied. Ensures the correct medication is being administered. Prevents preparation and administration errors.
Review *Australian Injectable Drugs Handbook* for compatibility with concurrent IV therapy. Prepare IV fluid/medication with a second nurse (RN) as per the *Australian Injectable Drugs Handbook* and calculate the correct dose. Ensure administration is according to manufacturer's instructions and organisation policy and procedure guidelines. Review high-risk medicines on facility/organisation APINCHS list. Table 20.4 Preparation of medications from ampoules and vials as per the *Australian Injectable Drugs Handbook*.	Promotes correct and safe administration of the IV fluid/medication. Prevents preparation errors. Review of *Australian Injectable Drugs Handbook* prevents incompatibilities and ensures correct mixing of IV fluid/medication. Review of APINCHS list alerts the nurse to checking procedures before, during and after high-risk medication delivery, decreasing the risk of toxic or adverse events from occurring.
Complete and attach additive label as per facility/organisation policy and the ACSQHC 2015 National Standard for User-applied Labelling of Injectable Medicines, Fluids and Lines.	Communicates to nurses the contents of the medication delivery systems.
Assess PIVC insertion site using VIPS for any signs of redness, warmth, swelling, pain or tenderness on palpation. Assess the patency of the cannula as per facility/organisation policy.	Assesses early signs of phlebitis to ascertain if PIVC needs replacing. Ensures safe administration of medication into venous system rather than into surrounding tissues.
Vigorously rub injection port with alcohol swab for 30 seconds and allow to dry for 30 seconds.	Prevents contamination.
Administer IV medication as per facility/organisation policy and the *Australian Injectable Drugs Handbook*.	Ensures the IV medication is administered correctly.
Large volume infusion—fluid bolus	
Check indication and IV fluid order for large volume IV bolus and calculate rate. Review FBC for fluid balance status. Check current IV fluid running to ensure it does not contain any additives such as potassium chloride.	Ensures large volume IV fluid bolus is being administered over the correct timeframe. Identifies a fluid volume deficit indicating the need for a fluid bolus. Ensures that individual is not given a bolus of IV potassium that could be fatal.
Pause current flow rate and set a secondary program using the medication library and set the bolus rate.	A secondary program once completed will revert to the original flow rate. Using the medication library in the volumetric pump reduces the risk of incorrect medication administration rates being programmed.
Check volumetric pump after completion of the large volume bolus timeframe and reduce VTBI by the fluid bolus amount. Record bolus on the FBC and IV fluid order chart.	Ensures large volume bolus has been delivered and has reverted back to original rate. Reducing VTBI reduces the risk of air in line. Allows review of fluid balance status.

Continued

CLINICAL SKILL 20.7 Administration of intravenous (IV) medications: Infusion and bolus—cont'd

Complete post bolus reviews—vital signs (BP), and FBC.	Large volume bolus should increase intravascular volume and improve blood pressure if individual was hypotensive. Large volume bolus can also cause fluid overload.

Intravenous medication bolus via IV cannula/IV line

Check compatibility of current IV fluid administration and medication in the *Australian Injectable Drugs Handbook.*	Prevents incompatibility reaction.
Prepare medication and two syringes with 5–10 mL of normal saline 0.9% each, for flushing the cannula/line before and after medication administration.	Prevents blockage of line and ensures medication has been injected completely, and prevents chemical irritation to the vein.
Take equipment to the individual in injection tray ensuring all sharps are contained/capped correctly. Select injection port closest to individual.	Ensures correct transporting of equipment and abides by infection control/ANTT procedures. Allows for easier aspiration for blood return to check placement.
Vigorously rub the injection port for 30 seconds with alcohol swab and allow to dry for 30 seconds.	Prevents introduction of microorganisms.
Pause pump program and occlude infusion line above port by pinching tubing or closing the roller clamp. Connect syringe containing normal saline 0.9% to needleless valve/injection port on IV line or PIVC. Gently pull back on syringe plunger to aspirate blood. Slowly inject 5–10 mL of normal saline 0.9% and remove syringe.	Prevents back flow of medication into IV line and ensures medication to be administered is into intravenous system. Checks position of cannula in vein. Clears reservoir of blood and checks patency of access port. Allows for access.
Attach IV medication syringe and inject medication as per the *Australian Injectable Drugs Handbook* guidelines or facility/organisation policy.	Ensures medication is given at the correct rate. Rapid administration may cause pain, phlebitis, adverse medication reactions, or could be fatal.
Attach second flush syringe and flush PIVC or line with 5–10 mL of normal saline 0.9%.	Flushes medication properly into the venous system preventing chemical irritation. Allows for medication clearance in the IV line and PIVC.
Release tubing and/or roller clamp and restart the pump infusion rate or gravity feed drip rate if required.	Re-establishes IV fluid delivery.
Vigorously rub the injection port for 30 seconds with alcohol swab and allow to dry for 30 seconds. If the port was capped, replace cap.	Prevents introduction of microorganisms.

Piggyback/tandem infusion

Check compatibility of current IV fluid administration and medication in the *Australian Injectable Drugs Handbook.*	Prevents incompatibility reaction.
Prepare medication by injecting medication into small volume IV fluid bag (e.g. 50–100 mL) through medication injection port. After withdrawing syringe, gently mix contents of infusion.	Ensures even distribution of medication throughout the infusion fluid and prevents medication pooling in the bottom of the IV bag, inadvertently giving the individual a concentrated dose.
Complete and attach an IV medication additive label, with details of medication added, fluid, date, time and two nurses' signatures (second nurse must be an RN).	Informs all staff of the contents of the infusion.
Close roller clamp on secondary giving set and correctly insert spike into medication IV bag using ANTT. Half fill the IV giving set chamber and then slowly prime the line by releasing the roller clamp, without introducing any air.	Prevents the introduction of microorganisms and cross-infection. Allows IV tubing to fill slowly preventing entry of air into the IV line. Prevents air embolus entering the individual.

CLINICAL SKILL 20.7 Administration of intravenous (IV) medications: Infusion and bolus—cont'd

Vigorously rub the injection port for 30 seconds with alcohol swab and allow to dry for 30 seconds.	Prevents introduction of microorganisms.
Hang IV medication bag on IV pole, insert into volumetric pump (if using) and connect IV giving set to infusion port on the primary infusion line.	Prepares IV medication for administration. IV fluid bag needs to be higher than the individual or the volumetric pump to prevent back flow into primary IV bag and aids drip rate via gravity feed.
Program the IV pump secondary line using the medication library with correct rate and VTBI or gravity feed with correct drip rate. Infuse medication as per manufacturer's recommendations and/or *Australian Injectable Drugs Handbook.*	Ensures medication is administered at the correct rate to maintain therapeutic levels and prevent toxicity or adverse reactions. Using the medication library in the volumetric pump reduces the risk of incorrect medication administration rates being programmed.
Remove and discard secondary infusion bag after completion of infusion, in a safe and appropriate manner. Connect a compatible IV fluid if required, to flush the giving set with 25 mL of normal saline 0.9%, then remove secondary line from the primary line. Return to primary infusion rate/drip rate.	Ensures complete infusion of medication. Ensures the return to the original infusion rate as ordered. IV giving set requires approx. 25 mL for priming, which ensures medication infuses correctly and totally in order to allow for therapeutic levels. Ensures no crystallisation of fluid occurs with any other medication or IV fluid delivery in the same line.
Ensure primary infusion is running at the correct pump/drip rate.	Secondary infusion may have interfered with the flow rate of the primary infusion. Prevents circulatory overload.
Burette	
Check compatibility of current IV fluid administration and medication in the *Australian Injectable Drugs Handbook.*	Prevents incompatibility reaction.
Fill burette with required amount of fluid from infusion bag as per the recommendations listed in the manufacturer's guidelines and/or *Australian Injectable Drugs Handbook.*	Ensures correct amount of diluent for the safe administration of the medication. Prevents the risk of circulatory overload. Prevents incompatibility reactions or toxicity.
Vigorously clean injection port on top of burette for 30 seconds with alcohol swab and allow to dry for 30 seconds.	Prevents introduction of microorganisms.
Attach syringe and inject medication into burette port and gently mix with fluid in burette.	Ensures even distribution of medication throughout fluid.
Label burette with medication administration label containing name of medication, total volume, time of starting administration, individual's details and two checking staff signature/initials.	Ensures all staff are aware of medication infusion occurring; prevents other medication being added to burette at same time. Abides by policy and procedure.
Calculate rate and program volumetric pump using the medication library with the correct rate as per the recommendations listed in the manufacturer's guidelines and/or *Australian Injectable Drugs Handbook.*	Ensures medication is administered at the correct rate to maintain therapeutic levels and prevent toxicity or adverse reactions. Using the medication library in the volumetric pump reduces the risk of incorrect medication administration rates being programmed.
On completion of infusion, fill burette to a minimum of 25 mL of normal saline 0.9% or fluid in primary bag and infuse over the same rate medication administered (ensure flush is enough to completely infuse total medication through the IV giving set). Once complete, remove label from burette and return infusion to previous rate.	IV giving set requires approx. 25 mL for priming, which ensures medication infuses correctly and totally in order to allow for therapeutic levels. Ensures no crystallisation of fluid occurs with any other medication or IV fluid delivery in the same line. Alerts staff that medication infusion is complete.

Continued

CLINICAL SKILL 20.7 Administration of intravenous (IV) medications: Infusion and bolus—cont'd

If more than one medication is to be administered, ensure that burette and line are 'flushed' with a minimum of 25 mL in between the medications, and wait the recommended time between the administration of medication as per the recommendations listed in the manufacturer's guidelines and/or *Australian Injectable Drugs Handbook*.	Prevents incompatible medications coming into contact with each other. Ensures that medication actions are adhered to and therapeutic outcomes are optimal.
Volumetric pump syringe driver	
Perform hand hygiene. Prepare 30–50 mL syringe with medication and diluent as per the recommendations listed in the manufacturer's guidelines and/or *Australian Injectable Drugs Handbook*.	Prevents cross-infection. Ensures correct amount of diluent for the safe administration of the medication. Prevents incompatibility reactions or toxicity.
Label syringe with medication additive label containing name of medication, diluent total volume, time of starting administration, individual's details and two checking staff signature/initials. Places label away from markings on syringe.	Ensures all staff are aware of medication being administered via the volumetric pump syringe driver. Abides by policy and procedure. Ensures syringe level can be easily visualised for assessment of delivery and documentation.
Open syringe driver module on the volumetric pump, lift plunger lock and insert syringe with volume numbers facing out, locking it in place.	Ensures syringe is correctly fitted. Ensures syringe level can be easily visualised for assessment of delivery and documentation.
Vigorously rub the cannula valve/injection port for 30 seconds with an alcohol swab and allow to dry for 30 seconds and attach syringe driver line using ANTT.	Prevents cross-contamination.
Calculate rate and program syringe module on volumetric pump using the medication library with the correct rate as per the recommendations and/or *Australian Injectable Drugs Handbook*.	Ensures medication is administered at the correct rate to maintain therapeutic levels and prevent toxicity or adverse reactions. Using the medication library in the volumetric pump reduces the risk of incorrect medication administration rates being programmed.

 AFTER THE SKILL

(Please refer to the Standard Steps on p. xii for related rationales.)
Communicate outcome to the individual, any ongoing care and to report any complications.
Restore the environment.
Report, record and document assessment findings, details of the skill performed and the individual's response.
Report, record and document any abnormalities and/or inability to perform the skill.
Reassess the individual to ensure there are no adverse effects/events from the skill.

Skill activity	Rationale
Record and sign for each medication administered on the NIMC/EMM system. Record volume of fluid in medication bag (used for piggyback/tandem administration) or burette on FBC.	Prompt documentation prevents medication errors. Sites should be rotated for long-term therapy such as insulin, as repeatedly using same site leads to thickening of skin and tissue atrophy. Prevents circulatory overload.
Safe medication management guidelines, outlined in Clinical Interest Box 20.3, should be incorporated into relevant aspects of this skill.	

(ACSQHC 2012; 2015; 2023; Gorski 2023; Queensland Health 2018; Rebeiro et al 2021; The SPHA 2023; Tollefson et al 2022; SESLHD 2019)

OBSERVATION CHECKLIST: ADMINISTRATION OF INTRAVE-NOUS (IV) MEDICATIONS: INFUSION AND BOLUS

STUDENT NAME: _____

CLINICAL SKILL 20.7: Administration of intravenous (IV) medications: infusion and bolus

DEMONSTRATION OF: The ability to safely and correctly administer intravenous medication via infusion and bolus

Independent (I)

Supervised (S)

Assisted (A)

Marginal (M)

Dependent (D)

If the observation checklist is being used as an assessment tool, the student will need to obtain a scale of independence for each of the performance criteria/evidence.

COMPETENCY ELEMENTS	PERFORMANCE CRITERIA/EVIDENCE	I	S	A	M	D
Preparation for the activity	Identifies indications and rationale for performing the IV therapy Identifies the individual using three individual identifiers: full name, DOB and UR number Ensures therapeutic interaction Gains the individual's consent Checks facility/organisation policy, resource material Validates the order on the individual's NIMC/EMM system Follows the 11 rights Locates and gathers equipment Prepares the work environment					
Performs activity informed by evidence	Reviews name of IV medication, dose, route, time of last administration and frequency of administration with NIMC/EMM system Verifies indication for the IV fluid/medication push with the medical officer/RN Considers any medication administration requirements, contraindications Performs and checks any necessary assessments related to the specific medication (vital signs, potassium/electrolyte levels, FBC) Prepares the individual's medication by first reading the name of medication on the container and the expiry date Compares the medication and expiry date with the name of medication on the NIMC/EMM system three times Checks for compatibility with IV fluid (if in progress) Prepares and administers medications as per facility/organisation policy Cleans injection port, flushes IV, administers medication over correct duration, re-cleans port and flushes again For intermittent infusion, connects and hangs piggyback container (with additive label in situ), sets rate for secondary infusion, monitors and returns to primary infusion when complete					

Continued

COMPETENCY ELEMENTS	PERFORMANCE CRITERIA/EVIDENCE	I	S	A	M	D
Applies critical thinking and reflective practice	Is able to link theory to practice Demonstrates current best practice in the care provided Assesses individual's knowledge regarding medication action and provides medication education as required Assesses the individual regarding the IV infusion and/or bolus for any reactions Assesses the individual's ability to cooperate with the procedure Assesses own performance Is able to link theory to practice Demonstrates current best practice in the care provided Assesses individual's knowledge regarding medication action and provides medication education as required Monitors individual for therapeutic effect of medication (if applicable) Monitors individual for any ADRs to the medication Assesses own performance					
Practises within safety and quality assurance guidelines	Reviews against facility/organisation policy and NSQHS Medication Standard Performs hand hygiene, dons appropriate PPE and uses ANTT principles Checks IV medication preparation and delivery process with second nurse (RN) Checks the expiry dates and performs calculations, as required Checks individual's allergies Cleans and disposes of equipment and waste appropriately					
Documentation and communication	Explains and communicates the medication delivery clearly to the individual Communicates outcome and ongoing care to individual and significant others Reports any complications and/or any reason for non-administration of medication to the RN and/or medical officer Documents all relevant information and any complications correctly in the healthcare record: • Documents and signs for medication • Records reasons for withholding any medication • Documents accurately on FBC if required Provides any special instructions Asks the individual to report any complications during and post procedure					

Educator/Facilitator Feedback:

Educator/Facilitator Score: Competent   Needs further development

How would you rate your overall performance while undertaking this clinical activity? (use a ✓ & initial)

Unsatisfactory   Satisfactory   Good   Excellent

Student Reflection: (discuss how you would approach your practice differently or more effectively)

EDUCATOR/FACILITATOR NAME/SIGNATURE:

STUDENT NAME/SIGNATURE: **DATE:**

CLINICAL SKILL 20.8 Removal of intravenous cannula

Please adhere to the policy and procedures of the facility/organisation prior to undertaking the skill. Ensure this skill is in your scope of practice.

NMBA Decision-making Framework considerations (refer to NMBA Decision-making framework for nursing and midwifery 2020):	Equipment:
1. Am I educated? 2. Am I authorised? 3. Am I competent? If you answer 'no' to any of these, do not perform that activity. Seek guidance and support from your teacher/a nurse team leader/clinical facilitator/educator.	Disposable gloves Dressing pack/sterile gauze (as per facility/organisation policy) Injection tray Antiseptic solution/swab (as per facility/organisation policy) Tape

 PREPARE FOR THE SKILL

(Please refer to the Standard Steps on p. xii for related rationales.)
Mentally review the steps of the skill.
Discuss the skill with your instructor/supervisor/team leader, if required.
Confirm correct facility/organisation policy/safe operating procedures.
Validate the order in the individual's record.
Identify indication and rationale for performing the activity.
Assess for any contraindications.
Locate and gather equipment.
Perform hand hygiene.
Ensure therapeutic interaction.
Identify the individual using three individual identifiers.
Gain the individual's consent.
Assess for pain relief.
Prepare the environment.
Provide and maintain privacy.
Assist the individual to assume an appropriate position of comfort.

 PERFORM THE SKILL

(Please refer to the Standard Steps on p. xii for related rationales.)
Perform hand hygiene.
Apply PPE: gloves, eyewear, mask and gown as appropriate.
Ensure the individual's safety and comfort throughout skill.
Promote independence and involvement of the individual if possible and/or appropriate.
Assess the individual's tolerance to the skill throughout.
Dispose of used supplies, equipment, waste and sharps appropriately.
Remove PPE and discard or store appropriately.
Perform hand hygiene.

Skill activity	Rationale
Gently remove tapes securing the IV and the occlusive dressing, ensuring no pulling of excess hair. Use scissors to cut away hair if required.	Decreases discomfort and helps prevent complications to the surrounding skin.
Clean with normal saline 0.9%/chlorhexidine after removal of tape/dressing according to facility/organisation policy and allow to dry. Place sterile gauze over insertion site (do not press) and gently remove cannula along the line of the vein. Place gauze and a strip of tape over site or pressure pad ensuring adequate pressure until there is no further bleeding from site. Inspect the PIVC for completeness.	Prevents the introduction of microorganisms. Prevents a haematoma or injury to the vein post removal. Ensures whole cannula was removed and no fragments are left behind.

CLINICAL SKILL 20.8 Removal of intravenous cannula—cont'd

 AFTER THE SKILL

(Please refer to the Standard Steps on p. xii for related rationales.)
Communicate outcome to the individual, any ongoing care and to report any complications.
Restore the environment.
Report, record and document assessment findings, details of the skill performed and the individual's response.
Report, record and document any abnormalities and/or inability to perform the skill.
Reassess the individual to ensure there are no adverse effects/events from the skill.

Skill activity	Rationale
Document date and time of removal, condition of site at time of removal and whether cannula and tip were complete and intact.	Any adverse effects can be managed promptly. Provides individual's healthcare data to the healthcare team.

Safe medication management guidelines, outlined in Clinical Interest Box 20.3, should be incorporated into relevant aspects of this skill.

(Gorski 2023; JBI 2022e; Queensland Health 2018)

OBSERVATION CHECKLIST: REMOVAL OF AN IV CANNULA

| Independent (I) |
| Supervised (S) |
| Assisted (A) |
| Marginal (M) |
| Dependent (D) |

STUDENT NAME: _____

CLINICAL SKILL 20.8: Removal of an IV cannula

DEMONSTRATION OF: The ability to safely and correctly remove an IV cannula

If the observation checklist is being used as an assessment tool, the student will need to obtain a scale of independence for each of the performance criteria/evidence.

COMPETENCY ELEMENTS	PERFORMANCE CRITERIA/EVIDENCE	I	S	A	M	D
Preparation for the activity	Identifies indications and rationale for performing removing the PIVC Identifies the individual using three individual identifiers: full name, DOB and UR number Ensures therapeutic interaction Gains the individual's consent Checks facility/organisation policy, resource material Validates the order in the individual's record Locates and gathers equipment Prepares the work environment					
Performs activity informed by evidence	Checks the PIVC site for any complications prior to removal using VIPs Follows medical officer's orders regarding the removal of the PIVC Ensures IV pump and/or IV therapy is discontinued/turned off Gently removes tapes securing the IV and the occlusive dressing ensuring no pulling of excess hair Cleanses site and allows to dry. Places sterile gauze over insertion site and gently removes cannula along the line of the vein Places gauze and a strip of tape over site ensuring adequate pressure until there is no further bleeding from site Inspects the PIVC for completeness					
Applies critical thinking and reflective practice	Is able to link theory to practice Demonstrates current best practice in the care provided Assesses the individual for any complications associated with the IV therapy Monitors the individual's anxiety related to the procedure Assesses the individual's ability to cooperate and assist with the procedure Assesses own performance Is able to link theory to practice Demonstrates current best practice in the care provided Assesses individual's knowledge regarding medication action and provides medication education as required Monitors individual for therapeutic effect of medication (if applicable) Monitors individual for any ADRs to the medication Assesses own performance					

COMPETENCY ELEMENTS	PERFORMANCE CRITERIA/EVIDENCE	I	S	A	M	D
Practises within safety and quality assurance guidelines	Reviews against facility/organisation policy and NSQHS Medication Standard Performs hand hygiene, dons appropriate PPE and uses ANTT principles Checks individual's allergies Cleans and disposes of equipment and waste appropriately					
Documentation and communication	Explains and communicates the activity clearly to the individual Communicates outcome and ongoing care to individual and significant others Reports any complications and/or any reason for non-administration to the RN and/or medical officer Documents all relevant information and any complications correctly in the healthcare record: • Documents accurately on IV fluid order chart/ EMM system fluid order, FBC and in progress notes that the IV therapy has been ceased and PIVC removed Provides any special instructions Asks the individual to report any complications during and after the procedure					
(Gorski 2023; JBI 2022e; Queensland Health 2018)						

Educator/Facilitator Feedback:

Educator/Facilitator Score: Competent   Needs further development

How would you rate your overall performance while undertaking this clinical activity? (use a ✓ & initial)

Unsatisfactory   Satisfactory   Good   Excellent

Student Reflection: (discuss how you would approach your practice differently or more effectively)

EDUCATOR/FACILITATOR NAME/SIGNATURE:

STUDENT NAME/SIGNATURE: **DATE:**

CLINICAL SKILL 20.9 Administration of intravenous (IV) blood or blood products

Please adhere to the policy and procedures of the facility/organisation prior to undertaking the skill. Ensure this skill is in your scope of practice.

NMBA Decision-making Framework considerations (refer to NMBA Decision-making framework for nursing and midwifery 2020):	Equipment:
1. Am I educated? 2. Am I authorised? 3. Am I competent? If you answer 'no' to any of these, do not perform that activity. Seek guidance and support from your teacher/a nurse team leader/clinical facilitator/educator.	Blood product prescription form Blood product administration consent form Blood component label Blood product Blood IV infusion giving set Antiseptic swabs Disposable gloves 10 mL syringe 10 mL normal saline 0.9% IV volumetric pump and fluid balance chart (FBC) Vital signs equipment Resource material (e.g. MIMS, *Australian Injectable Drugs Handbook*)

 PREPARE FOR THE SKILL

(Please refer to the Standard Steps on p. xii for related rationales.)
Mentally review the steps of the skill.
Discuss the skill with your instructor/supervisor/team leader, if required.
Confirm correct facility/organisation policy/safe operating procedures.
Validate the order in the individual's record.
Identify indication and rationale for performing the activity.
Assess for any contraindications.
Locate and gather equipment.
Perform hand hygiene.
Ensure therapeutic interaction.
Identify the individual using three individual identifiers.
Gain the individual's consent.
Assess for pain relief.
Prepare the environment.
Provide and maintain privacy.
Assist the individual to assume an appropriate position of comfort.

Skill activity	Rationale
General procedures for administration of IV blood or blood product transfusions	
Ensure correct blood or blood product is administered by following the '11 rights' throughout preparation and administration.	Identifies issues, which can be addressed prior to administration. Prevents transfusion errors from occurring and promotes correct and safe administration of blood and blood products.
Ensure blood or blood product orders are correctly prescribed and written. Verify indication for the administration of the blood or blood product. Assess for any contraindications: check individual's ABO and compare with the blood product ordered; ensure a dedicated IV line. Review all necessary information about the blood or blood product, including rationale, haemolytic and non-haemolytic reactions, any special administration information. Check blood product prescription form for signed consent.	Ensures correct blood or blood product administration is about to take place. Ensures the nurse understands why the individual is receiving the blood or blood product and is able to ask for a review by the medical officer if the individual's health status changes. Ensures compatibility of blood or blood product. Promotes correct and safe administration of the blood or blood product and prevents incorrect blood transfusion. Ensures individual has been fully informed and consents to the blood or blood product transfusion.

Continued

CLINICAL SKILL 20.9 Administration of intravenous (IV) blood or blood products—cont'd

Review name of blood or blood product on the blood product prescription form: blood product, route, time of last administration and frequency of administration.	Ensures that the right blood product is being given at the right frequency and time, via the correct route. Prevents medication errors from occurring.

 PERFORM THE SKILL

(Please refer to the Standard Steps on p. xii for related rationales.)
Perform hand hygiene.
Apply PPE: gloves, eyewear, mask and gown as appropriate.
Ensure the individual's safety and comfort throughout skill.
Promote independence and involvement of the individual if possible and/or appropriate.
Assess the individual's tolerance to the skill throughout.
Dispose of used supplies, equipment, waste and sharps appropriately.
Remove PPE and discard or store appropriately.
Perform hand hygiene.

Skill activity	Rationale
All blood checking processes independently verified by two nurses (one must be an RN). Check the blood product prescription form for the individual's identifiers, including asking the individual to state their full name, date of birth (DOB) and then check these as well as the UR number with the ID band and the blood product prescription form and blood product label. Check batch number, blood group (ABO & Rh(D)), blood or blood product expiry date and cross match expiry date with the blood product prescription form and blood product label according to safe administration of blood products and facility/organisation policy. **Note:** Blood should not exceed the maximum time of 30 minutes away from the fridge; platelets should continue to be agitated by hand prior to administration.	Nurses checking individually the blood product prescription form and blood product label with the individual's ID ensures accuracy of information once compared, instead of one nurse trusting the other nurse that the information is correct as they read it out. Promotes safety prior to blood product administration. Confirms the individual's identity and prevents incorrect blood or blood product being transfused. Promotes safety prior to blood product administration. Ensures the correct blood product is being administered to the correct person.
Calculate the correct volumetric pump rate according to the rate documented on the blood product prescription form and volume recorded on the blood bag.	Ensures the blood product is administered at the correct rate and reduces the risk of transfusion reactions.
Check PIVC insertion site using the VIPS for any signs of redness, warmth, swelling, pain or tenderness on palpation.	Assesses early signs of phlebitis to ascertain if PIVC needs replacing.
Perform pre-blood administration vital signs check before, during and after infusion of blood or blood product according to facility/organisation policy.	Allows nurse to monitor individual's response to blood product and allows for identification of blood transfusion reactions. Ensures safety of the individual during the administration of the blood or blood product.
Vigorously rub injection port with alcohol swab for 30 seconds and allow to dry for 30 seconds.	Prevents contamination.
Attach syringe and flush with 10 mL of normal saline 0.9%. Identify patency.	Ensures safe administration of medication into venous system rather than into surrounding tissues. Assesses the patency of the cannula as per facility/organisation policy and procedure guidelines.
Prime a dedicated blood product IV volumetric giving set with the blood or blood product. Connect line to IV cannula.	Protocol is for blood not to be transfused with any other IV fluid or medication. Prevents incompatibility reaction from occurring by using a new IV giving set dedicated for blood.

CLINICAL SKILL 20.9 Administration of intravenous (IV) blood or blood products—cont'd

Commence volumetric pump administration rate as per protocol.	Some organisations required that blood transfusions commence at a slower rate to minimise transfusion reactions.
Commence blood transfusion at a slower rate for the first 15 minutes as per organisational protocol (if required).	Indicates afebrile non-haemolytic or haemolytic reaction or circulatory overload.
Perform and record routine blood observations as per protocol: 15-minutely, then hourly until the transfusion finishes, and at conclusion of the blood transfusion according to facility/organisation policy and individual health status.	Different actions may be implemented depending on the reaction and medical officer's orders. Allows medical officer to stop or change blood product promptly if a transfusion reaction occurs, and to treat the symptoms or manage blood transfusion administration.
Observe and remain with the individual for the first 15 minutes.	**Note:** Platelets, plasma (FFP), serum albumin and cryoprecipitate generally do not require regular observations, but refer to facility/organisation policy for
Observe closely and report any transfusion reactions such as:	further information.
• Fever, chills, headache, malaise	Minimises risk of bacterial infection and contamination.
• Flushing of the skin, urticaria, wheezing, itchy rash	
• Restlessness, anxiety, chest pain, tachypnoea, tachycardia, nausea, shock, haematuria, back pain.	
Stop the blood transfusion if you suspect a reaction.	
Notify RN and medical officer, follow facility/organisation policy.	
Complete the transfusion when the blood unit is empty (or if four hours has elapsed since unit of blood removed from the blood fridge).	

 ## AFTER THE SKILL

(Please refer to the Standard Steps on p. xii for related rationales.)
Communicate outcome to the individual, any ongoing care and to report any complications.
Restore the environment.
Report, record and document assessment findings, details of the skill performed and the individual's response.
Report, record and document any abnormalities and/or inability to perform the skill.
Reassess the individual to ensure there are no adverse effects/events from the skill.

Skill activity	Rationale
Immediately record and sign blood administration commencement on blood product prescription form (two nurses to sign).	Ensures that blood or blood product administration is correctly recorded on the relevant charts.
Record blood volume on the fluid balance chart.	Ensures accurate recording of input.
Instruct the person to report any sudden chills, nausea, dyspnoea, fever, rash, itch, loin/flank pain.	Promotes participation in care and understanding of health status. Reduces risk of allergic reaction.
On completion of each blood transfusion, medical officer notified to complete a review of the individual. Flush line via secondary spike with normal saline 0.9%. Change the giving set as per facility/organisation policy.	Ensures the safety of the individual and detects fluid overload and any delayed transfusion reaction. Medical officer may prescribe diuretics to prevent fluid overload. To ensure all blood or blood product is administered. Decreases risk of bacterial contamination, and retains efficiency of filter.
Safe medication management guidelines, outlined in Clinical Interest Box 20.3, should be incorporated into relevant aspects of this skill.	

(ACSQHC 2012; 2015; Australian & New Zealand Society of Blood Transfusion Ltd 2019; Department of Health 2018; 2021; Gorski 2023; JBI 2021e; Rebeiro et al 2021; SESLHD 2019)

OBSERVATION CHECKLIST: ADMINISTRATION OF INTRAVENOUS BLOOD PRODUCTS

Independent (I)

Supervised (S)

Assisted (A)

Marginal (M)

Dependent (D)

STUDENT NAME: _____

CLINICAL SKILL 20.9: Administration of intravenous (IV) blood products

DEMONSTRATION OF: The ability to safely and correctly manage IV blood product administration

If the observation checklist is being used as an assessment tool, the student will need to obtain a scale of independence for each of the performance criteria/evidence.

COMPETENCY ELEMENTS	PERFORMANCE CRITERIA/EVIDENCE	I	S	A	M	D
Preparation for the activity	Identifies indications and rationale for safely and correctly managing blood product administration Identifies the individual using three individual identifiers: full name, DOB and UR number using the blood product prescription form Ensures therapeutic interaction Gains the individual's consent Checks facility/organisation policy, resource material Verifies the blood order in the individual's blood product prescription form and blood product label Checks the previous fluid or blood product orders and frequency with the blood product prescription form Follows the 11 rights Locates and gathers equipment Prepares the work environment Performs pre-blood vital signs observations					
Performs activity informed by evidence	Reviews blood or blood product type, blood label, batch number, written consent, blood group (ABO, Rh(D)) and expiry date with the blood product prescription form and blood label independently and with a second nurse (RN) Checks the volume of the blood product and calculates the pump rate Assesses the PIVC site and individual for any complications using the VIP score and checks patency Reviews FBC and fluid volume status Ensures IV volumetric pump is programmed with the correct rate and VTBI Ensures PIVC and IV line are secured correctly, and the insertion site is visible Stabilises limb as required Performs routine blood observations as per protocol and remains with the person for the first 15 minutes					

COMPETENCY ELEMENTS	PERFORMANCE CRITERIA/EVIDENCE	I	S	A	M	D
Applies critical thinking and reflective practice	Is able to link theory to practice Demonstrates current best practice in the care provided according to BloodSafe guidelines Assesses individual's knowledge regarding IV blood product administration and provides education as required Aware of haemolytic and non-haemolytic transfusion reactions to be able to act promptly if a transfusion reaction occurs Assesses own performance Is able to link theory to practice Demonstrates current best practice in the care provided Assesses individual's knowledge regarding medication action and provides medication education as required Monitors individual for therapeutic effect of medication (if applicable) Monitors individual for any ADRs to the medication Assesses own performance					
Practises within safety and quality assurance guidelines	Reviews against facility/organisation policy and NSQHS Medication Standard Performs hand hygiene, dons appropriate PPE and uses ANTT principles Checks the expiry dates and performs calculations, as required Checks individual's allergies Cleans and disposes of blood product and equipment and waste appropriately					
Documentation and communication	Explains and communicates the IV blood product administration procedure clearly to the individual Communicates outcome and ongoing care to individual and significant others Reports any complications and/or any reason for non-administration of IV blood product to the RN and/or medical officer Documents all relevant information and any complications correctly in the healthcare record: • Documents accurately the blood checks and observations on blood product prescription form, FBC and in progress notes • The PIVC site must be inspected and VIPS assessed as per facility/organisation policy Provides any special instructions Asks the individual to report any signs and symptoms throughout the blood product administration					

Educator/Facilitator Feedback:

Educator/Facilitator Score: Competent   Needs further development

How would you rate your overall performance while undertaking this clinical activity? (use a ✓ & initial)

Unsatisfactory   Satisfactory   Good   Excellent

Student Reflection: (discuss how you would approach your practice differently or more effectively)

EDUCATOR/FACILITATOR NAME/SIGNATURE:

STUDENT NAME/SIGNATURE: **DATE:**

CLINICAL SKILL 20.10 Administration of subcutaneous (subcut) medications: Infusion

Please adhere to the policy and procedures of the facility/organisation prior to undertaking the skill. Ensure this skill is in your scope of practice.

NMBA Decision-making Framework considerations (refer to NMBA Decision-making framework for nursing and midwifery 2020):	Equipment:
1. Am I educated? 2. Am I authorised? 3. Am I competent? If you answer 'no' to any of these, do not perform that activity. Seek guidance and support from your teacher/a nurse team leader/clinical facilitator/educator.	NIMC/EMM system medication orders (e.g. subcut continuous infusion chart) Prescribed medication/s Diluent Subcutaneous infusion set (extension tubing line) Syringe driver and appropriate size syringe Needleless device (butterfly) and vial access (if applicable) Subcutaneous additive and line label Antiseptic swabs Disposable gloves Injection tray Resource material (e.g. MIMS, *Australian Injectable Drugs Handbook*, APINCHS list)

 PREPARE FOR THE SKILL

(Please refer to the Standard Steps on p. xii for related rationales.)
Mentally review the steps of the skill.
Discuss the skill with your instructor/supervisor/team leader, if required.
Confirm correct facility/organisation policy/safe operating procedures.
Validate the order in the individual's record.
Identify indication and rationale for performing the activity.
Assess for any contraindications.
Locate and gather equipment.
Perform hand hygiene.
Ensure therapeutic interaction.
Identify the individual using three individual identifiers.
Gain the individual's consent.
Assess for pain relief.
Prepare the environment.
Provide and maintain privacy.
Assist the individual to assume an appropriate position of comfort.

Skill activity	Rationale
General procedures for administration of all subcutaneous medications	
Ensure correct medication is given by following the '11 rights' throughout preparation and administration.	Identifies issues, which can be addressed prior to administration. Prevents medication errors from occurring and promotes correct and safe administration of medication/s.

Continued

CLINICAL SKILL 20.10 Administration of subcutaneous (subcut) medications: Infusion—cont'd

Ensure medication orders are correctly prescribed and written. Verify indication for the medication on the NIMC/EMM system. Review name of medication on the NIMC/EMM system, dose, route, time of last administration and frequency of administration. Review high-risk medicines on facility/organisation APINCHS list. Assess for any medication contraindications; check allergy status on the medication chart and with the individual; compare with the medication ordered; check for medication interactions. Review all necessary information about the medication, including action, purpose, normal dose, side effects, any special administration information.	Ensures correct medication administration is about to take place. Ensures the nurse understands why the individual is receiving the medication and is able to ask for a review by the medical officer if the individual's health status changes. Ensures that the right medication is being given at the right frequency and time, via the correct route. Review of APINCHS list alerts the nurse to checking procedures before, during and after high-risk medication delivery decreasing the risk of toxic or adverse events from occurring. Prevents medication errors from occurring. Ensures all medication allergies are recorded and determines if a medication should be given. Reduces risk of allergic reactions occurring. Promotes correct and safe administration of the medication and enables the nurse to monitor the therapeutic effects of the medication.
Assess individual's ability to receive the medication in the prescribed form via the prescribed route.	Before administering morphine, the nurse must check the individual's sedation score to ascertain conscious state as further administration may increase the risk of complications.
Check medication orders for the individual's identifiers, including asking the individual to state their full name, date of birth (DOB) and then check these as well as the UR number with the ID band and NIMC/EMM system.	Confirms the individual's identity.
Perform any necessary assessments related to the medication such as sedation score (AVPU), respiratory rate (RR), blood glucose level (BGL).	Allows nurse to monitor individual's response to the medication. If any abnormalities are found, the nurse should not administer medication and should contact nurse in charge and medical officer.

 PERFORM THE SKILL

(Please refer to the Standard Steps on p. xii for related rationales.)
Perform hand hygiene.
Apply PPE: gloves, eyewear, mask and gown as appropriate.
Ensure the individual's safety and comfort throughout skill.
Promote independence and involvement of the individual if possible and/or appropriate.
Assess the individual's tolerance to the skill throughout.
Dispose of used supplies, equipment, waste and sharps appropriately.
Remove PPE and discard or store appropriately.
Perform hand hygiene.

CLINICAL SKILL 20.10 Administration of subcutaneous (subcut) medications: Infusion—cont'd

Skill activity	Rationale
Calculate correct dose and prepare medication according to Table 20.4 Preparation of medications from ampoules and vials and as per the *Australian Injectable Drugs Handbook*. Check the label and expiry date. Have two nurses check (one must be an RN) according to safe administration guidelines and the facility/organisation policy. Compare the medication container with the order on the subcutaneous infusion chart. Ensure right medication is being administered by comparing the label of the medication vial/ampoule and expiry date with the name of medication on the NIMC/EMM system three times: • First check: Before removing from the medication room • Second check: Before removing medication from the vial/ampoule • Third check: Before discarding medication vial/ampoule.	Promotes safety during administration. Ensures the correct medication is being administered. Prevents preparation errors. Prevents chemical reaction occurring, which may result in clouding or crystallisation of the medication in the syringe. Ensures medication order is the same as the medication supplied. Ensures the correct medication is being administered. Prevents preparation and administration errors.
Assess subcutaneous butterfly insertion site for any signs of redness, warmth, swelling, pain or tenderness on palpation. Assess the patency of the subcutaneous butterfly as per facility/organisation policy.	Ensures safe administration of medication into the subcutaneous tissue.
Attach the extension tubing line to the end of the syringe and prime the line. Insert the syringe into the syringe driver locking it into place. Clean butterfly port with antiseptic swab for 30 seconds and allow to dry for 30 seconds. Attach the extension tubing line to the port on the end of the subcutaneous butterfly, maintaining ANTT.	Prevents cross-infection.
Attach additive label to the syringe and line label to the line. Avoid placing additive label over syringe volume markings. Program the syringe driver to required rate/hr or mm/24 hours. Place a locking canister over syringe driver.	Ensures correct and safe administration of medication. To secure syringe and rate buttons preventing accidental administration of increased volume.
If necessary, check vital signs before, during and after subcutaneous infusion of medication as recommended and/or as per continuous infusion chart and facility/organisation policy.	Allows nurse to monitor individual's response to medication. Ensures safety of the individual during the administration of the medication.

AFTER THE SKILL

(Please refer to the Standard Steps on p. xii for related rationales.)
Communicate outcome to the individual, any ongoing care and to report any complications.
Restore the environment.
Report, record and document assessment findings, details of the skill performed and the individual's response.
Report, record and document any abnormalities and/or inability to perform the skill.
Reassess the individual to ensure there are no adverse effects/events from the skill.

Continued

CLINICAL SKILL 20.10 Administration of subcutaneous (subcut) medications: Infusion—cont'd

Skill activity	Rationale
Record medication administration promptly on medication/subcutaneous continuous infusion administration chart.	Prevents medication errors from occurring (e.g. dose being duplicated).
Record volume of fluid in syringe in mm or volume on the continuous infusion chart.	Allows for monitoring of delivery of medication through the syringe driver over a 24-hour period.

Safe medication management guidelines, outlined in Clinical Interest Box 20.3, should be incorporated into relevant aspects of this skill.

(ACSQHC 2012; 2015; 2023; Gorski 2023; Queensland Health 2018; Rebeiro et al 2021; The SPHA 2023; Tollefson et al 2022)

OBSERVATION CHECKLIST: ADMINISTRATION OF SUBCUTANEOUS (SUBCUT) MEDICATIONS: INFUSION

| Independent (I) |
| Supervised (S) |
| Assisted (A) |
| Marginal (M) |
| Dependent (D) |

STUDENT NAME: _____

CLINICAL SKILL 20.10: Administration of subcutaneous (subcut) medications: infusion

DEMONSTRATION OF: The ability to safely and correctly administer subcutaneous medication via infusion

If the observation checklist is being used as an assessment tool, the student will need to obtain a scale of independence for each of the performance criteria/evidence.

COMPETENCY ELEMENTS	PERFORMANCE CRITERIA/EVIDENCE	I	S	A	M	D
Preparation for the activity	Identifies indications and rationale for performing subcut medication infusion Identifies the individual using three individual identifiers: full name, DOB and UR number Ensures therapeutic interaction Gains the individual's consent Checks facility/organisation policy, resource material Validates the order on the individual's NIMC/EMM system Follows the 11 rights Locates and gathers equipment Prepares the work environment					
Performs activity informed by evidence	Reviews name of medication, dose, route, time of last administration and frequency of administration with NIMC/EMM system Verifies indication for medication Considers any medication administration requirements, contraindications Performs and checks any necessary assessments related to the specific medication (vital signs) Compares the medication and expiry date with the name of medication on the NIMC/EMM system three times Checks for compatibility with other medications to be delivered concurrently Prepares syringe and volumetric pump syringe driver module Attaches subcutaneous additive and line label Programs settings and administers subcut medications as per facility/organisation policy Checks subcut medication preparation and delivery process with subcut order chart and with a second nurse (RN) Checks compatibility of medications being delivered concurrently Assesses subcut cannula insertion site					

Continued

COMPETENCY ELEMENTS	PERFORMANCE CRITERIA/EVIDENCE	I	S	A	M	D
Applies critical thinking and reflective practice	Is able to link theory to practice Demonstrates current best practice in the care provided Assesses individual's knowledge regarding medication action and provides medication education as required Assesses the individual regarding the subcutaneous infusion and for any reactions Assesses the individual's ability to cooperate with the procedure Assesses own performance Is able to link theory to practice Demonstrates current best practice in the care provided Assesses individual's knowledge regarding medication action and provides medication education as required Monitors individual for therapeutic effect of medication (if applicable) Monitors individual for any ADRs to the medication Assesses own performance					
Practises within safety and quality assurance guidelines	Reviews against facility/organisation policy and NSQHS Medication Standard Performs hand hygiene, dons appropriate PPE and uses ANTT principles Checks the expiry dates and performs calculations, as required Checks individual's allergies Cleans and disposes of equipment and waste appropriately					
Documentation and communication	Explains and communicates the medication delivery clearly to the individual Communicates outcome and ongoing care to individual and significant others Reports any complications and/or any reason for non-administration of medication on the NIMC/EMM system, and to the RN and/or medical officer Documents all relevant information and any complications correctly in the healthcare record: • Documents and signs for medication • Records reasons for withholding any medication • Documents accurately on FBC if required Provides any special instructions Asks the individual to report any signs or symptoms during and post procedure					

Educator/Facilitator Feedback:

Educator/Facilitator Score: Competent   Needs further development

How would you rate your overall performance while undertaking this clinical activity? (use a ✓ & initial)

Unsatisfactory   Satisfactory   Good   Excellent

Student Reflection: (discuss how you would approach your practice differently or more effectively)

EDUCATOR/FACILITATOR NAME/SIGNATURE:

STUDENT NAME/SIGNATURE: **DATE:**

CLINICAL SKILL 20.11 Administration of a topical medication

Please adhere to the policy and procedures of the facility/organisation prior to undertaking the skill. Ensure this skill is in your scope of practice.

NMBA Decision-making Framework considerations (refer to NMBA Decision-making framework for nursing and midwifery 2020):	Equipment:
1. Am I educated? 2. Am I authorised? 3. Am I competent? If you answer 'no' to any of these, do not perform that activity. Seek guidance and support from your teacher/a nurse team leader/clinical facilitator/educator.	NIMC/EMM system medication order Prescribed medication Disposable gloves Resource material (e.g. MIMS)

 PREPARE FOR THE SKILL

(Please refer to the Standard Steps on p. xii for related rationales.)
Mentally review the steps of the skill.
Discuss the skill with your instructor/supervisor/team leader, if required.
Confirm correct facility/organisation policy/safe operating procedures.
Validate the order in the individual's record.
Identify indication and rationale for performing the activity.
Assess for any contraindications.
Locate and gather equipment.
Perform hand hygiene.
Ensure therapeutic interaction.
Identify the individual using three individual identifiers.
Gain the individual's consent.
Assess for pain relief.
Prepare the environment.
Provide and maintain privacy.
Assist the individual to assume an appropriate position of comfort.

Skill activity	Rationale
Ensure correct medication is given by following the '11 rights' throughout preparation and administration.	Identifies issues, which can be addressed prior to administration. Prevents medication errors from occurring and promotes correct and safe administration of medication/s.
Ensure medication orders are correctly prescribed and written. Verify indication for the medication on the NIMC/EMM system. Review name of medication on the NIMC/EMM system, dose, route, time of last administration and frequency of administration. Assess for any medication contraindications; check allergy status on the medication chart and with the individual; compare with the medication ordered; check for medication interactions. Review all necessary information about the medication, including action, purpose, normal dose, side effects, any special administration information.	Ensures correct medication administration is about to take place. Ensures the nurse understands why the individual is receiving the medication and is able to ask for a review by the medical officer if the individual's health status changes. Ensures that the right medication is being given at the right frequency and time, via the correct route and prevents medication errors from occurring. Ensures all medication allergies are recorded and determines if a medication should be given. Reduces risk of allergic reactions occurring. Promotes correct and safe administration of the medication and enables the nurse to monitor the therapeutic effects of the medication.
Assess the individual's ability to receive the medication in the prescribed form via the prescribed route.	If the individual has a skin rash, infection, bruising at the site, a review will need to occur to reassess the ordered route.
Check medication chart for the individual's identifiers, including asking the individual to state their full name, date of birth (DOB) and then check these as well as the UR number with the ID band and NIMC/EMM system.	Confirms the individual's identity.

CLINICAL SKILL 20.11 Administration of a topical medication—cont'd

 PERFORM THE SKILL

(Please refer to the Standard Steps on p. xii for related rationales.)
Perform hand hygiene.
Apply PPE: gloves, eyewear, mask and gown as appropriate.
Ensure the individual's safety and comfort throughout skill.
Promote independence and involvement of the individual if possible and/or appropriate.
Assess the individual's tolerance to the skill throughout.
Dispose of used supplies, equipment, waste and sharps appropriately.
Remove PPE and discard or store appropriately.
Perform hand hygiene.

Skill activity	Rationale
Prepare medication as per administration guidelines and calculate the correct dose. Ensure the right medication is being administered by comparing the label of the medication and expiry date with the name on the NIMC/EMM system three times: • First check: Before removing from the trolley or cupboard • Second check: Before removing from the container • Third check: Before returning to the trolley or cupboard, or discarding.	Following administration guidelines ensures the medication's effectiveness and the correct dosage of medication is being administered. Ensures medication order is the same as the medication supplied. Ensures the correct medication is being administered. Prevents preparation and administration errors.
Apply required amount of topical medication onto the individual's skin as per administration guidelines.	The amount of topical medication applied depends on the type of medication being applied. For example, for applying a corticosteroid the fingertip unit is used as a guide to determine how much product to apply. Other treatments such as emollients may require more generous application of the product.

 AFTER THE SKILL

(Please refer to the Standard Steps on p. xii for related rationales.)
Communicate outcome to the individual, any ongoing care and to report any complications.
Restore the environment.
Report, record and document assessment findings, details of the skill performed and the individual's response.
Report, record and document any abnormalities and/or inability to perform the skill.
Reassess the individual to ensure there are no adverse effects/events from the skill.

Skill activity	Rationale
Record and sign for each medication administered on NIMC/EMM system.	Prompt documentation prevents medication errors.

Safe medication management guidelines, outlined in Clinical Interest Box 20.3, should be incorporated into relevant aspects of this skill.

(ACSQHC 2012; 2019; JBI 2022g; Rebeiro et al 2021; Tollefson et al 2022)

OBSERVATION CHECKLIST: ADMINISTRATION OF A TOPICAL MEDICATION

Independent (I)	
Supervised (S)	
Assisted (A)	
Marginal (M)	
Dependent (D)	

STUDENT NAME: _____

CLINICAL SKILL 20.11: Administration of a topical medication

DEMONSTRATION OF: The ability to safely and correctly administer a topical medication

If the observation checklist is being used as an assessment tool, the student will need to obtain a scale of independence for each of the performance criteria/evidence.

COMPETENCY ELEMENTS	PERFORMANCE CRITERIA/EVIDENCE	I	S	A	M	D
Preparation for the activity	Identifies indications and rationale for medication administration Identifies the individual using three individual identifiers: full name, DOB and UR number Ensures therapeutic interaction Gains the individual's consent Checks facility/organisation policy, resource material Validates the order on the individual's NIMC/EMM system Validates the order in the individual's record Follows the 11 rights Locates and gathers equipment Prepares the work environment					
Performs activity informed by evidence	Reviews name of medication, dose, route, time of last administration and frequency of administration with NIMC/EMM system Verifies indication for medication Considers any medication administration requirements, contraindications Compares the medication and expiry date with the name of medication on the NIMC/EMM system three times Selects appropriate site for medication delivery Applies the required amount of topical medication onto the individual's skin					

COMPETENCY ELEMENTS	PERFORMANCE CRITERIA/EVIDENCE	I	S	A	M	D
Applies critical thinking and reflective practice	Is able to link theory to practice Demonstrates current best practice in the care provided Assesses individual's knowledge regarding medication action and provides medication education as required and ability to self-administer Applies the appropriate amount of the product Monitors individual for medication effectiveness (if applicable) Monitors individual for any adverse effects to the medication Assesses own performance Is able to link theory to practice Demonstrates current best practice in the care provided Assesses individual's knowledge regarding medication action and provides medication education as required Monitors individual for therapeutic effect of medication (if applicable) Monitors individual for any ADRs to the medication Assesses own performance					
Practises within safety and quality assurance guidelines	Reviews against facility/organisation policy and NSQHS Medication Standard Performs hand hygiene, dons appropriate PPE and uses ANTT principles Checks the expiry dates and performs calculations, as required Checks individual's allergies Cleans and disposes of equipment and waste appropriately					
Documentation and communication	Explains and communicates the activity clearly to the individual Communicates outcome and ongoing care to individual and significant others Reports any complications and/or any reason for non-administration on the NIMC/EMM system, and to the RN and/or medical officer Documents all relevant information and any complications correctly in the healthcare record: • Documents and signs for medication • Records reasons for withholding any medication Provides any special instructions Asks the individual to report any complications during and after the procedure					

Educator/Facilitator Feedback:

Educator/Facilitator Score: Competent   Needs further development

How would you rate your overall performance while undertaking this clinical activity? (use a ✓ & initial)

Unsatisfactory   Satisfactory   Good   Excellent

Student Reflection: (discuss how you would approach your practice differently or more effectively)

EDUCATOR/FACILITATOR NAME/SIGNATURE:

STUDENT NAME/SIGNATURE: **DATE:**

CLINICAL SKILL 20.12 Applying transdermal medications

Please adhere to the policy and procedures of the facility/organisation prior to undertaking the skill. Ensure this skill is in your scope of practice.

NMBA Decision-making Framework considerations (refer to NMBA Decision-making framework for nursing and midwifery 2020):	Equipment:
1. Am I educated? 2. Am I authorised? 3. Am I competent? If you answer 'no' to any of these, do not perform that activity. Seek guidance and support from your teacher/a nurse team leader/clinical facilitator/educator.	NIMC/EMM system medication order Prescribed medication Resource material (e.g. MIMS) Disposable gloves

 PREPARE FOR THE SKILL

(Please refer to the Standard Steps on p. xii for related rationales.)
Mentally review the steps of the skill.
Discuss the skill with your instructor/supervisor/team leader, if required.
Confirm correct facility/organisation policy/safe operating procedures.
Validate the order in the individual's record.
Identify indication and rationale for performing the activity.
Assess for any contraindications.
Locate and gather equipment.
Perform hand hygiene.
Ensure therapeutic interaction.
Identify the individual using three individual identifiers.
Gain the individual's consent.
Assess for pain relief.
Prepare the environment.
Provide and maintain privacy.
Assist the individual to assume an appropriate position of comfort.

Skill activity	Rationale
Ensure correct medication is given by following the '11 rights' throughout preparation and administration.	Identifies issues, which can be addressed prior to administration. Prevents medication errors from occurring and promotes correct and safe administration of medication/s.
Ensure medication orders are correctly prescribed and written. Verify indication for the medication on the NIMC/EMM system. Review name of medication on the NIMC/EMM system, dose, route, time of last administration and frequency of administration. Assess for any medication contraindications; check allergy status on the medication chart and with the individual; compare with the medication ordered; check for medication interactions. Review all necessary information about the medication, including action, purpose, normal dose, side effects, any special administration information.	Ensures correct medication administration is about to take place. Ensures the nurse understands why the individual is receiving the medication and is able to ask for a review by the medical officer if the individual's health status changes. Ensures that the right medication is being given at the right frequency and time, via the correct route and prevents medication errors from occurring. Ensures all medication allergies are recorded and determines if a medication should be given. Reduces risk of allergic reactions occurring. Promotes correct and safe administration of the medication and enables the nurse to monitor the therapeutic effects of the medication.
Assess individual's ability to receive the medication in the prescribed form via the prescribed route.	If the individual has a skin rash, infection, bruising at the site, a review will need to occur to reassess the ordered route.
Check medication chart for the individual's identifiers, including asking the individual to state their full name, date of birth (DOB) and then check these as well as the UR number with the ID band and NIMC/EMM system.	Confirms the individual's identity.

Continued

CLINICAL SKILL 20.12 Applying transdermal medications—cont'd

 PERFORM THE SKILL

(Please refer to the Standard Steps on p. xii for related rationales.)
Perform hand hygiene.
Apply PPE: gloves, eyewear, mask and gown as appropriate.
Ensure the individual's safety and comfort throughout skill.
Promote independence and involvement of the individual if possible and/or appropriate.
Assess the individual's tolerance to the skill throughout.
Dispose of used supplies, equipment, waste and sharps appropriately.
Remove PPE and discard or store appropriately.
Perform hand hygiene.

Skill activity	Rationale
Prepare medication as per administration guidelines and calculate the correct dose. Ensure the right medication is being administered by comparing the label of the medication and expiry date with the name on the NIMC/EMM system three times: • First check: Before removing from the trolley or cupboard • Second check: Before removing from the container • Third check: Before returning to the trolley or cupboard, or discarding.	Following administration guidelines ensures the medication's effectiveness and the correct dosage of medication is being administered. Ensures medication order is the same as the medication supplied. Ensures the correct medication is being administered. Prevents preparation and administration errors.
Inspect skin to ensure that it is intact. Identify previous application site and rotate site.	Broken skin can affect the medication's absorption. Rotating site reduces irritation. Increased absorption may occur if applied to the same site.
Ensure any previous transdermal patches in situ are removed before applying next patch. Patches that contain opioid agents must be folded with adhesive sides sticking together and disposed of in a sharps container.	Ensures the individual receives the correct dose of the medication. Ensures that these patches cannot be inappropriately used by another individual.
Write date and time on the patch. Remove the adhesive backing and apply the patch onto a dry, hairless area of the individual's skin. The patch cannot be cut into smaller pieces.	It can be clearly seen the date the patch was applied. Cutting the patch into smaller pieces can affect the dose of the medication that the individual receives.

 AFTER THE SKILL

(Please refer to the Standard Steps on p. xii for related rationales.)
Communicate outcome to the individual, any ongoing care and to report any complications.
Restore the environment.
Report, record and document assessment findings, details of the skill performed and the individual's response.
Report, record and document any abnormalities and/or inability to perform the skill.
Reassess the individual to ensure there are no adverse effects/events from the skill.

Skill activity	Rationale
Record and sign for each medication administered on the NIMC/EMM system.	Prompt documentation prevents medication errors.

Safe medication management guidelines, outlined in Clinical Interest Box 20.3, should be incorporated into relevant aspects of this skill.

(ACSQHC 2012; 2019; Rebeiro et al 2021; Tollefson et al 2022)

OBSERVATION CHECKLIST: APPLYING TRANSDERMAL MEDICATIONS

STUDENT NAME: _____

CLINICAL SKILL 20.12: Applying transdermal medications

DEMONSTRATION OF: The ability to safely and correctly apply transdermal medication

If the observation checklist is being used as an assessment tool, the student will need to obtain a scale of independence for each of the performance criteria/evidence.

Independent (I)						
Supervised (S)						
Assisted (A)						
Marginal (M)						
Dependent (D)						

COMPETENCY ELEMENTS	PERFORMANCE CRITERIA/EVIDENCE	I	S	A	M	D
Preparation for the activity	Identifies indications and rationale for performing medication administration Identifies the individual using three individual identifiers: full name, DOB and UR number Ensures therapeutic interaction Gains the individual's consent Checks facility/organisation policy, resource material Validates the order on the individual's NIMC/EMM system Follows the 11 rights Locates and gathers equipment Prepares the work environment					
Performs activity informed by evidence	Reviews name of medication, dose, route, time of last administration and frequency of administration with NIMC/EMM system Verifies indication for medication Considers any medication administration requirements, contraindications Compares the medication and expiry date with the name of medication on the NIMC/EMM system three times Selects appropriate site for medication delivery Ensures that any old patches/discs that are in situ are removed before applying another patch/disc Disposes of used patches appropriately Writes the date and time on the patch Removes the adhesive backing and applies the patch onto a dry, hairless area of the individual's skin					
Applies critical thinking and reflective practice	Is able to link theory to practice Demonstrates current best practice in the care provided Assesses individual's knowledge regarding medication action and provides medication education as required and ability for self-administration Monitors individual for medication effectiveness (if applicable) Monitors individual for any adverse effects to the medication Assesses own performance Is able to link theory to practice Demonstrates current best practice in the care provided Assesses individual's knowledge regarding medication action and provides medication education as required Monitors individual for therapeutic effect of medication (if applicable) Monitors individual for any ADRs to the medication Assesses own performance					

Continued

COMPETENCY ELEMENTS	PERFORMANCE CRITERIA/EVIDENCE	I	S	A	M	D
Practises within safety and quality assurance guidelines	Reviews against facility/organisation policy and NSQHS Medication Standard Performs hand hygiene, dons appropriate PPE and uses ANTT principles Checks the expiry dates and performs calculations, as required Checks individual's allergies Cleans and disposes of equipment and waste appropriately					
Documentation and communication	Explains and communicates the activity clearly to the individual Communicates outcome and ongoing care to individual and significant others Reports any complications and/or any reason for non-administration on the NIMC/EMM system, and to the RN and/or medical officer Documents all relevant information and any complications correctly in the healthcare record: • Documents and signs for medication • Records reasons for withholding any medication • Documents in accordance with state legislation for drug of dependency Provides any special instructions Asks the individual to report any complications during and after the procedure					

Educator/Facilitator Feedback:

Educator/Facilitator Score: Competent   Needs further development

How would you rate your overall performance while undertaking this clinical activity? (use a ✓ & initial)

Unsatisfactory   Satisfactory   Good   Excellent

Student Reflection: (discuss how you would approach your practice differently or more effectively)

EDUCATOR/FACILITATOR NAME/SIGNATURE:

STUDENT NAME/SIGNATURE: **DATE:**

CLINICAL SKILL 20.13 Instilling eye drops or ointment

Please adhere to the policy and procedures of the facility/organisation prior to undertaking the skill. Ensure this skill is in your scope of practice.

NMBA Decision-making Framework considerations (refer to NMBA Decision-making framework for nursing and midwifery 2020):	Equipment:
1. Am I educated? 2. Am I authorised? 3. Am I competent? If you answer 'no' to any of these, do not perform that activity. Seek guidance and support from your teacher/a nurse team leader/clinical facilitator/educator.	NIMC/EMM system medication order Eye drops/ointment Gauze Normal saline 0.9% (if required) Disposable gloves Resource material (e.g. MIMS)

 PREPARE FOR THE SKILL

(Please refer to the Standard Steps on p. xii for related rationales.)
Mentally review the steps of the skill.
Discuss the skill with your instructor/supervisor/team leader, if required.
Confirm correct facility/organisation policy/safe operating procedures.
Validate the order in the individual's record.
Identify indication and rationale for performing the activity.
Assess for any contraindications.
Locate and gather equipment.
Perform hand hygiene.
Ensure therapeutic interaction.
Identify the individual using three individual identifiers.
Gain the individual's consent.
Assess for pain relief.
Prepare the environment.
Provide and maintain privacy.
Assist the individual to assume an appropriate position of comfort.

Skill activity	Rationale
Ensure correct medication is given by following the '11 rights' throughout preparation and administration.	Identifies issues, which can be addressed prior to administration. Prevents medication errors from occurring and promotes correct and safe administration of medication/s.
Ensure medication orders are correctly prescribed and written. Verify indication for the medication on the NIMC/EMM system. Review name of medication on the NIMC/EMM system, dose, route, time of last administration and frequency of administration. Assess for any medication contraindications; check allergy status on the medication chart and with the individual; compare with the medication ordered; check for medication interactions. Review all necessary information about the medication, including action, purpose, normal dose, side effects, any special administration information.	Ensures correct medication administration is about to take place. Ensures the nurse understands why the individual is receiving the medication and is able to ask for a review by the medical officer if the individual's health status changes. Ensures that the right medication is being given at the right frequency and time, via the correct route and prevents medication errors from occurring. Ensures all medication allergies are recorded and determines if a medication should be given. Reduces risk of allergic reactions occurring. Promotes correct and safe administration of the medication and enables the nurse to monitor the therapeutic effects of the medication.
Check medication chart for the individual's identifiers, including asking the individual to state their full name, date of birth (DOB) and then check these as well as the UR number with the ID band and NIMC/EMM system.	Confirms the individual's identity.

CLINICAL SKILL 20.13 Instilling eye drops or ointment—cont'd

 PERFORM THE SKILL

(Please refer to the Standard Steps on p. xii for related rationales.)
Perform hand hygiene.
Apply PPE: gloves, eyewear, mask and gown as appropriate.
Ensure the individual's safety and comfort throughout skill.
Promote independence and involvement of the individual if possible and/or appropriate.
Assess the individual's tolerance to the skill throughout.
Dispose of used supplies, equipment, waste and sharps appropriately.
Remove PPE and discard or store appropriately.
Perform hand hygiene.

Skill activity	Rationale
Prepare medication as per administration guidelines and calculate the correct dose. Document opening date on the container. Ensure the right medication is being administered by comparing the label of the medication and expiry date with the name on the NIMC/EMM system three times: • First check: Before removing from the trolley or cupboard • Second check: Before removing from the container • Third check: Before returning to the trolley or the cupboard, or discarding.	Following administration guidelines ensures the medication's effectiveness and the correct dosage of medication is being administered. Ocular medications are required to be discarded in a certain timeframe after opening. Ensures medication order is the same as the medication supplied. Ensures the correct medication is being administered. Prevents preparation and administration errors.
Assist the individual to a position with the head tilted well back (if possible).	Facilitates correct instillation of medication.
If eye contains any discharge or crusting, it should be cleaned with normal saline and gauze swabs before instilling drops or ointment.	Discharge or crusting prevents adequate absorption of medication.
Remove the cap of the container and hold the dropper or tube slightly away from the eye.	Avoids contacting any part of the eye and contaminating the nozzle.
Gently pull down the lower lid to form a pouch.	Facilitates correct instillation of medication.
Instil prescribed medication into the pouch of the lower lid (e.g. 1 drop BE). Five minutes should be left between administering multiple eye drops.	Medications should be instilled correctly (e.g. into the pouch of the lower lid and not directly onto the eyeball). If eye drops are administered too quickly the previous eye drops may be washed away and not absorbed.
Advise individual to close their eye and place index finger against the side of nose near the eye and apply light pressure for 60 seconds after the drop has been administered.	This helps the drop to spread over the eye and be absorbed and prevents the drops running into the nose and being swallowed.
If ointment is being instilled, the eye drops should be administered first.	Ointment waterproofs the eye.
Discard 1.25 cm of ointment onto a swab. Direct nozzle of the tube near the lid, and apply a ribbon of ointment along the rim of the lower lid.	Reduces the risk of instilling contaminated ointment.
Give individual any special instructions related to medications. Instruct to close the eyelid gently. Wipe away any excess with a gauze swab. Instruct individual to blink gently several times. Ask individual to report any side effects/complications.	Facilitates even distribution of the medication over the eye's surface. Keeps individual informed and creates an opportunity to initiate medication education. Monitors for adverse effects and ensures that complications can be prevented or addressed early.
Apply eye pad if required (see Clinical Skill 34.1).	A pad may be prescribed for comfort or protection.

Continued

CLINICAL SKILL 20.13 Instilling eye drops or ointment—cont'd

 AFTER THE SKILL

(Please refer to the Standard Steps on p. xii for related rationales.)
Communicate outcome to the individual, any ongoing care and to report any complications.
Restore the environment.
Report, record and document assessment findings, details of the skill performed and the individual's response.
Report, record and document any abnormalities and/or inability to perform the skill.
Reassess the individual to ensure there are no adverse effects/events from the skill.

Skill activity	Rationale
Record and sign for each medication administered on the NIMC/EMM system.	Prompt documentation prevents medication errors.
Safe medication management guidelines, outlined in Clinical Interest Box 20.3, should be incorporated into relevant aspects of this skill.	

(ACSQHC 2012; 2019; JBI 2021b; Rebeiro et al 2021; Tollefson et al 2022)

OBSERVATION CHECKLIST: INSTILLING EYE DROPS OR OINTMENT

STUDENT NAME: _____

CLINICAL SKILL 20.13: Instilling eye drops or ointment

DEMONSTRATION OF: The ability to safely and correctly administer eye drops or ointment

If the observation checklist is being used as an assessment tool, the student will need to obtain a scale of independence for each of the performance criteria/evidence.

	Independent (I)
	Supervised (S)
	Assisted (A)
	Marginal (M)
	Dependent (D)

COMPETENCY ELEMENTS	PERFORMANCE CRITERIA/EVIDENCE	I	S	A	M	D
Preparation for the activity	Identifies indications and rationale for performing the medication administration Identifies the individual using three individual identifiers: full name, DOB and UR number Ensures therapeutic interaction Gains the individual's consent Checks facility/organisation policy, resource material Validates the order on the individual's NIMC or EMM system Checks the 11 rights Locates and gathers equipment					
Performs activity informed by evidence	Reviews name of medication, dose, route, time of last administration and frequency of administration with NIMC/EMM system Verifies indication for medication Considers any medication administration requirements, contraindications Compares the medication and expiry date with the name of medication on the NIMC/EMM system three times Positions individual's head appropriately Cleanses the eye if required Administers the prescribed number of drops into the lower pouch of the eye Leaves five minutes between administering multiple eye drops Administers drops before eye ointment Wipes excess medication from eye					
Applies critical thinking and reflective practice	Is able to link theory to practice Demonstrates current best practice in the care provided Assesses individual's knowledge regarding medication action and provides medication education as required and ability to self-administer Monitors individual for medication effectiveness (if applicable) Monitors individual for any adverse effects to the medication Assesses own performance Is able to link theory to practice Demonstrates current best practice in the care provided Assesses individual's knowledge regarding medication action and provides medication education as required Monitors individual for therapeutic effect of medication (if applicable) Monitors individual for any ADRs to the medication Assesses own performance					

Continued

COMPETENCY ELEMENTS	PERFORMANCE CRITERIA/EVIDENCE	I	S	A	M	D
Practises within safety and quality assurance guidelines	Reviews against facility/organisation policy and NSQHS Medication Standard Performs hand hygiene, dons appropriate PPE and uses ANTT principles Checks the expiry dates and performs calculations, as required Checks individual's allergies Cleans and disposes of equipment and waste appropriately					
Documentation and communication	Explains and communicates the activity clearly to the individual Communicates outcome and ongoing care to individual and significant others Reports any complications and/or any reason for non-administration on the NIMC/EMM system, and to the RN and/or medical officer Documents all relevant information and any complications correctly in the healthcare record: • Documents and signs for medication • Records reasons for withholding any medication Provides any special instructions Asks the individual to report any complications during and post procedure					

Educator/Facilitator Feedback:

Educator/Facilitator Score: Competent   Needs further development

How would you rate your overall performance while undertaking this clinical activity? (use a ✓ & initial)

Unsatisfactory   Satisfactory   Good   Excellent

Student Reflection: (discuss how you would approach your practice differently or more effectively)

EDUCATOR/FACILITATOR NAME/SIGNATURE:

STUDENT NAME/SIGNATURE: DATE:

CLINICAL SKILL 20.14 Instilling ear drops

Please adhere to the policy and procedures of the facility/organisation prior to undertaking the skill. Ensure this skill is in your scope of practice.

NMBA Decision-making Framework considerations (refer to NMBA Decision-making framework for nursing and midwifery 2020):	Equipment:
1. Am I educated? 2. Am I authorised? 3. Am I competent? If you answer 'no' to any of these, do not perform that activity. Seek guidance and support from your teacher/a nurse team leader/clinical facilitator/educator.	NIMC/EMM system medication order Ear drops Cotton balls Cotton-tipped applicator Resource material (e.g. MIMS)

PREPARE FOR THE SKILL

(Please refer to the Standard Steps on p. xii for related rationales.)
Mentally review the steps of the skill.
Discuss the skill with your instructor/supervisor/team leader, if required.
Confirm correct facility/organisation policy/safe operating procedures.
Validate the order in the individual's record.
Identify indication and rationale for performing the activity.
Assess for any contraindications.
Locate and gather equipment.
Perform hand hygiene.
Ensure therapeutic interaction.
Identify the individual using three individual identifiers.
Gain the individual's consent.
Assess for pain relief.
Prepare the environment.
Provide and maintain privacy.
Assist the individual to assume an appropriate position of comfort.

Skill activity	Rationale
Ensure correct medication is given by following the '11 rights' throughout preparation and administration.	Identifies issues, which can be addressed prior to administration. Prevents medication errors from occurring and promotes correct and safe administration of medication/s.
Ensure medication orders are correctly prescribed and written. Verify indication for the medication on the NIMC/EMM system. Review name of medication on the NIMC/EMM system, dose, route, time of last administration and frequency of administration. Assess for any medication contraindications; check allergy status on the medication chart and with the individual; compare with the medication ordered; check for medication interactions. Review all necessary information about the medication, including action, purpose, normal dose, side effects, any special administration information.	Ensures correct medication administration is about to take place. Ensures the nurse understands why the individual is receiving the medication and is able to ask for a review by the medical officer if the individual's health status changes. Ensures that the right medication is being given at the right frequency and time, via the correct route and prevents medication errors from occurring. Ensures all medication allergies are recorded and determines if a medication should be given. Reduces risk of allergic reactions occurring. Promotes correct and safe administration of the medication and enables the nurse to monitor the therapeutic effects of the medication.
Assess individual's ability to receive the medication in the prescribed form via the prescribed route.	If the individual has an ear infection, pain, ear wax build-up or occlusion such as no ear canal, a review will need to occur to reassess the ordered route.
Check medication chart for the individual's identifiers, including asking the individual to state their full name, date of birth (DOB) and then check these as well as the UR number with the ID band and NIMC/EMM system.	Confirms the individual's identity.

CLINICAL SKILL 20.14 Instilling ear drops—cont'd

 PERFORM THE SKILL

(Please refer to the Standard Steps on p. xii for related rationales.)
Perform hand hygiene.
Apply PPE: gloves, eyewear, mask and gown as appropriate.
Ensure the individual's safety and comfort throughout skill.
Promote independence and involvement of the individual if possible and/or appropriate.
Assess the individual's tolerance to the skill throughout.
Dispose of used supplies, equipment, waste and sharps appropriately.
Remove PPE and discard or store appropriately.
Perform hand hygiene.

Skill activity	Rationale
Prepare medication as per administration guidelines and calculate the correct dose Ensure the right medication is being administered by comparing the label of the medication and expiry date with the name on the NIMC/EMM system three times: • First check: Before removing from the trolley or cupboard • Second check: Before removing from the container • Third check: Before returning to the trolley or cupboard, or discarding.	Following administration guidelines ensures the medication's effectiveness and the correct dosage of medication is being administered. Ensures medication order is the same as the medication supplied. Ensures the correct medication is being administered. Prevents preparation and administration errors.
Assist the individual to lie on the side with affected ear facing upward.	Facilitates instillation of the drops into the ear.
Inspect the ear for any wax or drainage. Wipe out gently using a cotton ball, ensuring that wax is not forced inwards.	Any occlusion will prevent drops from being evenly distributed.
Pull auricle gently up and back. For a child under three years, the earlobe is pulled down and back.	Straightens the ear canal.
Ensure drops are at room temperature. Instil prescribed number of drops ensuring they fall against the sides of the ear canal and not onto the tympanic membrane.	Cold drops may cause vertigo and nausea. Avoids discomfort.
Massage gently or apply pressure to the projection in front of the meatus (the tragus).	Ensures that the drops flow into the canal.
Wipe the outer ear free of excess drops. Place a cotton wool swab loosely into the meatus if instructed.	Promotes comfort. Prevents the medication from leaking out.

 AFTER THE SKILL

(Please refer to the Standard Steps on p. xii for related rationales.)
Communicate outcome to the individual, any ongoing care and to report any complications.
Restore the environment.
Report, record and document assessment findings, details of the skill performed and the individual's response.
Report, record and document any abnormalities and/or inability to perform the skill.
Reassess the individual to ensure there are no adverse effects/events from the skill.

Skill activity	Rationale
Instruct to lie with affected ear upwards for 10 minutes.	Prevents the medication from leaking out.
Record and sign for each medication administered on the NIMC/EMM system.	Prompt documentation prevents medication errors.
Safe medication management guidelines, outlined in Clinical Interest Box 20.3, should be incorporated into relevant aspects of this skill.	

(ACSQHC 2012; 2019; JBI 2023; Rebeiro et al 2021; Tollefson et al 2022)

OBSERVATION CHECKLIST: INSTILLING EAR DROPS

STUDENT NAME: _____

CLINICAL SKILL 20.14: Instilling ear drops

DEMONSTRATION OF: The ability to safely and correctly administer ear drops

If the observation checklist is being used as an assessment tool, the student will need to obtain a scale of independence for each of the performance criteria/evidence.

Independent (I)
Supervised (S)
Assisted (A)
Marginal (M)
Dependent (D)

COMPETENCY ELEMENTS	PERFORMANCE CRITERIA/EVIDENCE	I	S	A	M	D
Preparation for the activity	Identifies indications and rationale for performing the medication administration Identifies the individual using three individual identifiers: full name, DOB and UR number Ensures therapeutic interaction Gains the individual's consent Checks facility/organisation policy, resource material Validates the order on the individual's NIMC/EMM system Follows the 11 rights Locates and gathers equipment Prepares the work environment					
Performs activity informed by evidence	Reviews name of medication, dose, route, time of last administration and frequency of administration with NIMC/EMM system Verifies indication for medication Considers any medication administration requirements, contraindications Compares the medication and expiry date with the name of medication on the NIMC/EMM system three times Inspects the ear for any wax or drainage. Wipes out gently using a cotton bud, ensuring that wax is not forced inwards Assists the individual into an appropriate position Gently pulls the auricle up and back. For a child under three years, pulls the earlobe down and back Ensures that the drops are at room temperature. Instils the prescribed number of drops so that they fall against the sides of the canal and not on the tympanic membrane Gently massages or applies pressure to the projection in front of the meatus (the tragus) Wipes the outer ear free of excess drops If prescribed, places a cotton wool swab loosely into the meatus, or instructs the individual to lie with affected ear upwards for 10 minutes					
Applies critical thinking and reflective practice	Is able to link theory to practice Demonstrates current best practice in the care provided Assesses individual's knowledge regarding medication action and provides medication education as required Monitors individual for medication effectiveness (if applicable) Monitors individual for any ADRs to the medication Assesses own performance					

COMPETENCY ELEMENTS	PERFORMANCE CRITERIA/EVIDENCE	I	S	A	M	D
Practises within safety and quality assurance guidelines	Reviews against facility/organisation policy, and NSQHS Medication Standard Performs hand hygiene, dons appropriate PPE and uses ANTT principles Checks the expiry dates and performs calculations, as required Checks individual's allergies Cleans and disposes of equipment and waste appropriately					
Documentation and communication	Explains and communicates the activity clearly to the individual Communicates outcome and ongoing care to individual and significant others Reports any complications and/or inability to administer the medication on the NIMC/EMM system, and to the RN and/or medical officer Documents all relevant information and any complications correctly in the healthcare record: • Documents and signs for medication • Records reasons for withholding any medication Provides any special instructions Asks the individual to report any complications during and after the procedure					

Educator/Facilitator Feedback:

Educator/Facilitator Score: Competent   Needs further development

How would you rate your overall performance while undertaking this clinical activity? (use a ✓ & initial)

Unsatisfactory   Satisfactory   Good   Excellent

Student Reflection: (discuss how you would approach your practice differently or more effectively)

EDUCATOR/FACILITATOR NAME/SIGNATURE:

STUDENT NAME/SIGNATURE: DATE:

CLINICAL SKILL 20.15 Administration of a vaginal medication

Please adhere to the policy and procedures of the facility/organisation prior to undertaking the skill. Ensure this skill is in your scope of practice.

NMBA Decision-making Framework considerations (refer to NMBA Decision-making framework for nursing and midwifery 2020):	Equipment:
1. Am I educated? 2. Am I authorised? 3. Am I competent? If you answer 'no' to any of these, do not perform that activity. Seek guidance and support from your teacher/a nurse team leader/clinical facilitator/educator.	NIMC/EMM system medication order Medication Applicator Disposable gloves Tissues Perineal pad Lubricant for a suppository/pessary Resource material (e.g. MIMS)

 PREPARE FOR THE SKILL

(Please refer to the Standard Steps on p. xii for related rationales.)
Mentally review the steps of the skill.
Discuss the skill with your instructor/supervisor/team leader, if required.
Confirm correct facility/organisation policy/safe operating procedures.
Validate the order in the individual's record.
Identify indication and rationale for performing the activity.
Assess for any contraindications.
Locate and gather equipment.
Perform hand hygiene.
Ensure therapeutic interaction.
Identify the individual using three individual identifiers.
Gain the individual's consent.
Assess for pain relief.
Prepare the environment.
Provide and maintain privacy.
Assist the individual to assume an appropriate position of comfort.

Skill activity	Rationale
Ensure correct medication is given by following the '11 rights' throughout preparation and administration.	Identifies issues, which can be addressed prior to administration. Prevents medication errors from occurring and promotes correct and safe administration of medication/s.
Ensure medication orders are correctly prescribed and written. Verify indication for the medication on the NIM/EMM system. Review name of medication on the NIMC/EMM system, dose, route, time of last administration and frequency of administration. Assess for any medication contraindications; check allergy status on the medication chart and with the individual; compare with the medication ordered; check for medication interactions. Review all necessary information about the medication, including action, purpose, normal dose, side effects, any special administration information.	Ensures correct medication administration is about to take place. Ensures the nurse understands why the individual is receiving the medication and is able to ask for a review by the medical officer if the individual's health status changes. Ensures that the right medication is being given at the right frequency and time, via the correct route and prevents medication errors from occurring. Ensures all medication allergies are recorded and determines if a medication should be given. Reduces risk of allergic reactions occurring. Promotes correct and safe administration of the medication and enables the nurse to monitor the therapeutic effects of the medication.
Assess individual's ability to receive the medication in the prescribed form via the prescribed route.	If the individual has PV discharge or is menstruating a review will need to occur to reassess the ordered route.
Prepares individual and directs to empty bladder.	If the bladder is emptied, the individual may experience less discomfort. Voiding after the medication is administered may result in the medication not being retained.

Continued

CLINICAL SKILL 20.15 Administration of a vaginal medication—cont'd

Assess the individual's ability to self-administer the medication in the prescribed form via the vaginal route.	Promotes independence and avoids embarrassment and loss of privacy and dignity.
Check the medication chart for the individual's identifiers, including asking the individual to state their full name, date of birth (DOB) and then check these as well as the UR number with the ID band and NIMC/EMM system.	Confirms the individual's identity.

 PERFORM THE SKILL

(Please refer to the Standard Steps on p. xii for related rationales.)
Perform hand hygiene.
Apply PPE: gloves, eyewear, mask and gown as appropriate.
Ensure the individual's safety and comfort throughout skill.
Promote independence and involvement of the individual if possible and/or appropriate.
Assess the individual's tolerance to the skill throughout.
Dispose of used supplies, equipment, waste and sharps appropriately.
Remove PPE and discard or store appropriately.
Perform hand hygiene.

Prepare medication as per administration guidelines and calculate the correct dose. Ensure the right medication is being administered by comparing the label of the medication and expiry date with the name on the NIMC/EMM system three times: • First check: Before removing from the trolley or cupboard • Second check: Before removing from the container • Third check: Before returning to the trolley or cupboard, or discarding.	Following administration guidelines ensures the medication's effectiveness and the correct dosage of medication is being administered. Ensures medication order is the same as the medication supplied. Ensures the correct medication is being administered. Prevents preparation and administration errors.
Ensure privacy and assist the individual into the dorsal recumbent position, with legs flexed and extended apart, using a privacy towel/cover.	Privacy reduces embarrassment. Position provides easy access to and adequate exposure of the vaginal canal.
Attach applicator to the tube of cream or place the pessary in the applicator. Apply lubricant to the applicator.	Promotes correct and safe administration of the medication. Lubrication facilitates insertion.
Retract the labial folds gently or instruct individual on technique of self-administering.	Exposes the vaginal orifice. Maintains independence, and privacy and dignity.
Insert applicator into the vagina in an upwards and backwards direction, about 7.5 cm. Push plunger to deposit medication.	Proper placement ensures equal distribution of medication along the walls of the vaginal cavity.
Withdraw applicator, offer individual tissues to wipe any residual cream from labia and apply a perineal pad.	Promotes comfort; perineal pad prevents staining of clothing.

 AFTER THE SKILL

(Please refer to the Standard Steps on p. xii for related rationales.)
Communicate outcome to the individual, any ongoing care and to report any complications.
Restore the environment.
Report, record and document assessment findings, details of the skill performed and the individual's response.
Report, record and document any abnormalities and/or inability to perform the skill.
Reassess the individual to ensure there are no adverse effects/events from the skill.

CLINICAL SKILL 20.15 Administration of a vaginal medication—cont'd

Skill activity	Rationale
Encourage individual to remain in a recumbent position for at least 10 minutes after administration.	Allows medication to melt and be absorbed into the vaginal mucosa. The vagina has no sphincters, and the medications may not be retained if the individual stands immediately after administration. Medication given via the vaginal route is best administered at night for this reason.
Wash applicator in warm soapy water, rinse and dry. The applicator is stored for future use by that individual only.	Cleans applicator for next administration.
Record and sign for administration on the NIMC/EMM system.	Prompt documentation prevents medication errors.
Safe medication management guidelines, outlined in Clinical Interest Box 20.3, should be incorporated into relevant aspects of this skill.	

(ACSQHC 2012; 2019; JBI 2021f; Rebeiro et al 2021; Tollefson et al 2022)

OBSERVATION CHECKLIST: ADMINISTRATION OF A VAGINAL MEDICATION

STUDENT NAME: _____

CLINICAL SKILL 20.15: Administration of a vaginal medication

DEMONSTRATION OF: The ability to safely and correctly administer a vaginal medication

Independent (I)

Supervised (S)

Assisted (A)

Marginal (M)

Dependent (D)

If the observation checklist is being used as an assessment tool, the student will need to obtain a scale of independence for each of the performance criteria/evidence.

COMPETENCY ELEMENTS	PERFORMANCE CRITERIA/EVIDENCE	I	S	A	M	D
Preparation for the activity	Identifies indications and rationale for performing the medication administration Identifies the individual using three individual identifiers: full name, DOB and UR number Ensures therapeutic interaction Gains the individual's consent Checks facility/organisation policy, resource material Validates the order on the individual's NIMC/EMM system Follows the 11 rights Locates and gathers appropriate equipment Prepares the work environment Advises individual to empty their bladder prior to medication administration					
Performs activity informed by evidence	Reviews name of medication, dose, route, time of last administration and frequency of administration with NIMC/EMM system Verifies indication for medication Considers any medication administration requirements, contraindications Verifies name of medication, dose, route, time of last administration and frequency of administration with NIMC or EMM system Compares the medication and expiry date with the name of medication on the NIMC/EMM system three times Assesses individual's ability to self-administer Dons non-sterile gloves Assists the individual into the dorsal recumbent position, with legs flexed and extended apart Attaches the applicator to the tube of cream or places the pessary in the applicator. Applies lubricant to the applicator Inserts the applicator into the vagina in an upwards and backwards direction, about 7.5 cm. Pushes the plunger to deposit the medication Withdraws the applicator, wipes any residual cream from the labia and applies a perineal pad Advises the individual to remain in the supine position for at least 10 minutes post medication administration					

COMPETENCY ELEMENTS	PERFORMANCE CRITERIA/EVIDENCE	I	S	A	M	D
Applies critical thinking and reflective practice	Is able to link theory to practice Demonstrates current best practice in the care provided Assesses individual's knowledge regarding medication action and provides medication education as required, assesses for self-administration Monitors individual for medication effectiveness (if applicable) Monitors individual for any adverse effects to the medication Assesses own performance					
Practises within safety and quality assurance guidelines	Reviews against facility/organisation policy and NSQHS Medication Standard Performs hand hygiene, dons appropriate PPE and uses ANTT principles Checks the expiry dates and performs calculations, as required Checks individual's allergies Cleans and disposes of equipment and waste appropriately					
Documentation and communication	Explains and communicates the activity clearly to the individual Communicates outcome and ongoing care to individual and significant others Reports any complications and/or any reason for non-administration on the NIMC/EMM system, and to the RN and/or medical officer Documents all relevant information and any complications correctly in the healthcare record: • Documents and signs for medication • Records reasons for withholding any medication Provides any special instructions Asks the individual to report any complications during and after the procedure					

Educator/Facilitator Feedback:

Educator/Facilitator Score: Competent   Needs further development

How would you rate your overall performance while undertaking this clinical activity? (use a ✓ & initial)

Unsatisfactory   Satisfactory   Good   Excellent

Student Reflection: (discuss how you would approach your practice differently or more effectively)

EDUCATOR/FACILITATOR NAME/SIGNATURE:

STUDENT NAME/SIGNATURE: **DATE:**

CLINICAL SKILL 20.16 Administration of a medication via nebuliser

Please adhere to the policy and procedures of the facility/organisation prior to undertaking the skill. Ensure this skill is in your scope of practice.

NMBA Decision-making Framework considerations (refer to NMBA Decision-making framework for nursing and midwifery 2020):	Equipment:
1. Am I educated? 2. Am I authorised? 3. Am I competent? If you answer 'no' to any of these, do not perform that activity. Seek guidance and support from your teacher/a nurse team leader/clinical facilitator/educator.	NIMC/EMM system medication order Prescribed medication Nebuliser mask Nebuliser bowl Oxygen tubing FiO_2 outlet or air outlet Appropriate PPE for droplet or airborne precautions: • Disposable gloves • Mask • Protective eyewear or face shield Resource material (e.g. MIMS)

PREPARE FOR THE SKILL

(Please refer to the Standard Steps on p. xii for related rationales.)
Mentally review the steps of the skill.
Discuss the skill with your instructor/supervisor/team leader, if required.
Confirm correct facility/organisation policy/safe operating procedures.
Validate the order in the individual's record.
Identify indication and rationale for performing the activity.
Assess for any contraindications.
Locate and gather equipment.
Perform hand hygiene.
Ensure therapeutic interaction.
Identify the individual using three individual identifiers.
Gain the individual's consent.
Assess for pain relief.
Prepare the environment.
Provide and maintain privacy.
Assist the individual to assume an appropriate position of comfort.

Skill activity	Rationale
Ensure the correct medication is given by following the '11 rights' throughout preparation and administration.	Identifies issues, which can be addressed prior to administration. Prevents medication errors from occurring and promotes correct and safe administration of medication/s.
Ensure medication orders are correctly prescribed and written. Verify indication for the medication on the NIMC/EMM system. Review name of medication on the NIMC/EMM system, dose, route, time of last administration and frequency of administration. Assess for any medication contraindications; check allergy status on the medication chart and with the individual; compare with the medication ordered; check for medication interactions. Review all necessary information about the medication, including action, purpose, normal dose, side effects, any special administration information.	Ensures correct medication administration is about to take place. Ensures the nurse understands why the individual is receiving the medication and is able to ask for a review by the medical officer if the individual's health status changes. Ensures that the right medication is being given at the right frequency and time, via the correct route and prevents medication errors from occurring. Ensures all medication allergies are recorded and determines if a medication should be given. Reduces risk of allergic reactions occurring. Promotes correct and safe administration of the medication and enables the nurse to monitor the therapeutic effects of the medication.
Assess individual's ability to receive the medication in the prescribed form via the prescribed route.	If the individual is vomiting, and is not able to tolerate a nebuliser mask, a review will need to occur to reassess the ordered route.

Continued

CLINICAL SKILL 20.16 Administration of a medication via nebuliser—cont'd

Check medication chart for the individual's identifiers, including asking the individual to state their full name, date of birth (DOB) and then check these as well as the UR number with the ID band and NIMC/EMM system.	Confirms the individual's identity.
Perform any necessary assessments related to the medication such as potassium levels, chest auscultation, pulse, respiratory rate (RR) and SpO_2. Check if individual is a CO_2 retainer.	Salbutamol drives potassium into the cells and individual may have hypokalaemia. Salbutamol causes tachycardia as it stimulates the beta cells in both the lungs and heart. Assessment of lung sounds may indicate a respiratory wheeze and further assessments post dose may need to occur. An increase in respiratory rate or decrease in SpO_2 may indicate a decreased intake of O_2. Will need to use the air outlet instead of O_2 outlet as level of FiO_2 required to mist medication can decrease the respiratory drive in a person who retains CO_2. If any abnormalities are found, the nurse should not administer medication and should contact nurse in charge and medical officer.
Assess for transmission-based precautions such as airborne or droplet and PPE required: gloves, mask, and protective eyewear/face shield.	The nurse is wearing the correct PPE if individual sneezes from medication insertion since the PPE prevents contact with body fluids.

 PERFORM THE SKILL

(Please refer to the Standard Steps on p. xii for related rationales.)
Perform hand hygiene.
Apply PPE: gloves, eyewear, mask and gown as appropriate.
Ensure the individual's safety and comfort throughout skill.
Promote independence and involvement of the individual if possible and/or appropriate.
Assess the individual's tolerance to the skill throughout.
Dispose of used supplies, equipment, waste and sharps appropriately.
Remove PPE and discard or store appropriately.
Perform hand hygiene.

Skill activity	Rationale
Prepare medication as per administration guidelines and calculate the correct dose. Ensure the right medication is being administered by comparing the label of the medication and expiry date with the name on the NIMC/EMM system three times: • First check: Before removing from the trolley or cupboard • Second check: Before removing from the container • Third check: Before returning to the trolley or cupboard, or discarding.	Following administration guidelines ensures the medication's effectiveness and the correct dosage of medication is being administered. Ensures medication order is the same as the medication supplied. Ensures the correct medication is being administered. Prevents preparation and administration errors.
Assist individual into a semi-Fowler's or high Fowler's position.	Position facilitates entry of the medication into the respiratory tract.
Attach oxygen tubing to the oxygen or air outlet (if CO_2 retainer). Open the nebuliser and add medication into the nebuliser bowl.	Nebuliser can be administered using the air or the oxygen outlet. Individuals who are CO_2 retainers must not be given high doses of FiO_2.
Attach nebuliser mask to the oxygen tubing. Turn the oxygen/air on to 6–8 L/min and check that mist is coming from the nebuliser mask, and apply mask to individual's face looping the elastic straps behind the individual's head.	Setting the oxygen/air delivery to 6 L/min ensures that the medication is nebulised. Holds mask in place while medication is administered.

CLINICAL SKILL 20.16 Administration of a medication via nebuliser—cont'd

Remove mask once medication has ceased misting. Check bowl if all medication has been delivered.	Mist will no longer come from the mask once the medication has been delivered. Mask may need repositioning to allow residual medication to mist.

 AFTER THE SKILL

(Please refer to the Standard Steps on p. xii for related rationales.)
Communicate outcome to the individual, any ongoing care and to report any complications.
Restore the environment.
Report, record and document assessment findings, details of the skill performed and the individual's response.
Report, record and document any abnormalities and/or inability to perform the skill.
Reassess the individual to ensure there are no adverse effects/events from the skill.

Skill activity	Rationale
Dispose of or clean mask as per facility/organisation policy.	It is imperative that the nurse follows the facility/ organisation policy in regards to the use of nebuliser masks to ensure standard or transmission-based precautions are adhered to.
Record and sign for each medication administered on the NIMC/EMM system.	Prompt documentation prevents medication errors.

Safe medication management guidelines, outlined in Clinical Interest Box 20.3, should be incorporated into relevant aspects of this skill.

(ACSQHC 2012; 2019; 2020; Department of Health 2021; JBI 2021c; Tollefson et al 2022)

OBSERVATION CHECKLIST: ADMINISTRATION OF A MEDICATION VIA NEBULISER

STUDENT NAME: _____

CLINICAL SKILL 20.16: Administration of a medication via nebuliser

DEMONSTRATION OF: The ability to safely and correctly administer a nebulised medication

If the observation checklist is being used as an assessment tool, the student will need to obtain a scale of independence for each of the performance criteria/evidence.

Independent (I)
Supervised (S)
Assisted (A)
Marginal (M)
Dependent (D)

COMPETENCY ELEMENTS	PERFORMANCE CRITERIA/EVIDENCE	I	S	A	M	D
Preparation for the activity	Identifies indications and rationale for performing medication administration Identifies the individual using three individual identifiers: full name, DOB and UR number Ensures therapeutic interaction Gains the individual's consent Checks facility/organisation policy, resource material Validates the order on the individual's NIMC/EMM system Follows the 11 rights Checks individual's CO_2 retainer status Locates and gathers equipment Prepares the work environment					
Performs activity informed by evidence	Reviews name of medication, dose, route, time of last administration and frequency of administration with NIMC/EMM system Verifies indication for medication Considers any medication administration requirements, contraindications Compares the medication and expiry date with the name of medication on the NIMC/EMM system three times Positions individual in a position that promotes lung expansion and medication delivery Attaches the oxygen tubing to the oxygen or air outlet Opens the nebuliser and adds the medication that is to be administered to the nebuliser bowl Attaches the nebuliser mask to the oxygen tubing Turns oxygen FiO_2 6 L/min to ensure medication is nebulised or air for CO_2 retainer Removes mask once medication has been delivered					
Applies critical thinking and reflective practice	Is able to link theory to practice Demonstrates current best practice in the care provided Assesses individual's knowledge regarding medication action and provides medication education as required Monitors individual for medication effectiveness (if applicable) Monitors individual for any adverse effects to the medication Assesses own performance					

COMPETENCY ELEMENTS	PERFORMANCE CRITERIA/EVIDENCE	I	S	A	M	D
Practises within safety and quality assurance guidelines	Reviews against facility/organisation policy and NSQHS Medication Standard, and follows aerosol or droplet transmission-based precautions if required Performs hand hygiene, dons appropriate PPE and uses ANTT principles Checks the expiry dates and performs calculations, as required Checks individual's allergies Cleans and disposes of equipment and waste appropriately					
Documentation and communication	Explains and communicates the activity clearly to the individual Communicates outcome and ongoing care to individual and significant others Reports any complications and/or any reason for non-administration on the NIMC/EMM system, and to the RN and/or medical officer Documents all relevant information and any complications correctly in the healthcare record: • Documents and signs for medication • Records reasons for withholding any medication Provides any special instructions Asks the individual to report any complications during and after the procedure					

Educator/Facilitator Feedback:

Educator/Facilitator Score: Competent   Needs further development

How would you rate your overall performance while undertaking this clinical activity? (use a ✓ & initial)

Unsatisfactory   Satisfactory   Good   Excellent

Student Reflection: (discuss how you would approach your practice differently or more effectively)

EDUCATOR/FACILITATOR NAME/SIGNATURE:

STUDENT NAME/SIGNATURE: DATE:

CLINICAL SKILL 20.17 Use of a hand-held inhaler and spacer

Please adhere to the policy and procedures of the facility/organisation prior to undertaking the skill. Ensure this skill is in your scope of practice.

NMBA Decision-making Framework considerations (refer to NMBA Decision-making framework for nursing and midwifery 2020):	Equipment:
1. Am I educated? 2. Am I authorised? 3. Am I competent? If you answer 'no' to any of these, do not perform that activity. Seek guidance and support from your teacher/a nurse team leader/clinical facilitator/educator.	NIMC/EMM system medication order Medication—MDI Spacer Appropriate PPE for droplet or airborne precautions: • Disposable gloves • Mask • Protective eyewear or face shield Resource material (e.g. MIMS)

 PREPARE FOR THE SKILL

(Please refer to the Standard Steps on p. xii for related rationales.)
Mentally review the steps of the skill.
Discuss the skill with your instructor/supervisor/team leader, if required.
Confirm correct facility/organisation policy/safe operating procedures.
Validate the order in the individual's record.
Identify indication and rationale for performing the activity.
Assess for any contraindications.
Locate and gather equipment.
Perform hand hygiene.
Ensure therapeutic interaction.
Identify the individual using three individual identifiers.
Gain the individual's consent.
Assess for pain relief.
Prepare the environment.
Provide and maintain privacy.
Assist the individual to assume an appropriate position of comfort.

Skill activity	Rationale
Ensure correct medication is given by following the '11 rights' throughout preparation and administration.	Identifies issues, which can be addressed prior to administration. Prevents medication errors from occurring and promotes correct and safe administration of medication/s.
Ensure medication orders are correctly prescribed and written. Verify indication for the medication on the NIMC/EMM system. Review name of medication on the NIMC/EMM system, dose, route, time of last administration and frequency of administration. Assess for any medication contraindications; check allergy status on the medication chart and with the individual; compare with the medication ordered; check for medication interactions. Review all necessary information about the medication, including action, purpose, normal dose, side effects, any special administration information.	Ensures correct medication administration is about to take place. Ensures the nurse understands why the individual is receiving the medication and is able to ask for a review by the medical officer if the individual's health status changes. Ensures that the right medication is being given at the right frequency and time, via the correct route and prevents medication errors from occurring. Ensures all medication allergies are recorded and determines if a medication should be given. Reduces risk of allergic reactions occurring. Promotes correct and safe administration of the medication and enables the nurse to monitor the therapeutic effects of the medication.
Assess the individual's ability to self-administer the medication in the prescribed form using MDI & spacer.	Promotes independence and confidence with administration.
Check the medication chart for the individual's identifiers, including asking the individual to state their full name, date of birth (DOB) and then check these as well as the UR number with the ID band and NIMC/EMM system.	Confirms the individual's identity.

Continued

CLINICAL SKILL 20.17 Use of a hand-held inhaler and spacer—cont'd

Assess for transmission-based precautions such as airborne or droplet and PPE required: gloves, mask, and protective eyewear/face shield.	The nurse is wearing the correct PPE if individual sneezes from medication insertion and the PPE prevents contact with body fluids.

 PERFORM THE SKILL

(Please refer to the Standard Steps on p. xii for related rationales.)
Perform hand hygiene.
Apply PPE: gloves, eyewear, mask and gown as appropriate.
Ensure the individual's safety and comfort throughout skill.
Promote independence and involvement of the individual if possible and/or appropriate.
Assess the individual's tolerance to the skill throughout.
Dispose of used supplies, equipment, waste and sharps appropriately.
Remove PPE and discard or store appropriately.
Perform hand hygiene.

Skill activity	Rationale
Prepare medication as per administration guidelines and calculate the correct dose. Ensure the right medication is being administered by comparing the label of the medication and expiry date with the name on the NIMC/EMM system three times: • First check: Before removing from the trolley or cupboard • Second check: Before removing from the container • Third check: Before returning to the trolley or cupboard, or discarding.	Following administration guidelines ensures the medication's effectiveness and the correct dosage of medication is being administered. Ensures medication order is the same as the medication supplied. Ensures the correct medication is being administered. Prevents preparation and administration errors.
Assist individual into a semi-Fowler's or high Fowler's position.	Position facilitates entry of the medication into the respiratory tract.
Load MDI with canister of medication. Remove mouthpiece cap and shake MDI.	Prepares the MDI for administration of the medication. Not shaking the MDI can cause sedimentation and affect the dosage delivered.
Attach mouthpiece of inhaler into spacer.	The use of a spacer is recommended to ensure more of the medication is delivered into the respiratory tract.
Instruct individual to: • Place the mouthpiece of the spacer well into mouth, close lips firmly around it and tilt head back slightly • Start to breathe in through mouth and to press canister to deliver one puff of medication • Breathe in and out normally for four to five breaths.	Tight seal is necessary to prevent the escape of medication into the air. Ensures the whole dose is delivered into the respiratory tract.
Repeat technique if necessary until the prescribed dose has been inhaled or if a different inhaler is also required. Time between inhalations depends on which medications are being inhaled.	Time between inhalations allows deeper penetration of the second inhalation.

 AFTER THE SKILL

(Please refer to the Standard Steps on p. xii for related rationales.)
Communicate outcome to the individual, any ongoing care and to report any complications.
Restore the environment.
Report, record and document assessment findings, details of the skill performed and the individual's response.
Report, record and document any abnormalities and/or inability to perform the skill.
Reassess the individual to ensure there are no adverse effects/events from the skill.

CLINICAL SKILL 20.17 Use of a hand-held inhaler and spacer—cont'd

Skill activity	Rationale
Instruct individual to rinse their mouth after administration.	Prevents hoarseness, irritated sore throat or oropharyngeal candidiasis.
Clean mouthpiece and spacer after each use with mild soap and water. Replace the cap on the mouthpiece.	Prevents contamination of mouthpiece.
Record and sign for each medication administered on the NIMC/EMM system.	Prompt documentation prevents medication errors.
Safe medication management guidelines, outlined in Clinical Interest Box 20.3, should be incorporated into relevant aspects of this skill.	

(ACSQHC 2012; 2019; 2020; Department of Health 2021; JBI 2021a; Rebeiro et al 2021; Tollefson et al 2022)

OBSERVATION CHECKLIST: USE OF A HAND-HELD INHALER AND SPACER

STUDENT NAME: _____

CLINICAL SKILL 20.17: Use of a hand-held inhaler and spacer

DEMONSTRATION OF: The ability to safely and correctly administer a medication using a hand-held inhaler and a spacer

Independent (I)

Supervised (S)

Assisted (A)

Marginal (M)

Dependent (D)

If the observation checklist is being used as an assessment tool, the student will need to obtain a scale of independence for each of the performance criteria/evidence.

COMPETENCY ELEMENTS	PERFORMANCE CRITERIA/EVIDENCE	I	S	A	M	D
Preparation for the activity	Identifies indications and rationale for performing the medication administration Identifies the individual using three individual identifiers: full name, DOB and UR number Ensures therapeutic interaction Gains the individual's consent Checks facility/organisation policy, resource material Validates the order on the individual's NIMC/EMM system Follows the 11 rights Locates and gathers equipment Prepares the work environment					
Performs activity informed by evidence	Reviews name of medication, dose, route, time of last administration and frequency of administration with NIMC/EMM system Verifies indication for medication Considers any medication administration requirements, contraindications Compares the medication and expiry date with the name of medication on the NIMC/EMM system three times Positions individual as required Shakes inhaler and inserts into opening on spacer Asks individual to place mouth around spacer mouthpiece Presses the canister to deliver one puff of medication. Informs the individual to breathe in and out for 4–5 breaths Repeats technique if necessary. Time between inhalations depends on which medications are being inhaled Instructs the individual to rinse their mouth after administration Promotes use of a spacer to ensure delivery of medication into the respiratory tract					
Applies critical thinking and reflective practice	Is able to link theory to practice Demonstrates current best practice in the care provided Assesses individual's knowledge regarding medication action and provides medication education as required Monitors individual for medication effectiveness (if applicable) Monitors individual for any ADRs to the medication Assesses own performance					

COMPETENCY ELEMENTS	PERFORMANCE CRITERIA/EVIDENCE	I	S	A	M	D
Practises within safety and quality assurance guidelines	Reviews against facility/organisation policy, NSQHS Medication Standard and follows aerosol or droplet transmission-based precautions if required Performs hand hygiene, dons appropriate PPE and uses ANTT principles Checks the expiry dates and performs calculations, as required Checks individual's allergies Cleans and disposes of equipment and waste appropriately					
Documentation and communication	Explains and communicates the activity clearly to the individual Communicates outcome and ongoing care to individual and significant others Reports any complications and/or any reason for non-administration on the NIMC/EMM system, and to the RN and/or medical officer Documents all relevant information and any complications correctly in the healthcare record: • Documents and signs for medication • Records reasons for withholding any medication Provides any special instructions Asks the individual to report any complications during and after the procedure					

Educator/Facilitator Feedback:

Educator/Facilitator Score: Competent   Needs further development

How would you rate your overall performance while undertaking this clinical activity? (use a ✓ & initial)

Unsatisfactory   Satisfactory   Good   Excellent

Student Reflection: (discuss how you would approach your practice differently or more effectively)

EDUCATOR/FACILITATOR NAME/SIGNATURE:

STUDENT NAME/SIGNATURE: **DATE:**

CLINICAL SKILL 20.18 Administering nasal sprays and drops

Please adhere to the policy and procedures of the facility/organisation prior to undertaking the skill. Ensure this skill is in your scope of practice.

NMBA Decision-making Framework considerations (refer to NMBA Decision-making framework for nursing and midwifery 2020):	Equipment:
1. Am I educated? 2. Am I authorised? 3. Am I competent? If you answer 'no' to any of these, do not perform that activity. Seek guidance and support from your teacher/a nurse team leader/clinical facilitator/educator.	NIMC/EMM system medication order Nasal spray/drops Tissues Appropriate PPE for droplet or airborne precautions: • Disposable gloves • Mask • Protective eyewear or face shield Resource material (e.g. MIMS)

 PREPARE FOR THE SKILL

(Please refer to the Standard Steps on p. xii for related rationales.)
Mentally review the steps of the skill.
Discuss the skill with your instructor/supervisor/team leader, if required.
Confirm correct facility/organisation policy/safe operating procedures.
Validate the order in the individual's record.
Identify indication and rationale for performing the activity.
Assess for any contraindications.
Locate and gather equipment.
Perform hand hygiene.
Ensure therapeutic interaction.
Identify the individual using three individual identifiers.
Gain the individual's consent.
Assess for pain relief.
Prepare the environment.
Provide and maintain privacy.
Assist the individual to assume an appropriate position of comfort.

Skill activity	Rationale
Ensure correct medication is given by following the '11 rights' throughout preparation and administration.	Identifies issues, which can be addressed prior to administration. Prevents medication errors from occurring and promotes correct and safe administration of medication/s.
Ensure medication orders are correctly prescribed and written. Verify indication for the medication on the NIMC/EMM system. Review name of medication on the NIMC/EMM system, dose, route, time of last administration and frequency of administration. Assess for any medication contraindications; check allergy status on the medication chart and with the individual; compare with the medication ordered; check for medication interactions. Review all necessary information about the medication, including action, purpose, normal dose, side effects, any special administration information.	Ensures correct medication administration is about to take place. Ensures the nurse understands why the individual is receiving the medication and is able to ask for a review by the medical officer if the individual's health status changes. Ensures that the right medication is being given at the right frequency and time, via the correct route and prevents medication errors from occurring. Ensures all medication allergies are recorded and determines if a medication should be given. Reduces risk of allergic reactions occurring. Promotes correct and safe administration of the medication and enables the nurse to monitor the therapeutic effects of the medication.
Assess the individual's ability to self-administer the medication in the prescribed form.	Promotes independence and confidence with administration. Avoids individual being startled during administration triggering a cough or sneeze.

Continued

CLINICAL SKILL 20.18 Administering nasal sprays and drops—cont'd

Check the medication chart for the individual's identifiers, including asking the individual to state their full name, date of birth (DOB) and then check these as well as the UR number with the ID band and NIMC/EMM system.	Confirms the individual's identity with the individual and documentation.
Assess for transmission-based precautions such as airborne or droplet and PPE required: gloves, mask, and protective eyewear/face shield.	Ensures the nurse is wearing the correct PPE if individual sneezes from medication insertion since the PPE prevents contact with body fluids.

 PERFORM THE SKILL

(Please refer to the Standard Steps on p. xii for related rationales.)
Perform hand hygiene.
Apply PPE: gloves, eyewear, mask and gown as appropriate.
Ensure the individual's safety and comfort throughout skill.
Promote independence and involvement of the individual if possible and/or appropriate.
Assess the individual's tolerance to the skill throughout.
Dispose of used supplies, equipment, waste and sharps appropriately.
Remove PPE and discard or store appropriately.
Perform hand hygiene.

Skill activity	Rationale
Prepare medication as per administration guidelines and calculate the correct dose. Ensure right medication is being administered by comparing the label of the medication and expiry date with the name of medication on the NIMC or EMM system three times: • First check: Before removing from the trolley or cupboard • Second check: Before removing from the container • Third check: Before returning to the trolley or cupboard, or discarding.	Following administration guidelines ensures the medication's effectiveness and the correct dosage of medication is being administered. Ensures medication order is the same as the medication supplied. Ensures the correct medication is being administered. Prevents preparation and administration errors.
Ask individual to gently blow their nose.	Clears the nasal passages of mucus that may inhibit absorption of the medication.
Assist individual into supine position with head tilted back.	Facilitates administration of the medication.
Instil the nasal medication, aiming for the midline of the nose. Drops: hold the dropper 1 cm above the nares and instil the prescribed number of drops. Pressurised container: hold the spray container just into the nostril and press down as the individual slowly breathes in. Pump bottle: squeeze the pump as the individual inhales. Use tissues to wipe away any excess fluid.	Promotes correct administration of the medication. Promotes comfort.

 AFTER THE SKILL

(Please refer to the Standard Steps on p. xii for related rationales.)
Communicate outcome to the individual, any ongoing care and to report any complications.
Restore the environment.
Report, record and document assessment findings, details of the skill performed and the individual's response.
Report, record and document any abnormalities and/or inability to perform the skill.
Reassess the individual to ensure there are no adverse effects/events from the skill.

CLINICAL SKILL 20.18 Administering nasal sprays and drops—cont'd

Skill activity	Rationale
Advise individual to not blow their nose and to remain in the supine position for a few minutes.	Promotes absorption of the medication.
Record and sign for each medication administered on the NIMC or EMM system.	Prompt documentation prevents medication errors.
Safe medication management guidelines, outlined in Clinical Interest Box 20.3, should be incorporated into relevant aspects of this skill.	

(ACSQHC 2012; 2019; Department of Health 2021; JBI 2022d; Rebeiro et al 2021; Tollefson et al 2022)

OBSERVATION CHECKLIST: ADMINISTERING NASAL SPRAYS AND DROPS

STUDENT NAME: _____

CLINICAL SKILL 20.18: Administering nasal sprays and drops

DEMONSTRATION OF: The ability to safely and correctly administer nasal sprays and drops

If the observation checklist is being used as an assessment tool, the student will need to obtain a scale of independence for each of the performance criteria/evidence.

Independent (I)
Supervised (S)
Assisted (A)
Marginal (M)
Dependent (D)

COMPETENCY ELEMENTS	PERFORMANCE CRITERIA/EVIDENCE	I	S	A	M	D
Preparation for the activity	Identifies indications and rationale for performing medication administration Identifies the individual using three individual identifiers: full name, DOB and UR number Ensures therapeutic interaction Gains the individual's consent Checks facility/organisation policy, resource material Validates the order on the individual's NIMC/EMM system Follows the 11 rights Locates and gathers equipment Prepares the work environment					
Performs activity informed by evidence	Reviews name of medication, dose, route, time of last administration and frequency of administration with NIMC/EMM system Verifies indication for medication Considers any medication administration requirements, contraindications Compares the medication and expiry date with the name of medication on the NIMC/EMM system three times Asks the individual to gently blow their nose Assists the individual into an appropriate position: supine with head tilted back Correctly administers nasal spray or drops Uses tissues to wipe away any excess fluid and advises the individual to not blow their nose and to remain in the supine position for a few minutes					
Applies critical thinking and reflective practice	Is able to link theory to practice Demonstrates current best practice in the care provided Assesses individual's knowledge regarding medication action and provides medication education as required Assesses individual's ability to receive medication or self-administer Monitors individual for medication effectiveness (if applicable) Monitors individual for any ADRs to the medication Assesses own performance					

COMPETENCY ELEMENTS	PERFORMANCE CRITERIA/EVIDENCE	I	S	A	M	D
Practises within safety and quality assurance guidelines	Reviews against facility/organisation policy and NSQHS Medication Standard Performs hand hygiene, dons appropriate PPE and uses ANTT principles Checks the expiry dates and performs calculations, as required Checks individual's allergies Cleans and disposes of equipment and waste appropriately					
Documentation and communication	Explains and communicates the activity clearly to the individual Communicates outcome and ongoing care to individual and significant others Reports any complications and/or any reason for non-administration on the NIMC/EMM system, and to the RN and/or medical officer Documents all relevant information and any complications correctly in the healthcare record: • Documents and signs for medication • Records reasons for withholding any medication Provides any special instructions Asks the individual to report any complications during and after the procedure					

Educator/Facilitator Feedback:

Educator/Facilitator Score:　　　Competent　　　　　Needs further development

How would you rate your overall performance while undertaking this clinical activity? (use a ✓ & initial)

Unsatisfactory　　　　　　　Satisfactory　　　　Good　　　　　　Excellent

Student Reflection: (discuss how you would approach your practice differently or more effectively)

EDUCATOR/FACILITATOR NAME/SIGNATURE:

STUDENT NAME/SIGNATURE:　　　　　　　　　　　　　　　　　　　　　**DATE:**

Evolve® Answer guide for the Critical Thinking Exercises and Critical Thinking Questions in Case Studies is hosted on Evolve: http://evolve.elsevier.com/AU/Koutoukidis/Tabbner/

References

Aseptic Non-Touch Technique (ANTT) n.d. ANTT Clinical Practice Framework. Available at: <https://www.antt.org/antt-practice-framework.html>.

Australian & New Zealand Society of Blood Transfusion Ltd, 2019. *Guidelines for the administration of blood products*, 3rd ed. Australian & New Zealand Society of Blood Transfusion Ltd, Sydney.

Australian Commission on Safety and Quality in Health Care (ACSQHC), 2012. Medication safety action guide. Available at: <https://www.safetyandquality.gov.au/sites/default/files/migrated/1.1-Medication-Safety.pdf>.

Australian Commission on Safety and Quality in Health Care (ACSQHC), 2015. National standard for user-applied labelling of injectable medicines, fluids and lines. Available at: <https://www.safetyandquality.gov.au/wp-content/uploads/2015/09/National-Standard-for-User-Applied-Labelling-Aug-2015.pdf>.

Australian Commission on Safety and Quality in Health Care (ACSQHC), 2016. National terminology, abbreviations, and symbols to be used in medicines documentation (2016). Available at: <https://www.safetyandquality.gov.au/wp-content/uploads/2017/01/Recommendations-for-terminology-abbreviations-and-symbols-used-in-medicines-December-2016.pdf>.

Australian Commission on Safety and Quality in Health Care (ACSQHC), 2019. NIMC user guide. Available at: <https://www.safetyandquality.gov.au/publications-and-resources/resource-library/national-inpatient-medication-chart-nimc-user-guide>.

Australian Commission on Safety and Quality in Health Care (ACSQHC), 2020. Managing intranasal administration of medicines for patients during COVID-19. Available at: <https://www.safetyandquality.gov.au/sites/default/files/2020-05/covid-19_-_position_statement_-_intranasal_medicines.pdf>.

Australian Commission on Safety and Quality in Health Care (ACSQHC), 2021. National Safety and Quality Health Service Standards, 2nd edn. ACSQHC, Sydney. Available at: <https://www.safetyandquality.gov.au/publications-and-resources/resource-library/national-safety-and-quality-health-service-standards-second-edition>.

Australian Commission on Safety and Quality in Health Care (ACSQHC), 2023. APINCHS classification of high risk medicines. Available at: <https://www.safetyandquality.gov.au/our-work/medication-safety/high-risk-medicines/apinchs-classification-high-risk-medicines>.

Department of Health, 2018. Royal Melbourne Hospital blood component prescription includes consent. Available at: <https://www.health.vic.gov.au/publications/royal-melbourne-hospital-blood-component-prescription-includes-consent-pdf>.

Department of Health, 2021. Infection control – standard and transmission-based precautions. Available at: <https://www.health.vic.gov.au/infectious-diseases/infection-control-standard-and-transmission-based-precautions>.

Frotjold, A., Bloomfield, J., 2021. Medication therapy. In: Crisp, J., Douglas, C., Rebeiro, G., et al. (eds.), *Potter and Perry's fundamentals of nursing*, ANZ ed, 6th ed. Elsevier, Chatswood.

Gorski, L.A., 2023. *Phillips's manual of IV therapeutics: Evidence-based practice for infusion therapy*, 8th ed. F.A. Davis Company, Philadelphia.

Joanna Briggs Institute (JBI), 2021a. Aerosol inhaler (puffer) techniques. (JBI2115.) Available at: <https://jbi.global/ebp>.

Joanna Briggs Institute (JBI), 2021b. Eye medication: Administration. (JBI2172.) Available at: <https://jbi.global/ebp>.

Joanna Briggs Institute (JBI), 2021c. Inhalation therapy (nebulizer). (JBI2149.) Available at: <https://jbi.global/ebp>.

Joanna Briggs Institute (JBI), 2021d. Intramuscular injection. (JBI2138.) Available at: <https://jbi.global/ebp>.

Joanna Briggs Institute (JBI), 2021e. Transfusion: Blood or blood product. (JBI1846.) Available at: <https://jbi.global/ebp>.

Joanna Briggs Institute (JBI), 2021f. Vaginal medication. (JBI1999.) Available at: <https://jbi.global/ebp>.

Joanna Briggs Institute (JBI), 2022a. Enema: Disposable (Older Adult). (JBI2129.) Available at: <https://jbi.global/ebp>.

Joanna Briggs Institute (JBI), 2022b. Enteral tube: Administration of medication. (JBI23655.) Available at: <https://jbi.global/ebp>.

Joanna Briggs Institute (JBI), 2022c. Medication administration: Oral. (JBI2144.) Available at: <https://jbi.global/ebp>.

Joanna Briggs Institute (JBI), 2022d. Nasal medications. (JBI1968.) Available at: <https://jbi.global/ebp>.

Joanna Briggs Institute (JBI), 2022e. Peripheral intravenous cannula: Removal. (JBI14047.) Available at: <https://jbi.global/ebp>.

Joanna Briggs Institute (JBI), 2022f. Subcutaneous injection. (JBI1964.) Available at: <https://jbi.global/ebp>.

Joanna Briggs Institute (JBI), 2022g. Topical medications. (JBI1962.) Available at: <https://jbi.global/ebp>.

Joanna Briggs Institute (JBI), 2023. Ear drops instillation. (JBI2337.) Available at: <https://jbi.global/ebp>.

Nursing and Midwifery Board of Australia (NMBA), 2020. Decision-making framework for nursing and midwifery. Available at: <https://www.nursingmidwiferyboard.gov.au/Codes-Guidelines-Statements/Frameworks.aspx>.

Queensland Health, 2018. Guideline: Peripheral Intravenous Catheter (PIVC). Available at: <https://www.health.qld.gov.au/__data/assets/pdf_file/0025/444490/icare-pivc-guideline.pdf>.

Rebeiro, G., Wilson, D., Fuller, S., 2021. *Potter and Perry's fundamentals of nursing workbook*, 4th ed. Elsevier, Chatswood.

South Eastern Sydney Local Health District (SESLHD), 2019. Infective complications – Mandatory reporting requirements of peripheral intravenous cannula (PIVC) or/central venous access device (CVAD) infections in the incident information management systems (IIMS). Available at: <https://www.seslhd.health.nsw.gov.au/sites/default/files/documents/SESLHDPD%20280.pdf>.

The Agency for Clinical Innovation and the Gastroenterological Nurses College of Australia, 2015. A clinician's guide: Caring for people with gastrostomy tubes and devices. Available at: <https://aci.health.nsw.gov.au/__data/assets/pdf_file/0017/251063/ACI-Clinicians-guide-caring-people-gastrostomy-tubes-devices.pdf>.

The Society of Hospital Pharmacists of Australia (SHPA), 2022. *Don't rush to crush*, 4th ed. SHPA, South Melbourne.

The Society of Hospital Pharmacists of Australia (SHPA), 2023. *Australian injectable drugs handbook*, 8th ed. SHPA, South Melbourne.

Tollefson, J., Watson, G., Jelly, E., et al., 2022. *Essential clinical skills: Enrolled Nurses*, 5th ed. Cengage Learning, Australia.

Williams, P.A., 2022. *deWit's fundamental concepts and skills for nursing*, 6th ed. Elsevier Saunders, Philadelphia.

World Health Organization, 2019. 10 facts on patient safety. Available at: <https://www.who.int/news-room/photo-story/photo-story-detail/10-facts-on-patient-safety>.

Online Resources and Recommended Reading

Australian Commission on Safety and Quality in Health Care (ACSQHC), 2020. Managing intranasal administration of medicines for patients during COVID-19. Available at <https://www.safetyandquality.gov.au/sites/default/files/2020-05/covid-19_-_position_statement_-_intranasal_medicines.pdf>.

Blood Safe e-learning Australia, 2018. Clinical transfusion practice. Available at: <https://learn.bloodsafelearning.org.au/course/details/ctp>.

Broyles, B., Reiss, B., Evans, M., et al., 2019. *Pharmacology in nursing: Australian and New Zealand edition*, 3rd ed. Cengage Learning Australia, Melbourne.

Department of Health and Aged Care, Therapeutic Goods Administration (TGA), 2023. Therapeutic Goods (Poisons Standard—February 2023) Instrument 2023. Available at: <https://www.tga.gov.au/publication/poisons-standard-susmp>.

Department of Health and Wellbeing, Government of South Australia, 2023. South Australian Paediatric Clinical Practice Guidelines. Available at: <https://www.sahealth.sa.gov.au/wps/wcm/connect/fbce826b-e137-4716-a2c0-72c7e70a0e3c/Intravenous+%28IV%29+Fluid+Management+in+Children_Paed_v1_0.pdf?MOD=AJPERES&CACHEID=ROOTWORKSPACE-fbce826b-e137-4716-a2c0-72c7e70a0e3c-ocQI.X2>.

MacDowell, P., Cabri, A., Davis. M., 2021. Medication Administration Errors. Available at: <https://psnet.ahrq.gov/primer/medication-administration-errors>.

National Institute of Standards and Technology (NIST), 2019. International system of units (SI). Available at: <https://physics.nist.gov/cuu/Units/index.html>.

Nursing and Midwifery Board of Australia (NMBA), 2016. Enrolled nurse standards for practice. Available at: <https://www.nursingmidwiferyboard.gov.au/Codes-Guidelines-Statements/Professional-standards/enrolled-nurse-standards-for-practice.aspx>.

World Health Organization, 2023. Promoting rational use of medicines. <https://www.who.int/activities/promoting-rational-use-of-medicines#:,:text=Rational%20use%20of%20medicines%20requires,to%20them%20and%20their%20community>.

CARDIOVASCULAR AND RESPIRATORY HEALTH

Kylie Porritt

Overview

Oxygen is an essential gas required by the human body to survive. The body's oxygen demands are supplied by the cardiovascular system (which transports oxygen to cells and tissue through the body's circulation) and the respiratory system (which is involved in the processes of ventilation, re-oxygenation, transport of respiratory gases and perfusion).

The process of oxygenation occurs as follows:
- De-oxygenated blood enters the right side of the heart via the venous circulation (the inferior and superior vena cava) and enters the pulmonary circulation via the pulmonary artery
- Through the process of respiration, carbon dioxide (CO_2) (excreted) and oxygen (O_2) (absorbed) are exchanged in the alveoli via the capillaries
- The oxygenated blood is then transported via the pulmonary vein to the left side of the heart, where it re-enters the circulation via the aorta and the arterial circulation.

Oxygen is a drug that is not routinely prescribed on a medication chart. It must be ordered (either written or verbal) by a medical officer: the amount (L/min), concentration (FiO_2) and the delivery method. However, oxygen can be administered based on a nurse's initiative in an emergency situation following consultation/collaboration with a Registered Nurse (RN) and based on the organisation's policies and procedures.

Oxygen should only be prescribed for hypoxaemia (low oxyhaemoglobin concentration in the arterial blood) and is routinely administered to individuals who are postoperative or experiencing the following signs of respiratory distress: dyspnoea, tachypnoea, bradypnoea, apnoea; pallor, cyanosis; lethargy or restlessness; use of accessory muscles—nasal flaring, intercostal or sternal recession, tracheal tug; chest pain.

Prior to any commencement of oxygen therapy a thorough health assessment must be undertaken and consideration given to the individual's past medical history, including any pulmonary or cardiac conditions (Crisp et al 2021). Individuals who are O_2 retainers should be approached with caution in regard to oxygen therapy due to their hypoxic drive, and any signs of hypercapnia (high O_2 concentrations in the blood) should be monitored. These signs include restlessness, headache, hypertension, lethargy and tremor. Health professionals may perform a set of arterial blood gases (ABGs) to gather baseline data in order to prescribe the correct concentration of oxygen to be delivered (Pinsky et al 2019).

CASE STUDY 25.2

Margaret, an 81-year-old female, has been admitted to the hospital due to atrial fibrillation. She has a history of ischemic heart disease, chronic obstructive pulmonary disease (COPD), and hypertension. This morning, she had managed to walk to the bathroom for her morning routine but is now complaining of increasing shortness of breath. Her respirations have increased, and she is speaking in short, 1–2-word sentences. Margaret's ankles are swollen, and her heart rate is elevated.

1. What are your first actions?
2. Who would you notify?
3. What test may be undertaken to assist with the management plan of this individual?

CRITICAL THINKING EXERCISE 25.1

A 25-year-old male is brought into the emergency department by ambulance following a motor vehicle accident. The paramedic reports that the male's oxygen saturation levels are currently within normal limits, but they have been decreasing, and he is experiencing increasing difficulty in breathing. Upon assessment, you observe that he has an elevated respiratory rate, unusual breathing patterns, shortness of breath and reports chest tightness. What nursing procedures would you implement to alleviate his respiratory distress?

CLINICAL SKILL 25.1 Performing an ECG

Please adhere to the policy and procedures of the facility/organisation prior to undertaking the skill. Ensure this skill is in your scope of practice.

NMBA Decision-making Framework considerations (refer to NMBA Decision-making framework for nursing and midwifery 2020):	Equipment:
1. Am I educated? 2. Am I authorised? 3. Am I competent? If you answer 'no' to any of these, do not perform that activity. Seek guidance and support from your teacher/a nurse team leader/clinical facilitator/educator.	ECG machine Electrodes Gauze squares/tissues Razor/hair clippers Conduction gel Covering to maintain privacy/modesty

 PREPARE FOR THE SKILL

(Please refer to the Standard Steps on p. xii for related rationales.)
Mentally review the steps of the skill.
Discuss the skill with your instructor/supervisor/team leader, if required.
Confirm correct facility/organisation policy/safe operating procedures.
Validate the order in the individual's record.
Identify indication and rationale for performing the activity.
Assess for any contraindications.
Locate and gather equipment.
Perform hand hygiene.
Ensure therapeutic interaction.
Identify the individual using three individual identifiers.
Gain the individual's consent.
Assess for pain relief.
Prepare the environment.
Provide and maintain privacy.
Assist the individual to assume an appropriate position of comfort.

Skill activity	Rationale
Position in supine position, head supported. Make note if the person has chest pain. Loosen or remove clothing above the waistline. Remove jewellery (including piercings). **Note:** If the individual has breathing difficulties position in the semi-Fowler's position.	Ensures an accurate ECG can be taken, and helps reduces the amount of artefact.

 PERFORM THE SKILL

(Please refer to the Standard Steps on p. xii for related rationales.)
Perform hand hygiene.
Apply PPE: gloves, eyewear, mask and gown as appropriate.
Ensure the individual's safety and comfort throughout skill.
Promote independence and involvement of the individual if possible and/or appropriate.
Assess the individual's tolerance to the skill throughout.
Dispose of used supplies, equipment, waste and sharps appropriately.
Remove PPE and discard or store appropriately.
Perform hand hygiene.

Skill activity	Rationale
Attach limb leads to clean, hair-free sites on arms and legs.	Area chosen should be over fleshy, not bony, tissue. Skin needs to be clean to ensure the best conduction of electrical impulses. If skin is unclean or wet, use an alcohol swab or soap and water to clean and dry the sites for electrode placement. Excess hair is removed as it prevents adequate contact with the skin.

Continued

CLINICAL SKILL 25.1 Performing an ECG—cont'd

Determine chest sites and attach electrodes to clean, dry, hair-free sites. V_1—4th intercostal space, right sternal border V_2—4th intercostal space, left sternal border V_3—5th intercostal space, left sternal border V_4—5th intercostal space, left mid-clavicular line V_5—5th intercostal space, left anterior axillary line V_6—5th intercostal space, left mid-axillary line	**Note:** Care must be taken that the electrodes are accurately placed, since errors in diagnosis can occur if the electrodes are incorrectly placed. If the individual has large breasts, place under the breasts.
Attach lead wires to all electrodes.	Attaching the electrodes to the leads ensures the electrical activity is conducted to the ECG machine.
Follow manufacturer's instructions for calibrating and preparing the ECG machine.	Machines may be single channel or multichannel. Familiarity with the machine will increase accuracy of recording and decrease individual and nurse stress.
Ask the individual to relax, refrain from moving and breathe normally. Record ECG and provide to RN for review.	Lack of experience and ability in interpreting an ECG recording might lead the nurse to overlook changes that are significant. RN can also compare ECG to any previous ECGs.
Remove electrodes and conduction gel.	Increases comfort.

 AFTER THE SKILL

(Please refer to the Standard Steps on p. xii for related rationales.)
Communicate outcome to the individual, any ongoing care and to report any complications.
Restore the environment.
Report, record and document assessment findings, details of the skill performed and the individual's response.
Report, record and document any abnormalities and/or inability to perform the skill.
Reassess the individual to ensure there are no adverse effects/events from the skill.

Skill activity	Rationale
Document on ECG—actual recording, noting name, medical record number, doctor, date and time. Some machines have the ability to program this information so that it is printed out on the ECG recording. Document if individual was pain free or had chest pain during procedure.	Medicolegal requirement. Allows for the planning and implementation of care.

(Aitken et al 2019; Menzies-Gow 2018; Perry et al 2022; Rebeiro et al 2021)

OBSERVATION CHECKLIST: PERFORMING AN ECG

STUDENT NAME: _____

CLINICAL SKILL 25.1: Performing an ECG

DEMONSTRATION OF: The ability to effectively and safely record an electrocardiograph (ECG) on an individual

If the observation checklist is being used as an assessment tool, the student will need to obtain a scale of independence for each of the performance criteria/evidence.

Independent (I)

Supervised (S)

Assisted (A)

Marginal (M)

Dependent (D)

COMPETENCY ELEMENTS	PERFORMANCE CRITERIA/EVIDENCE	I	S	A	M	D
Preparation for the activity	Identifies indications and rationale for performing the activity Identifies the individual using three individual identifiers Ensures therapeutic interaction Gains the individual's consent Checks facility/organisation policy Validates the order in the individual's record Locates and gathers equipment Assists the individual into an appropriate position					
Performs activity informed by evidence	Applies electrodes in correct placement Connects ECG leads to correct electrodes Enters person's details as per manufacturer's settings Records ECG and reports to experienced RN/medical officer Removes electrodes and conduction gel Cleans used equipment Ensures person's comfort and informs of procedure result Restores environment to pre-procedure state					
Applies critical thinking and reflective practice	Is able to link theory to practice Demonstrates current best practice in the care provided Demonstrates critical thinking (e.g. is the individual able to lie flat; if amputated limbs, modifies the limb leads and documents accordingly; places electrodes under breast tissue to obtain correct anatomical position; shaves large amounts of hair on chest to ensure correct attachment of electrodes) Assesses own performance					
Practises within safety and quality assurance guidelines	Reviews against facility/organisation policy Performs hand hygiene, dons appropriate PPE as per infection control protocols Raises the bed to the appropriate working position based on nurse's height and lowers at completion of activity Cleans and disposes of equipment and waste appropriately					
Documentation and communication	Explains and communicates the activity clearly to the individual Communicates abnormal findings to appropriate personnel Reports and documents all relevant information and any complications correctly in the healthcare record: Documents procedure and associated complications (pain) Reports any complications and/or inability to perform the procedure to the RN and/or medical officer Records and prints ECG with person's name, date of birth (DOB), sex and medical record number Asks the individual to report any complications during and post procedure					

Educator/Facilitator Feedback:

Educator/Facilitator Score: Competent Needs further development

How would you rate your overall performance while undertaking this clinical activity? (use a ✓ & initial)

Unsatisfactory Satisfactory Good Excellent

Student Reflection: (discuss how you would approach your practice differently or more effectively)

EDUCATOR/FACILITATOR NAME/SIGNATURE:

STUDENT NAME/SIGNATURE: DATE:

CLINICAL SKILL 25.2 Incentive spirometry

Please adhere to the policy and procedures of the facility/organisation prior to undertaking the skill. Ensure this skill is in your scope of practice.

NMBA Decision-making Framework considerations (refer to NMBA Decision-making framework for nursing and midwifery 2020):	Equipment:
1. Am I educated? 2. Am I authorised? 3. Am I competent? If you answer 'no' to any of these, do not perform that activity. Seek guidance and support from your teacher/a nurse team leader/clinical facilitator/educator.	Incentive spirometer Disposable mouthpiece/tube

 ### PREPARE FOR THE SKILL

(Please refer to the Standard Steps on p. xii for related rationales.)
Mentally review the steps of the skill.
Discuss the skill with your instructor/supervisor/team leader, if required.
Confirm correct facility/organisation policy/safe operating procedures.
Validate the order in the individual's record.
Identify indication and rationale for performing the activity.
Assess for any contraindications.
Locate and gather equipment.
Perform hand hygiene.
Ensure therapeutic interaction.
Identify the individual using three individual identifiers.
Gain the individual's consent.
Assess for pain relief.
Prepare the environment.
Provide and maintain privacy.
Assist the individual to assume an appropriate position of comfort .

Skill activity	Rationale
Sit individual into an upright position (if able) and lean forwards either on side of the bed or in a chair.	Facilitates breathing and lung expansion.

 ### PERFORM THE SKILL

(Please refer to the Standard Steps on p. xii for related rationales.)
Perform hand hygiene.
Apply PPE: gloves, eyewear, mask and gown as appropriate.
Ensure the individual's safety and comfort throughout skill.
Promote independence and involvement of the individual if possible and/or appropriate.
Assess the individual's tolerance to the skill throughout.
Dispose of used supplies, equipment, waste and sharps appropriately.
Remove PPE and discard or store appropriately.
Perform hand hygiene.

Skill activity	Rationale
Instruct the individual to practise inhaling and exhaling three times, letting all of their last breath out. Ask them to place their lips over the mouthpiece of the spirometer.	Enables the person to practise inhaling and exhaling. Allows for more accurate results.
Instruct the individual to inhale slowly (elevating the balls or cylinder) and hold their breath for 2–3 seconds, then exhale slowly.	Slow breathing prevents or minimises pain from sudden pressure change in the chest Holding their breath and slowing exhalation helps to maintain maximal inspiration and reduces the risk of progressive collapse of individual alveoli. Prevents anxiety.

Continued

CLINICAL SKILL 25.2 Incentive spirometry—cont'd

Ask the person to remove the mouthpiece, and relax and breathe slowly for a few seconds.	Alleviates anxiety and relaxes chest.
Repeat for a total of 10 times every hour or as indicated by the doctor/physiotherapist If they feel light-headed or dizzy, ask the individual to slow down their breathing and wait longer intervals between cycles. Once 10 cycles have been completed ask the individual to cough up and expectorate any sputum.	Allows for chest clearance and proper expansion of the lungs and prevents atelectasis. Coughing can facilitate removal of any secretions. Feeling light-headed and dizzy is a normal reaction; provide reassurance to alleviate anxiety.

 AFTER THE SKILL

(Please refer to the Standard Steps on p. xii for related rationales.)
Communicate outcome to the individual, any ongoing care and to report any complications.
Restore the environment.
Report, record and document assessment findings, details of the skill performed and the individual's response.
Report, record and document any abnormalities and/or inability to perform the skill.
Reassess the individual to ensure there are no adverse effects/events from the skill.

(Crisp et al 2021; Perry et al 2022)

OBSERVATION CHECKLIST: INCENTIVE SPIROMETRY

STUDENT NAME: _____

CLINICAL SKILL 25.2: Incentive spirometry

DEMONSTRATION OF: The ability to effectively and safely perform incentive spirometry

If the observation checklist is being used as an assessment tool, the student will need to obtain a scale of independence for each of the performance criteria/evidence.

Independent (I)
Supervised (S)
Assisted (A)
Marginal (M)
Dependent (D)

COMPETENCY ELEMENTS	PERFORMANCE CRITERIA/EVIDENCE	I	S	A	M	D
Preparation for the activity	Identifies indications and rationale for performing the activity Identifies the individual using three individual identifiers Ensures therapeutic interaction Gains the individual's consent Checks facility/organisation policy Validates the order in the individual's record Locates and gathers equipment Assists the individual into an appropriate position					
Performs activity informed by evidence	Instructs the individual to practise inhaling and exhaling three times, letting all of their last breath out Asks individual to place their lips over the mouthpiece of the spirometer Instructs the individual to inhale slowly (elevating the balls or cylinder), hold their breath for 2–3 seconds, then exhale slowly Asks the person to remove the mouthpiece and relax and breathe slowly for a few seconds Instructs to repeat for a total of 10 times every hour or as indicated by the medical officer/physiotherapist Asks the individual to slow down their breathing and wait longer intervals between cycles if they feel light-headed or dizzy Asks the individual to cough up and expectorate any sputum once 10 cycles have been completed Cleans used equipment Ensures person's comfort and informs of procedure result Restores environment to pre-procedure state					
Applies critical thinking and reflective practice	Is able to link theory to practice Demonstrates current best practice in the care provided Assesses own performance					
Practises within safety and quality assurance guidelines	Reviews against facility/organisation policy Performs hand hygiene Raises the bed to the appropriate working position based on nurse's height and lowers at completion of activity Cleans and disposes of equipment and waste appropriately					
Documentation and communication	Explains and communicates the activity clearly to the individual Communicates outcome and ongoing care to individual and significant others Reports and documents all relevant information and any complications correctly in the healthcare record Communicates abnormal findings to appropriate personnel Reports any complications and/or inability to perform the procedure to the RN and/or medical officer					

Educator/Facilitator Feedback:

Educator/Facilitator Score: Competent   Needs further development

How would you rate your overall performance while undertaking this clinical activity? (use a ✓ & initial)

Unsatisfactory   Satisfactory   Good   Excellent

Student Reflection: (discuss how you would approach your practice differently or more effectively)

EDUCATOR/FACILITATOR NAME/SIGNATURE:

STUDENT NAME/SIGNATURE: **DATE:**

CLINICAL SKILL 25.3 Collection of sputum

Please adhere to the policy and procedures of the facility/organisation prior to undertaking the skill. Ensure this skill is in your scope of practice.

NMBA Decision-making Framework considerations (refer to NMBA Decision-making framework for nursing and midwifery 2020):	Equipment:
1. Am I educated? 2. Am I authorised? 3. Am I competent? If you answer 'no' to any of these, do not perform that activity. Seek guidance and support from your teacher/a nurse team leader/clinical facilitator/educator.	Disposable gloves Sterile specimen container Tissues Biohazard bag Pathology form—completed by the medical officer Mouth care equipment

 PREPARE FOR THE SKILL

(Please refer to the Standard Steps on p. xii for related rationales.)
Mentally review the steps of the skill.
Discuss the skill with your instructor/supervisor/team leader, if required.
Confirm correct facility/organisation policy/safe operating procedures.
Validate the order in the individual's record.
Identify indication and rationale for performing the activity.
Assess for any contraindications.
Locate and gather equipment. Perform hand hygiene.
Ensure therapeutic interaction.
Identify the individual using three individual identifiers.
Gain the individual's consent.
Assess for pain relief.
Prepare the environment.
Provide and maintain privacy.
Assist the individual to assume an appropriate position of comfort.

Skill activity	Rationale
Check the pathology form, ensuring that it is completed, and verify details with the individual.	Ensures need for the procedure and prevents errors.
Assist the person to a sitting position. Offer mouth care/rinse out the mouth with water.	Facilitates coughing and expectoration. Reduces contamination of the specimen with any debris in the mouth.

 PERFORM THE SKILL

(Please refer to the Standard Steps on p. xii for related rationales.)
Perform hand hygiene.
Apply PPE: gloves, eyewear, mask and gown as appropriate.
Ensure the individual's safety and comfort throughout skill.
Promote independence and involvement of the individual if possible and/or appropriate.
Assess the individual's tolerance to the skill throughout.
Dispose of used supplies, equipment, waste and sharps appropriately.
Remove PPE and discard or store appropriately.
Perform hand hygiene.

Skill activity	Rationale
Ask the person to start deep breathing and coughing to help facilitate sputum expectoration.	Facilitates coughing and expectoration. A normal saline nebuliser (if ordered) may be required to help loosen sputum and facilitate expectoration.
Instruct the person to cough and to expectorate 15–30 mL of sputum into a sterile specimen container.	A sterile container ensures that the specimen is not contaminated.

Continued

CLINICAL SKILL 25.3 Collection of sputum—cont'd

Place the lid on the container, wipe the outside of the container if contaminated.	Prevents cross-infection.
Ensure that the container is clearly labelled with the relevant information. Specimen container is placed in the zip lock section of the plastic biohazard bag.	Ensures the correct person's sputum is tested to avoid errors.
Pathology request form is checked for the person's details. The pathology request form is placed in the other section of the bag.	Ensures correct form and specimen are sent to pathology department and correct test will be undertaken in the pathology department.
Offer/perform oral hygiene using a mouth swab and/or mouth rinse.	Reduces bad taste or halitosis in mouth. Clears the mouth of residual secretions.

 AFTER THE SKILL

(Please refer to the Standard Steps on p. xii for related rationales.)
Communicate outcome to the individual, any ongoing care and to report any complications.
Restore the environment.
Report, record and document assessment findings, details of the skill performed and the individual's response.
Report, record and document any abnormalities and/or inability to perform the skill.
Reassess the individual to ensure there are no adverse effects/events from the skill.

Skill activity	Rationale
The specimen should be transported to the laboratory as soon as possible, or stored in a refrigerator until transport can be arranged.	Proliferation of microorganisms occurs if the specimen is not dispatched as soon as possible after collection.

(Carter & Notter 2024; Perry et al 2022)

OBSERVATION CHECKLIST: COLLECTION OF SPUTUM

STUDENT NAME: _____

CLINICAL SKILL 25.3: Collection of sputum

DEMONSTRATION OF: The ability to effectively and safely collect sputum

If the observation checklist is being used as an assessment tool, the student will need to obtain a scale of independence for each of the performance criteria/evidence.

Independent (I)

Supervised (S)

Assisted (A)

Marginal (M)

Dependent (D)

COMPETENCY ELEMENTS	PERFORMANCE CRITERIA/EVIDENCE	I	S	A	M	D
Preparation for the activity	Identifies indications and rationale for performing the activity Checks pathology request form Identifies the individual using three individual identifiers Ensures therapeutic interaction Gains the individual's consent Checks facility/organisation policy Validates the order in the individual's record Locates and gathers equipment					
Performs activity informed by evidence	Assists the individual to a sitting position Offers mouth care/rinses out the mouth with water Asks the individual to start deep breathing and coughing to help facilitate sputum expectoration Instructs the individual to cough and to expectorate 15–30 mL of sputum into a sterile specimen container Labels the specimen and dispatches correctly					
Applies critical thinking and reflective practice	Is able to link theory to practice Demonstrates current best practice in the care provided Assesses the individual's ability to expectorate sputum without suction Ensures individual is in upright position Monitors the individual's anxiety related to the procedure Assesses the individual's ability to cooperate with the procedure Assesses own performance					
Practises within safety and quality assurance guidelines	Reviews against facility/organisation policy Performs hand hygiene, dons appropriate PPE as per infection control protocols Cleans and disposes of equipment and waste appropriately					
Documentation and communication	Explains and communicates the activity clearly to the individual Communicates outcome and ongoing care to individual and significant others Communicates abnormal findings to appropriate personnel Reports and documents all relevant information and any complications correctly in the healthcare record Reports any complications and/or inability to perform the procedure to the RN and/or medical officer Asks the individual to report any complications during procedure if able					

Educator/Facilitator Feedback:

Educator/Facilitator Score: Competent Needs further development

How would you rate your overall performance while undertaking this clinical activity? (use a ✓ & initial)

Unsatisfactory Satisfactory Good Excellent

Student Reflection: (discuss how you would approach your practice differently or more effectively)

EDUCATOR/FACILITATOR NAME/SIGNATURE:

STUDENT NAME/SIGNATURE: DATE:

CLINICAL SKILL 25.4 Collecting a nasopharyngeal (nasal) or nasalpharynx (throat) swab

Please adhere to the policy and procedures of the facility/organisation prior to undertaking the skill. Ensure this skill is in your scope of practice.

NMBA Decision-making Framework considerations (refer to NMBA Decision-making framework for nursing and midwifery 2020):	Equipment:
1. Am I educated? 2. Am I authorised? 3. Am I competent? If you answer 'no' to any of these, do not perform that activity. Seek guidance and support from your teacher/a nurse team leader/clinical facilitator/educator.	Disposable gloves Pathology form completed by medical officer Tissues Biohazard bag Normal saline 0.9% Penlight torch Tongue depressor Throat swab

PREPARE FOR THE SKILL

(Please refer to the Standard Steps on p. xii for related rationales.)
Mentally review the steps of the skill.
Discuss the skill with your instructor/supervisor/team leader, if required.
Confirm correct facility/organisation policy/safe operating procedures.
Validate the order in the individual's record.
Identify indication and rationale for performing the activity.
Assess for any contraindications.
Locate and gather equipment.
Perform hand hygiene.
Ensure therapeutic interaction.
Identify the individual using three individual identifiers.
Gain the individual's consent.
Assess for pain relief.
Prepare the environment.
Provide and maintain privacy.
Assist the individual to assume an appropriate position of comfort.

Skill activity	Rationale
Check the pathology form, ensuring that it is completed, and verify details with the individual.	Ensures need for the procedure and prevents errors.
Inform the individual that they may experience the urge to sneeze or gag during the swabbing.	Reduces anxiety/apprehension and gains trust and cooperation. Promotes participation in care and understanding of health status.
Assist the person, if possible, to a sitting position.	Facilitates collection of the specimen.

PERFORM THE SKILL

(Please refer to the Standard Steps on p. xii for related rationales.)
Perform hand hygiene.
Apply PPE: gloves, eyewear, mask and gown as appropriate.
Ensure the individual's safety and comfort throughout skill.
Promote independence and involvement of the individual if possible and/or appropriate.
Assess the individual's tolerance to the skill throughout.
Dispose of used supplies, equipment, waste and sharps appropriately.
Remove PPE and discard or store appropriately.
Perform hand hygiene.

Continued

CLINICAL SKILL 25.4 Collecting a nasopharyngeal (nasal) or nasalpharynx (throat) swab—cont'd

Skill activity	Rationale
For a nasopharyngeal (nose) swab: Request the person to blow their nose. If the nasal passage is dry, dip the tip of the swab into the normal saline. Request the individual to tilt their head back. Insert the swab 2 cm into each nostril, rotating against the anterior nasal mucosa.	Clears the nasal passages. Prevents trauma. Normal saline prevents degradation of viruses or bacteria. Facilitates collection of the specimen.
For a swab of the nasopharynx (throat): Request the individual to open their mouth, depress the tongue with a tongue depressor and use a torch to illuminate the throat. If the throat is dry, dip the tip of the swab into normal saline. Ask the person to say 'ah'. Pass the swab over the tonsils, posterior pharyngeal wall and posterior edge of the soft palate.	Gentle insertion prevents tissue damage. Do not force the swab. Facilitates access and visualisation. Prevents trauma and facilitates the collection of microorganisms. Normal saline prevents degradation of viruses or bacteria. Raises the uvula to expose proper site of collection.
Ensure that the container is clearly labelled with the relevant information. Specimen container is placed in the zip lock section of the plastic biohazard bag.	Ensures the correct specimen is tested to avoid errors.
Pathology request form is checked for the person's details. The pathology request form is placed in the other section of the bag.	Ensures correct form and specimen are sent to pathology department and correct test will be undertaken in the pathology department.

 AFTER THE SKILL

(Please refer to the Standard Steps on p. xii for related rationales.)
Communicate outcome to the individual, any ongoing care and to report any complications.
Restore the environment.
Report, record and document assessment findings, details of the skill performed and the individual's response.
Report, record and document any abnormalities and/or inability to perform the skill.
Reassess the individual to ensure there are no adverse effects/events from the skill.

Skill activity	Rationale
The specimen should be transported to the laboratory as soon as possible.	Proliferation of microorganisms occurs if the specimen is not dispatched as soon as possible after collection.

(Perry et al 2022)

OBSERVATION CHECKLIST: NASOPHARYNGEAL (NASAL) OR NASOPHARYNX (THROAT) SWAB COLLECTION

Independent (I)

Supervised (S)

Assisted (A)

Marginal (M)

Dependent (D)

STUDENT NAME: _____

CLINICAL SKILL 25.4: Collecting a nasopharyngeal (nasal) or nasopharynx (throat) swab

DEMONSTRATION OF: The ability to effectively and safely collect a nasopharyngeal or nasopharynx swab

If the observation checklist is being used as an assessment tool, the student will need to obtain a scale of independence for each of the performance criteria/evidence.

COMPETENCY ELEMENTS	PERFORMANCE CRITERIA/EVIDENCE	I	S	A	M	D
Preparation for the activity	Identifies indications and rationale for performing the activity Checks pathology request form Identifies the individual using three individual identifiers Ensures therapeutic interaction Gains the individual's consent Checks facility/organisation policy Validates the order in the individual's record Locates and gathers equipment					
Performs activity informed by evidence	Assists the individual to a sitting position If a *nasopharyngeal* (nasal) swab is to be obtained, requests the individual to blow their nose If the nasal passage is dry, dips the tip of the swab into the normal saline Inserts the swab 2 cm into each nostril, rotating against the anterior nasal mucosa If a swab of the *nasopharynx* (throat) is to be obtained, requests the individual to open their mouth, depresses the tongue with a tongue depressor and uses a torch to illuminate the throat If the throat is dry, dips the tip of the swab into normal saline Asks the person to say 'ah'. Passes the swab over the tonsils, posterior pharyngeal wall and posterior edge of the soft palate Places the swab in the culture tube/container Labels the specimen and dispatches correctly					
Applies critical thinking and reflective practice	Is able to link theory to practice Demonstrates current best practice in the care provided Assesses the individual's ability to tolerate their position and ability to obtain a nasopharyngeal or throat swab Ensures individual is in upright position Monitors the individual's anxiety related to the procedure Assesses the individual's ability to cooperate with the procedure and report any adverse outcomes Assesses own performance					
Practises within safety and quality assurance guidelines	Reviews against facility/organisation policy Performs hand hygiene, dons appropriate PPE as per infection control protocols Cleans and disposes of equipment and waste appropriately					
Documentation and communication	Explains and communicates the activity clearly to the individual Communicates abnormal findings to appropriate personnel Reports and documents all relevant information and any complications correctly in the healthcare record Reports any complications and/or inability to perform the procedure to the RN and/or medical officer Asks the individual to report any complications during procedure if able					

Educator/Facilitator Feedback:

Educator/Facilitator Score: Competent   Needs further development

How would you rate your overall performance while undertaking this clinical activity? (use a ✓ & initial)

Unsatisfactory   Satisfactory   Good   Excellent

Student Reflection: (discuss how you would approach your practice differently or more effectively)

EDUCATOR/FACILITATOR NAME/SIGNATURE:

STUDENT NAME/SIGNATURE: **DATE:**

CLINICAL SKILL 25.5 Oronasopharyngeal suction

Please adhere to the policy and procedures of the facility/organisation prior to undertaking the skill. Ensure this skill is in your scope of practice.

NMBA Decision-making Framework considerations (refer to NMBA Decision-making framework for nursing and midwifery 2020):	Equipment:
1. Am I educated? 2. Am I authorised? 3. Am I competent? If you answer 'no' to any of these, do not perform that activity. Seek guidance and support from your teacher/a nurse team leader/clinical facilitator/educator.	Suction catheter Suction apparatus Suction tubing Yankauer suction catheter Disposable gloves Oronasopharyngeal tube Sterile water and infectious waste bag Normal saline 0.9% (if ordered) Waterproof pad Goggles or face shield (if appropriate)

 PREPARE FOR THE SKILL

(Please refer to the Standard Steps on p. xii for related rationales.)
Mentally review the steps of the skill.
Discuss the skill with your instructor/supervisor/team leader, if required.
Confirm correct facility/organisation policy/safe operating procedures.
Validate the order in the individual's record.
Identify indication and rationale for performing the activity.
Assess for any contraindications.
Locate and gather equipment.
Perform hand hygiene.
Ensure therapeutic interaction.
Identify the individual using three individual identifiers.
Gain the individual's consent.
Assess for pain relief.
Prepare the environment.
Provide and maintain privacy.
Assist the individual to assume an appropriate position of comfort.

Skill activity	Rationale
Perform an assessment of the individual, ensuring their vital signs are stable and their oxygen saturations are adequate to allow for the suctioning. If possible, position the individual in a sitting position or with the neck extended. Place a waterproof pad across individual's chest.	Ensures the individual is stable so as to prevent complications. A burst of oxygen or normal saline nebuliser may be required prior (if ordered) to help loosen secretions and allow for better clearance of mucus during suctioning. Promotes lung expansion and effective coughing.

 PERFORM THE SKILL

(Please refer to the Standard Steps on p. xii for related rationales.)
Perform hand hygiene.
Apply PPE: gloves, eyewear, mask and gown as appropriate.
Ensure the individual's safety and comfort throughout skill.
Promote independence and involvement of the individual if possible and/or appropriate.
Assess the individual's tolerance to the skill throughout.
Dispose of used supplies, equipment, waste and sharps appropriately.
Remove PPE and discard or store appropriately.
Perform hand hygiene.

Skill activity	Rationale
Remove oxygen mask or nasal cannulae if in situ.	Facilitates catheter insertion. **Note:** If suctioning required due to a mucus plug this will facilitate better oxygen saturations.
Attach collection bottle to the suction unit, attach connecting tubing, connector and catheter.	Equipment must be assembled and checked for function before the procedure starts.

Continued

CLINICAL SKILL 25.5 Oronasopharyngeal suction—cont'd

Turn on the suction and dip the tip of the catheter into sterile water.	Lubricates the catheter to facilitate insertion. Prevents the introduction of microorganisms.
With the suction off (e.g. by using the Y-connector), gently introduce the catheter into the mouth or nostril. If the oral route is used, the individual's tongue may be depressed with a tongue depressor.	Suction during insertion may damage the mucosa. Facilitates insertion of the suction catheter. Do not put the catheter into the nose and then the mouth. Ensure it is cleaned between suctions.
Ensure that suction pressure is below 120 mmHg. Apply suction as the catheter is withdrawn, rotating the catheter as it is being withdrawn.	Pressure above 120 mmHg may damage the mucosa. Rotating motion prevents tissue trauma and obtains maximal volume of secretions. **Note:** Do not force the catheter into the nasal cavity as this can cause trauma. When suctioning neonates, infants or children, ensure correct measurement is obtained of their nasal cavity to ensure the catheter is not inserted too far, which may cause irreversible damage.
Apply suction for a maximum of 5–10-second intervals, or less in the young or critically unwell individual, then remove from the airway. Allow the individual time to rest (30 seconds) between suctioning.	Suctioning for longer than 10 seconds can cause tissue trauma and hypoxia. Allows the individual time to rest and replace oxygen until the next suction.
If secretions are tenacious, dip the tip of the catheter into the sterile water and apply suction. If a specimen is required for virology or bacterial studies, use of normal saline is recommended.	Clears the lumen of catheter. Normal saline prevents degradation of viruses or bacteria.
Repeat the procedure, if necessary, until the mucus obstruction has been removed.	Promotes a clear airway.
After suctioning, instruct the individual (if able) to take several slow deep breaths.	Relieves hypoxia and promotes relaxation. Facilitates coughing.
Dip the catheter into the sterile water and apply suction.	Clears catheter and connecting tubing. Prevents the reintroduction of microorganisms and contamination.

 AFTER THE SKILL

(Please refer to the Standard Steps on p. xii for related rationales.)
Communicate outcome to the individual, any ongoing care and to report any complications.
Restore the environment.
Report, record and document assessment findings, details of the skill performed and the individual's response.
Report, record and document any abnormalities and/or inability to perform the skill.
Reassess the individual to ensure there are no adverse effects/events from the skill.

(Perry et al 2022; Rebeiro et al 2021)

OBSERVATION CHECKLIST: ORONASOPHARYNGEAL SUCTION

STUDENT NAME: _____

CLINICAL SKILL 25.5: Oronasopharyngeal suction

DEMONSTRATION OF: The ability to effectively and safely perform oronasopharyngeal suctioning

If the observation checklist is being used as an assessment tool, the student will need to obtain a scale of independence for each of the performance criteria/evidence.

Independent (I)

Supervised (S)

Assisted (A)

Marginal (M)

Dependent (D)

COMPETENCY ELEMENTS	PERFORMANCE CRITERIA/EVIDENCE	I	S	A	M	D
Preparation for the activity	Identifies indications and rationale for performing the activity Identifies the individual using three individual identifiers Ensures therapeutic interaction Gains the individual's consent Checks facility/organisation policy Validates the order in the individual's record Locates and gathers equipment Assists the individual into an appropriate position					
Performs activity informed by evidence	Attaches collection bottle to the suction unit; attaches connecting tubing, connector and catheter Ensures wall or portable suction working Ensures that suction pressure is below 120 mmHg or on lowest setting Turns on the suction and dips the tip of the catheter into sterile water With the suction off (e.g. by using the Y-connector), gently introduces the catheter into the mouth or nostril Applies suction as the catheter is withdrawn, rotating the catheter as it is being withdrawn; repeats if required After suctioning, instructs the individual (if able) to take several slow deep breaths Dips the catheter into the sterile water and applies suction					
Applies critical thinking and reflective practice	Is able to link theory to practice Demonstrates current best practice in the care provided Performs an assessment of the individual, ensuring their vital signs are stable and their oxygen saturations are adequate to allow for the suctioning Monitors the individual's anxiety related to the procedure Assesses the individual's ability to cooperate with the procedure and reports any adverse outcomes Assesses own performance					
Practises within safety and quality assurance guidelines	Reviews against facility/organisation policy Performs hand hygiene, dons appropriate PPE as per infection control protocols Adheres to infection control/ANTT principles Cleans and disposes of equipment and waste appropriately					
Documentation and communication	Explains and communicates the activity clearly to the individual Communicates outcome and ongoing care to individual and significant others Communicates abnormal findings to appropriate personnel Reports and documents all relevant information and any complications correctly in the healthcare record Reports any complications and/or inability to perform the procedure to the RN and/or medical officer Asks the individual to report any complications during and post procedure if able					

Educator/Facilitator Feedback:

Educator/Facilitator Score: Competent   Needs further development

How would you rate your overall performance while undertaking this clinical activity? (use a ✓ & initial)

Unsatisfactory   Satisfactory   Good   Excellent

Student Reflection: (discuss how you would approach your practice differently or more effectively)

EDUCATOR/FACILITATOR NAME/SIGNATURE:

STUDENT NAME/SIGNATURE: **DATE:**

CLINICAL SKILL 25.6 Tracheostomy suctioning and tracheal stoma care

Please adhere to the policy and procedures of the facility/organisation prior to undertaking the skill. Ensure this skill is in your scope of practice.

NMBA Decision-making Framework considerations (refer to NMBA Decision-making framework for nursing and midwifery 2020):	Equipment:
1. Am I educated? 2. Am I authorised? 3. Am I competent? If you answer 'no' to any of these, do not perform that activity. Seek guidance and support from your teacher/a nurse team leader/clinical facilitator/educator. Tracheostomy suctioning and tracheal stoma care is an advanced skill for an Enrolled Nurse (EN).	Sterile gloves Disposable gloves Plastic apron Protective eyewear Waterproof pad Sterile dressing pack Sterile gauze squares Sterile cotton tip applicators Normal saline Clean tapes cut to the correct length Suction apparatus Suction catheter Sterile water Swedish nose or equivalent humidification filter and inner tube

 PREPARE FOR THE SKILL

(Please refer to the Standard Steps on p. xii for related rationales.)
Mentally review the steps of the skill.
Discuss the skill with your instructor/supervisor/team leader, if required.
Confirm correct facility/organisation policy/safe operating procedures.
Validate the order in the individual's record.
Identify indication and rationale for performing the activity.
Assess for any contraindications.
Locate and gather equipment.
Perform hand hygiene.
Ensure therapeutic interaction.
Identify the individual using three individual identifiers.
Gain the individual's consent.
Assess for pain relief.
Prepare the environment.
Provide and maintain privacy.
Assist the individual to assume an appropriate position of comfort.

Skill activity	Rationale
Tracheostomy suctioning	
Perform an assessment of the individual, ensuring their vital signs are stable and their oxygen saturations are adequate to allow for the suctioning. The individual should be informed that suctioning may cause transient coughing or gagging.	Ensures the individual is stable so as to prevent complications. A burst of oxygen or normal saline nebuliser may be required prior (if ordered) to help loosen secretions and allow for better clearance of mucus during suctioning. **Note:** If suctioning required due to a mucus plug, this will facilitate better oxygen saturations.
If possible, position the individual in a sitting position or with the head hyperextended Place a waterproof pad across individual's chest.	Reduces stimulation of gag reflex, assists secretion drainage. Reduces transmission of microorganisms.

Continued

CLINICAL SKILL 25.6 Tracheostomy suctioning and tracheal stoma care—cont'd

 PERFORM THE SKILL

(Please refer to the Standard Steps on p. xii for related rationales.)
Perform hand hygiene.
Apply PPE: gloves, eyewear, mask and gown as appropriate.
Ensure the individual's safety and comfort throughout skill.
Promote independence and involvement of the individual if possible and/or appropriate.
Assess the individual's tolerance to the skill throughout.
Dispose of used supplies, equipment, waste and sharps appropriately.
Remove PPE and discard or store appropriately.
Perform hand hygiene.

Skill activity	Rationale
Open procedure pack using corners. Assemble the required equipment, using aseptic technique. Drop sterile equipment into sterile field.	Facilitates performance of the procedure and promotes functional body alignment and body mechanics while the procedure is being performed. Prevents contamination of sterile items.
Remove any humidification (or ventilation) device (i.e. Swedish nose). Inner tube may also need to be removed and cleaned prior to suctioning.	Allows access to the tracheostomy tube. Prevents a mucus plug from forming and allows for proper removal of secretions.
Attach the catheter to the suction tubing and set suction pressure to 80–120 mmHg. Catheter size must be smaller than the diameter of the tracheostomy/inner tube.	Pressure above 120 mmHg may damage the tracheal mucosa. Prevents obstruction of airway.
Ask the individual to cough and breathe slowly and deeply.	Coughing helps loosen secretions, and deep breathing helps to minimise hypoxia.
If necessary, or prescribed, the individual's lungs are hyperoxygenated before aspiration.	Helps to prevent hypoxia.
Insert the catheter without suction into the tracheostomy tube just past the correct length of the tracheostomy tube.	Prevents hypoxia and tracheal mucosa trauma. Suctioning to the xiphoid process can cause trauma and permanent damage to the cartilage, especially in neonates, infants and children; it also prevents discomfort.
Apply suction and withdraw the catheter, rotating it gently. Suction for no longer than 5–10 seconds at a time. Allow the individual to take four to five breaths between each aspiration. If secretions are thick, dip the catheter into sterile water and apply suction.	Rotating motion avoids tissue trauma. Short-term suctioning limits the amount of oxygen removed and prevents hypoxia. Helps to clear the lumen of the catheter. **Note:** In neonates and infants do not rotate catheter but simply insert in and out to the required measurement.
Report immediately if there is any difficulty in inserting the catheter into the tube.	The tube may be partially blocked with secretions.
When suctioning is completed, the individual may need to be hyperoxygenated again. Replace any humidification device (unless tracheal stoma care/dressing is to be performed). Reinsert the clean inner tube. Clear suction catheter and tubing with sterile water.	Prevents hypoxia and promotes relaxation. Re-establishes delivery of humidity. Prevents the reintroduction of microorganisms. **Note:** Suction catheters can be used for up to 24 hours prior to disposal if cleaned thoroughly after use.
Tracheal stoma care	
Open procedure pack and prepare equipment using ANTT.	Prevents contamination of sterile items.
Remove and discard the tracheostomy dressing into a suitable waste receptacle. Ensure ties secure around tracheostomy tube.	Correct disposal prevents cross-infection and abides by infection prevention policies and procedures. Prevents dislodgement of tracheostomy tube.

CLINICAL SKILL 25.6 Tracheostomy suctioning and tracheal stoma care—cont'd

Perform hand hygiene and don sterile gloves. For a newly formed stoma, use a sterile drape around the tracheostomy site.	Prevents cross-infection. Provides a sterile field around the stoma.
Cleanse the skin around the stoma and the flanges of the tube using gauze and normal saline. Take care not to let normal saline or strands of gauze to enter the tube or stoma. Use cotton tip applicators dipped in normal saline for hard-to-reach areas of the stoma.	Removes accumulated secretions and crusts. Prevents aspiration and the risk of infection.
Inspect the surrounding area and stoma site for inflammation or skin breakdown. Inspect for the formation of a granuloma, especially in older tracheostomy stoma sites.	Signs of impaired healing or infection require immediate attention. Granulomas are generally a collection of macrophages forming a nodular area around the stoma site. These are quite common, especially in older stomas, and can be treated with silver nitrate.
Apply a sterile tracheostomy dressing using aseptic non-touch technique.	Protects the stoma site and reduces transmission of microorganisms.
Replace the tracheostomy tapes if they are soiled or loose. Two people are required to change the tapes (one must be an RN who has achieved competency; the EN would assist with the procedure).	Tracheostomy tube must be secured in position. Soiled tapes predispose the person to infection. Prevents accidental dislodgement of the tube.
Replace any humidification device (Swedish nose). Change to a new one if the old one is soiled.	Re-establishes delivery of humidity and helps filter the air to prevent the introduction of microorganisms.

AFTER THE SKILL

(Please refer to the Standard Steps on p. xii for related rationales.)
Communicate outcome to the individual, any ongoing care and to report any complications.
Restore the environment.
Report, record and document assessment findings, details of the skill performed and the individual's response.
Report, record and document any abnormalities and/or inability to perform the skill.
Reassess the individual to ensure there are no adverse effects/events from the skill.

Skill activity	Rationale
Document the time of suctioning, the type and amount of aspirate and the individual's response. Document and report on the dressing change.	Appropriate care can be planned and implemented.

(Berman et al 2020; Carter & Notter 2024; Perry et al 2022; Rebeiro et al 2021)

OBSERVATION CHECKLIST: TRACHEOSTOMY SUCTIONING AND TRACHEAL STOMA CARE

STUDENT NAME: _____

CLINICAL SKILL 25.6: Tracheostomy suctioning and tracheal stoma care

DEMONSTRATION OF: Tracheostomy suctioning and the ability to effectively and safely care for a tracheal stoma

If the observation checklist is being used as an assessment tool, the student will need to obtain a scale of independence for each of the performance criteria/evidence.

Independent (I)
Supervised (S)
Assisted (A)
Marginal (M)
Dependent (D)

COMPETENCY ELEMENTS	PERFORMANCE CRITERIA/EVIDENCE	I	S	A	M	D
Preparation for the activity	Identifies indications and rationale for performing the activity Identifies the individual using three individual identifiers Ensures therapeutic interaction Gains the individual's consent Checks facility/organisation policy Validates the order in the individual's record Locates and gathers equipment Assists the individual into an appropriate position					
Performs activity informed by evidence	Performs an assessment of the individual, ensuring their vital signs are stable and their oxygen saturations are within range as specified by the medical officer Assesses for any pain at the insertion site Checks for bilateral rise and fall of the chest and that there is no respiratory distress Ensures the individual is nursed in a semi-Fowler's or high-Fowler's position Assesses the tracheostomy tube for any patency and secretions Checks wall suction Assesses the indications for a dressing change around stoma and tape change					
Applies critical thinking and reflective practice	Is able to link theory to practice Demonstrates current best practice in the care provided Assesses the individual's ability to tolerate the tracheostomy tube Monitors the individual's anxiety and pain level related to the tracheostomy Assesses the individual's ability to cooperate with tracheal suctioning and care of the tracheostomy site Assesses own performance					
Practises within safety and quality assurance guidelines	Reviews against facility/organisation policy Performs hand hygiene, dons appropriate PPE as per infection control protocols Adheres to infection control/ANTT principles Raises the bed to the appropriate working position based on nurse's height and lowers at completion of activity Cleans and disposes of equipment and waste appropriately					
Documentation and communication	Explains and communicates the activity clearly to the individual Communicates outcome and ongoing care to individual and significant others Communicates abnormal findings to appropriate personnel Reports and documents all relevant information and any complications correctly in the healthcare record Reports any complications and/or inability to perform the procedure to the RN and/or medical officer Asks the individual to report any complications during procedure if able					

Educator/Facilitator Feedback:

Educator/Facilitator Score: Competent Needs further development

How would you rate your overall performance while undertaking this clinical activity? (use a ✓ & initial)

Unsatisfactory Satisfactory Good Excellent

Student Reflection: (discuss how you would approach your practice differently or more effectively)

EDUCATOR/FACILITATOR NAME/SIGNATURE:

STUDENT NAME/SIGNATURE: **DATE:**

CLINICAL SKILL 25.7 Care of chest tube/drainage and dressing change

Please adhere to the policy and procedures of the facility/organisation prior to undertaking the skill. Ensure this skill is in your scope of practice.

NMBA Decision-making Framework considerations (refer to NMBA Decision-making framework for nursing and midwifery 2020):	Equipment:
1. Am I educated? 2. Am I authorised? 3. Am I competent? If you answer 'no' to any of these, do not perform that activity. Seek guidance and support from your teacher/a nurse team leader/clinical facilitator/educator.	Disposable and sterile gloves Sterile dressing pack Approved antiseptic solution (2% chlorhexidine gluconate in 70% isopropyl, 10% povidone-iodine or 70% alcohol) Normal saline 0.9% Split dressing/gauze Occlusive dressing Fluid balance chart or chest drain observation chart Two artery forceps

 PREPARE FOR THE SKILL

(Please refer to the Standard Steps on p. xii for related rationales.)
Mentally review the steps of the skill.
Discuss the skill with your instructor/supervisor/team leader, if required.
Confirm correct facility/organisation policy/safe operating procedures.
Validate the order in the individual's record.
Identify indication and rationale for performing the activity.
Assess for any contraindications.
Locate and gather equipment.
Perform hand hygiene.
Ensure therapeutic interaction.
Identify the individual using three individual identifiers.
Gain the individual's consent.
Assess for pain relief.
Prepare the environment.
Provide and maintain privacy.
Assist the individual to assume an appropriate position of comfort.

Skill activity	Rationale
Care of chest tube/drainage	
Ensure the individual is nursed in a semi-Fowler's or high Fowler's position. Perform an assessment of the individual, ensuring their vital signs are stable and their oxygen saturations are within range as specified by the medical officer. Assess for any pain during inspiration or expiration and/or at the insertion site. Check for bilateral rise and fall of the chest and that there is no respiratory distress.	Allows for adequate chest expansion and better respiration. Semi-Fowler's position is preferred for pneumothorax to evacuate air. High Fowler's is preferred for haemothorax to drain fluid. Reduces anxiety and embarrassment. Ensures individual is stable so as to prevent any complications.
Provide two artery forceps for each chest tube, attached at top of bed with adhesive tape.	Chest tubes are clamped only under specific circumstances and with medical orders. Double-clamp close to the individual's chest for as short a time as possible only in the following circumstances: a. To assess air leak. b. To quickly change the disposable under water seal drain (UWSD), which should only be performed by a nurse who has received training in this procedure. c. To assess if the individual is ready to have chest tube removed (which is done by medical order); the nurse must monitor for re-accumulation of pneumothorax. d. During drainage of large volumes to reduce shock (on doctor's orders). e. To prepare for removal (on doctor's orders). f. When the system may have to be raised above chest level.

CLINICAL SKILL 25.7 Care of chest tube/drainage and dressing change—cont'd

 PERFORM THE SKILL

(Please refer to the Standard Steps on p. xii for related rationales.)
Perform hand hygiene.
Apply PPE: gloves, eyewear, mask and gown as appropriate.
Ensure the individual's safety and comfort throughout skill.
Promote independence and involvement of the individual if possible and/or appropriate.
Assess the individual's tolerance to the skill throughout.
Dispose of used supplies, equipment, waste and sharps appropriately.
Remove PPE and discard or store appropriately.
Perform hand hygiene.

Skill activity	Rationale
Assess the chest tube dressing and insertion site to ensure the dressing is dry and intact and observe for any signs of infection. Report any signs of infection to the RN/medical officer.	Prevents complications from arising and prevents the introduction of microorganisms. Appropriate care can be planned and implemented.
Assess the drain tube and drainage for any bubbling, swing and drainage. Observe the tubing for kinks, clots or dependent loops. Check wall suction and connection to underwater sealed drain (UWSD) is intact. Ensure the UWSD is upright and below the level of the chest.	Increased bubbling indicates an air leak, which may mean the connection to the person and the tube is faulty. This can lead to a pneumothorax if not sealed properly. Swing refers to oscillation of the fluid in the tubing. Ensures the tubing is patent. Wall suction should be set at >80 mmHg with the suction on the UWSD unit being set at 20 cmH$_2$O for adults (5 cmH$_2$O for neonates and 10–20 cmH$_2$O for children) or as prescribed by the doctor. Suction helps facilitate the reinflation of the lung. Prevents the introduction of microorganisms. Prevents fluid from flowing back into the pleural cavity.
Chest tube dressing change	
Open procedure pack and prepare equipment using ANTT.	Prevents contamination of sterile items.
Gently remove the old dressing ensuring that there is a little slack on the tube.	Prevents the accidental dislodgement of the tube. Tautness of the tube can cause discomfort and pull on the sutures, causing trauma to the area. **Note:** Chest tubes are usually sutured in place.
Perform hand hygiene and don sterile gloves. Use normal saline 0.9% to cleanse area, ensuring the tubing is also cleaned well.	Prevents cross-infection and the introduction of microorganisms.
Apply approved skin antiseptic solution and allow to dry. 2% chlorhexidine gluconate in 70% isopropyl is the preferred choice, or 10% povidone-iodine or 70% alcohol as the alternative.	Prevents cross-infection and eliminates the introduction of microorganisms.
Apply split gauze around the insertion site and then place a sandwich dressing over the area (two large pieces of occlusive dressing).	Helps collect any exudate. Ensures the insertion site and surrounding skin can be seen readily and secures tubing to prevent irritation.

 AFTER THE SKILL

(Please refer to the Standard Steps on p. xii for related rationales.)
Communicate outcome to the individual, any ongoing care and to report any complications.
Restore the environment.
Report, record and document assessment findings, details of the skill performed and the individual's response.
Report, record and document any abnormalities and/or inability to perform the skill.
Reassess the individual to ensure there are no adverse effects/events from the skill.

Continued

CLINICAL SKILL 25.7 Care of chest tube/drainage and dressing change—cont'd

Skill activity	Rationale
Document observations, pain, drain tube assessment and drainage hourly or as per policy and procedure on the relevant observation and/or fluid balance chart. Document the respiratory status of the individual, the amount, colour and consistency of drainage, the presence of swinging and bubbling.	Ensures the safety of the individual. Abides by facility/organisation policy. Monitors for any complications and excessive drainage. **Note:** The individual may be on a patient-controlled analgesia (PCA) infusion for analgesia maintenance, which will also need to be documented hourly as per policy.

(Carter & Notter 2024; Knapp 2019; Perry et al 2022; Rebeiro et al 2021)

OBSERVATION CHECKLIST: CARE OF CHEST TUBE/ DRAINAGE AND DRESSING CHANGE

STUDENT NAME: _____

CLINICAL SKILL 25.7: Care of chest tube/drainage and dressing change

DEMONSTRATION OF: The ability to effectively and safely care for a chest drain including checking for drainage and dressing change

If the observation checklist is being used as an assessment tool, the student will need to obtain a scale of independence for each of the performance criteria/evidence.

Independent (I)
Supervised (S)
Assisted (A)
Marginal (M)
Dependent (D)

COMPETENCY ELEMENTS	PERFORMANCE CRITERIA/EVIDENCE	I	S	A	M	D
Preparation for the activity	Identifies indications and rationale for performing the activity Identifies the individual using three individual identifiers Ensures therapeutic interaction Gains the individual's consent Checks facility/organisation policy Validates the order in the individual's record Locates and gathers equipment					
Performs activity informed by evidence	Performs an assessment of the individual, ensuring their vital signs are stable and their oxygen saturations are within range as specified by the medical officer Assesses for any pain during inspiration or expiration and/or at the insertion site Ensures the individual is nursed in a semi-Fowler's or high-Fowler's position Checks for bilateral rise and fall of the chest and that there is no respiratory distress Assesses the drain tube and drainage for any bubbling, swing and drainage. Observes the tubing for kinks, clots or dependent loops Checks wall suction and connection to UWSD is intact Fills the water chamber of the UWSD to the required level with sterile water Ensures the UWSD is upright and below the level of the chest Assesses the indications for a dressing change and replaces as per facility/organisation policy					
Applies critical thinking and reflective practice	Is able to link theory to practice Demonstrates current best practice in the care provided Assesses the individual's ability to tolerate the chest drain Monitors the individual's anxiety and pain level related to the chest drain Assesses own performance					
Practises within safety and quality assurance guidelines	Reviews against facility/organisation policy Performs hand hygiene, dons appropriate PPE as per infection control protocols Adheres to infection control/ANTT principles Raises the bed to the appropriate working position based on nurse's height and lowers at completion of activity Cleans and disposes of equipment and waste appropriately					
Documentation and communication	Explains and communicates the activity clearly to the individual Communicates outcome and ongoing care to individual and significant others Communicates abnormal findings to appropriate personnel Reports and documents all relevant information and any complications correctly in the healthcare record Reports any complications and/or inability to perform the procedure to the RN and/or medical officer Asks the individual to report any complications during procedure if able					

Educator/Facilitator Feedback:

Educator/Facilitator Score: Competent   Needs further development

How would you rate your overall performance while undertaking this clinical activity? (use a ✓ & initial)

Unsatisfactory   Satisfactory   Good   Excellent

Student Reflection: (discuss how you would approach your practice differently or more effectively)

EDUCATOR/FACILITATOR NAME/SIGNATURE:

STUDENT NAME/SIGNATURE: **DATE:**

CLINICAL SKILL 25.8 Oxygen therapy—nasal, mask

Please adhere to the policy and procedures of the facility/organisation prior to undertaking the skill. Ensure this skill is in your scope of practice.

NMBA Decision-making Framework considerations (refer to NMBA Decision-making framework for nursing and midwifery 2020):	Equipment:
1. Am I educated? 2. Am I authorised? 3. Am I competent? If you answer 'no' to any of these, do not perform that activity. Seek guidance and support from your teacher/a nurse team leader/clinical facilitator/educator.	Oxygen source (wall outlet, cylinder) Flow meter Humidifier and sterile water (if indicated) Oxygen tubing Oxygen delivery system (if FiO$_2$ required) Nasal cannula Oxygen mask (or required mask) Pulse oximeter

📋 PREPARE FOR THE SKILL

(Please refer to the Standard Steps on p. xii for related rationales.)
Mentally review the steps of the skill.
Discuss the skill with your instructor/supervisor/team leader, if required.
Confirm correct facility/organisation policy/safe operating procedures.
Validate the order in the individual's record.
Identify indication and rationale for performing the activity.
Assess for any contraindications.
Locate and gather equipment.
Perform hand hygiene.
Ensure therapeutic interaction.
Identify the individual using three individual identifiers.
Gain the individual's consent.
Assess for pain relief.
Prepare the environment.
Provide and maintain privacy.
Assist the individual to assume an appropriate position of comfort.

Skill activity	Rationale
Perform an assessment of the person, record their vital signs and oxygen saturations. Assess indications for oxygen requirement: • Dyspnoea, tachypnoea, bradypnoea, apnoea • Pallor, cyanosis • Lethargy or restlessness • Use of accessory muscles: nasal flaring, intercostal or sternal recession, tracheal tug.	Baseline observations attended to assess for initiation of oxygen therapy. Enables safe administration of oxygen therapy.
Sit person into an upright or semi-Fowler's position (if able).	Facilitates breathing and lung expansion.

PERFORM THE SKILL

(Please refer to the Standard Steps on p. xii for related rationales.)
Perform hand hygiene.
Apply PPE: gloves, eyewear, mask and gown as appropriate.
Ensure the individual's safety and comfort throughout skill.
Promote independence and involvement of the individual if possible and/or appropriate.
Assess the individual's tolerance to the skill throughout.
Dispose of used supplies, equipment, waste and sharps appropriately.
Remove PPE and discard or store appropriately.
Perform hand hygiene.

Continued

CLINICAL SKILL 25.8 Oxygen therapy—nasal, mask—cont'd

Skill activity	Rationale
Attach oxygen delivery device to oxygen tubing and attach to oxygen source at prescribed rate. Apply the appropriate delivery device to the individual.	Oxygen delivery devices change the amount and the concentration of oxygen being delivered: **Low-flow delivery devices** • Nasal cannulae: 1–6 L/min (24–44%) • Simple face mask: 6–12 L/min (35–50%) • Reservoir mask (non-rebreathing mask): 10–15 L/min (60–90%) **High-flow delivery devices** • Venturi system (used in high-flow oxygen): FiO_2 and amount of oxygen determined as per dialled amount (24–50%) • High-flow nasal cannula or mask (adjustable FiO_2 (21–100%) with modifiable low flow (up to 60 L/min)) • Continuous positive airway pressure (CPAP) and bilevel positive airway pressure (BiPAP) (21–100%)
Monitor the individual's response to oxygen and their observations as indicated by the medical officer until stable (usually every 15 minutes to hourly). Ensure tubing is not kinked, check mask or cannula stay in correct position.	Prevents complications and ensures treatment is working.
Offer/perform oral hygiene using a mouth swab and/or mouth rinse. Wash face masks daily with warm soapy water. Observe the nares and top of the individual's ears for skin breakdown.	Reduces bad taste or halitosis in mouth. Provides comfort and maintains moist mucosa. Oxygen therapy can dry the nares and the cannula tubing or elastic can cause skin irritation.

 AFTER THE SKILL

(Please refer to the Standard Steps on p. xii for related rationales.)
Communicate outcome to the individual, any ongoing care and to report any complications.
Restore the environment.
Report, record and document assessment findings, details of the skill performed and the individual's response.
Report, record and document any abnormalities and/or inability to perform the skill.
Reassess the individual to ensure there are no adverse effects/events from the skill.

(Carter & Notter 2024; Perry et al 2022; Rebeiro et al 2021)

OBSERVATION CHECKLIST: OXYGEN THERAPY—NASAL, MASK

STUDENT NAME: _____

CLINICAL SKILL 25.8: Administration of oxygen therapy via mask and nasal prongs

DEMONSTRATION OF: The ability to effectively and safely administer oxygen therapy

If the observation checklist is being used as an assessment tool, the student will need to obtain a scale of independence for each of the performance criteria/evidence.

Independent (I)

Supervised (S)

Assisted (A)

Marginal (M)

Dependent (D)

COMPETENCY ELEMENTS	PERFORMANCE CRITERIA/EVIDENCE	I	S	A	M	D
Preparation for the activity	Identifies indications and rationale for commencing oxygen therapy Identifies the individual using three individual identifiers Ensures therapeutic interaction Gains the individual's consent Checks facility/organisation policy Validates the order in the individual's record Locates and gathers equipment Assists the individual into an appropriate position					
Performs activity informed by evidence	Attaches oxygen meter to wall outlet and attaches mask or nasal prongs Ensures wall or portable oxygen working Ensures correct oxygen delivery device used Monitors the individual's response to oxygen and their observations as indicated by the medical officer until stable (usually 15 minutely to hourly) Ensures tubing is not kinked; checks mask or cannula stays in correct position Offers/performs oral hygiene using a mouth swab and/or mouth rinse Washes face masks daily with warm soapy water Observes the nares and top of the individual's ears for skin breakdown					
Applies critical thinking and reflective practice	Is able to link theory to practice Demonstrates current best practice in the care provided Assesses indications for oxygen requirement: • Dyspnoea, tachypnoea, bradypnoea, apnoea • Pallor, cyanosis • Lethargy or restlessness, use of accessory muscles: nasal flaring, intercostal or sternal recession, tracheal tug Ensures individual is in upright position Monitors the individual's anxiety related to the procedure Assesses the individual's ability to cooperate with the procedure Assesses own performance					
Practises within safety and quality assurance guidelines	Reviews against facility/organisation policy Performs hand hygiene, dons appropriate PPE as per infection control protocols Cleans and disposes of equipment and waste appropriately					
Documentation and communication	Explains and communicates the activity clearly to the individual Communicates outcome and ongoing care to individual and significant others Communicates abnormal findings to appropriate personnel Reports and documents all relevant information and any complications correctly in the healthcare record Reports any complications and/or inability to perform the procedure to the RN and/or medical officer Asks the individual to report any complications during and after the procedure if able					

Educator/Facilitator Feedback:

Educator/Facilitator Score: Competent   Needs further development

How would you rate your overall performance while undertaking this clinical activity? (use a ✓ & initial)

Unsatisfactory   Satisfactory   Good   Excellent

Student Reflection: (discuss how you would approach your practice differently or more effectively)

EDUCATOR/FACILITATOR NAME/SIGNATURE:

STUDENT NAME/SIGNATURE: **DATE:**

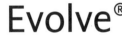 ® Answer guide for the Critical Thinking Exercises and Critical Thinking Questions in Case Studies is hosted on Evolve: http://evolve.elsevier.com/AU/Koutoukidis/Tabbner/

References

Aitken, L.M., Marshall, A., Chaboyer, W. (eds.), 2019. *Critical care nursing*, 4th ed. Elsevier Australia, Chatswood.

Berman, A., Kozier, B., Erb, G.L., 2020. *Kozier and Erb's fundamentals of nursing: Concepts, process and practice*, 5th ed. Pearson Australia, Melbourne.

Carter, C., Notter, J., 2024. *Handbook for registered nurses*. Elsevier.

Crisp, J., Douglas, C., Rebeiro, G., et al. (eds.), 2021. *Potter and Perry's fundamentals of nursing*, 65th ed. Elsevier, Australia and New Zealand, Sydney.

Knapp, R. (ed.), 2019. *Respiratory care made incredibly easy!*, 2nd ed. Wolters Kluwer, Philadelphia.

Menzies-Gow, E., 2018. How to record a 12-lead electrocardiogram. *Nursing Standard* 33(2) 38–42. doi: 10.7748/ns.2018.e11066.

Nursing and Midwifery Board of Australia (NMBA), 2020. Decision-making framework for nursing and midwifery. Available at: <https://www.nursingmidwiferyboard.gov.au/Codes-Guidelines-Statements/Frameworks.aspx>.

Pinsky, M., Teboul, J., Vincent J. (eds.), 2019. *Hemodynamic monitoring*. Springer International Publishing, Cham.

Perry, A.G., Potter, P.A., Ostendorf, W., Laplante, N., 2022. *Nursing interventions and clinical skills*, 10th ed. Elsevier, St Louis.

Rebeiro, G., Wilson, D., Fuller, S., 2021. *Potter and Perry's fundamentals of nursing workbook*, 4th ed. Elsevier, Chatswood.

Recommended Reading

Andriolo, B.N.G., Andriolo, R.B., Saconato, H., et al., 2015. Early versus late tracheostomy for critically ill patients. *Cochrane Database of Systematic Reviews* 1(1), CD007271. doi: 10.1002/14651858.CD007271.pub3.

Broaddus, V., Mason, R., Ernst, J., et al., 2015. *Murray & Nadel's textbook of respiratory medicine*. Elsevier Health Sciences, Philadelphia.

Global Initiative for Asthma (GINA), 2023. Global strategy for asthma management and prevention: Updated 2023. Available at: <https://ginasthma.org/reports/>.

Heart Failure Guidelines Working Group, 2018. National Heart Foundation of Australia and Cardiac Society of Australia and New Zealand: Guidelines for the prevention, detection, and management of heart failure in Australia 2018. *Heart Lung and Circulation* 27(10), 1123–1208. Available at: <https://doi.org/10.1016/j.hlc.2018.06.1042>.

Millar, F., Hillman, T., 2018. Managing chest drains on medical wards. *BMJ* 363, k4639.

National Heart Foundation of Australia, 2016. Guideline for the diagnosis and management of hypertension in adults. National Heart Foundation of Australia, Melbourne. Available at: <https://www.heartfoundation.org.au/getmedia/c83511ab-835a-4fcf-96f5->.

NSW Agency for Clinical Innovation, 2021. Care of adult patients in acute care facilities with a tracheostomy: Clinical Practice Guide. Sydney: (accessed 31/07/2023) Available at: <https://aci.health.nsw.gov.au/__data/assets/pdf_file/0004/685300/ACI-CPG-Tracheostomy.pdf>.

Pahal, P., Avula, A., Sharma, S., 2023. Emphysema. In: StatPearls [Internet]. StatPearls Publishing, Treasure Island (FL).

Patel, S., Mohiuddin, S., 2019. Physiology, oxygen transport and carbon dioxide dissociation curve. In: StatPearls [Internet]. StatPearls Publishing, Treasure Island (FL).

Pilcher, J., Beasley, R., 2015. Acute use of oxygen therapy. *Australian Prescriber* 38, 98–100.

Sajadi-Ernazarova, K., Martin, J., Gupta, N., 2022. Acute pneumothorax evaluation and treatment. In: StatPearls [Internet]. StatPearls Publishing, Treasure Island (FL).

Saleh, M., Ambrose, J.A., 2018. Understanding myocardial infarction. *F1000Research* 7, 1378.

World Health Organization (WHO), 2020. A guide to EHO's Guidance on COVID-19. WHO, Geneva. Available at: <https://www.who.int/emergencies/diseases/novel-coronavirus-2019/technical-guidance>.

FLUIDS AND ELECTROLYTES

Kalpana Raghunathan

Overview

Meeting fluid, electrolyte and acid–base needs helps maintain equilibrium within the human body. This state of equilibrium is known as homeostasis, and it is essential for a healthy internal environment. The nurse has a vital role in helping to maintain and restore an individual's homeostasis, and understanding the individual's fluid and electrolyte status can give an indication of overall health. This is especially important for individuals who are unwell or have pathological conditions that affect proper regulation of fluid and electrolyte status.

The average adult's fluid intake per day is approximately 2.5 L (1.5 L is in the form of fluids consumed; the other 1 L is from food consumed during the metabolic process). Fluid imbalances occur through either isotonic or osmolar means. Isotonic fluid imbalances occur when fluid and electrolytes are either lost or gained in equal proportions, whereas osmolar imbalances occur when there is a loss or gain of water only (Berman et al 2020).

Common medications, food consumption, fluid intake and output, illness, exertion levels and the environment contribute to an individual's change in homeostasis. Uncorrected or untreated fluid and electrolyte imbalances can lead to life-threatening complications. In a healthy body, water and molecules containing electrolytes consist of 60% of the body's total volume of fluid in men; 50% in women. Two-thirds of the body's fluid is intracellular (ICF) and one-third is extracellular (ECF). However, there is also transcellular fluid (TCF), which is contained in body cavities or cerebrospinal fluid (CSF) (Brown et al 2020).

In a healthy person, fluid balance fluctuates from day to day, but has no major impact on health or homeostasis. Individuals who are acutely ill or have ongoing issues with maintaining fluid balance are at risk of complications requiring admission to a healthcare facility. It is the nurse's role to maintain an accurate fluid balance record to ensure correct management and prevent further complications. However, a fluid balance chart (FBC) in isolation is not sufficient to assess the fluid status of a person. Daily weight, physical assessment findings and electrolyte monitoring (blood chemistry) are also required for accurately assessing hydration status (Sivapuram 2022).

When assessing fluid balance, the nurse should:
- Perform a physical assessment
- Review the fluid balance chart
- Review blood chemistry results.

A physical assessment is crucial in assessing fluid status. It includes assessing vital signs, under- or overload, capillary refill, skin elasticity, weight changes and urine output. Urine output of at least 0.5 mL/kg/hour is reflective of normal urine production (Brown et al 2020). Reviewing the fluid balance chart (if accurate) allows for a numerical balance in determining an individual's fluid status, and reviewing the blood chemistry results determines any electrolyte imbalances, primarily in potassium and sodium, especially if there has been a large diuresis or loss of fluid in another form.

It is important that the fluid balance chart is completed hourly and as accurately as possible over the 24-hour period. Where possible, the individual should be involved, and made aware of fluid balance charting so that they can inform the nurse to record any fluid intake/output (Simpson & McIntosh 2021). Accurate fluid intake and output measurement can ensure the best outcome for the individual and enable effective management.

 CASE STUDY 26.1

Administering intravenous fluids

Jean, an 80-year-old female, is admitted to the medical ward. Jean lives at a residential aged-care home. Jean had become increasingly confused and developed a fever of 38.2°C. Medical diagnosis on admission: urinary tract infection, dehydration and fever. Medical history of stroke affecting her ability to self-care, atrial fibrillation and myo-congestive failure. Treatment and management plan were for slow rehydration (intravenous Hartmann's solution, 12-hourly rate), oral intake as tolerated, intravenous antibiotics stat order (1 g Ceftriaxone) while waiting for urine and blood culture sensitivities. Vital signs 4-hourly, monitor BP, urine output and daily weight. Referral to dietitian, physio and occupational therapist.

1. What risk factors could have contributed to Jean's dehydration?
2. What risk factors could have contributed to Jean developing a urinary tract infection?
3. What are some possible nursing diagnoses for Jean?
4. How will you manage Jean's infusion of IV fluid? What are some important considerations?
5. What will your ongoing assessment of Jean consist of and what potential complications will you be monitoring Jean for?
6. Why is Jean prescribed Hartmann's solution at the 12-hourly rate to treat and manage dehydration?

CRITICAL THINKING EXERCISE 26.3

Fluid balance

A 78-year-old man was having multiple IV antibiotics throughout the day. Each dose was administered with 100 mL 0.9% sodium chloride six times a day. Nursing care included 6-hourly vital signs observations to be recorded, daily weight, fluid balance chart, total fluid restriction of 1200 mL daily and a low-salt diet. The person has renal impairment. After 24 hours, the individual is exhibiting signs of swollen ankles and shortness of breath. The fluid balance chart shows oral intake is 1200 mL and output is 800 mL over 24 hours. What has caused the person's symptoms and fluid retention in this case? What is the critical issue with the fluid balance charting for this person?

CLINICAL SKILL 26.1 Fluid balance charting

Please adhere to the policy and procedures of the facility/organisation prior to undertaking the skill. Ensure this skill is in your scope of practice.

An accurate fluid balance chart (FBC) should be completed using the correct equipment listed below. Charting should be completed immediately post meals; it includes oral intake, nasogastric, percutaneous endoscopic gastrostomy (PEG) and liquid medicines. Intravenous (IV) fluid should be recorded hourly and any IV medications and accompanying flush should be recorded on the FBC. All sensible (measurable) losses (urine, faeces, emesis, nasogastric aspirates/drainage and drain tubes) should be recorded. Accurate measurements of urine, drainage and aspirates should be recorded. Fluid input and output is measured and recorded hourly over a 24-hour period. Six-hourly subtotals should be recorded, which will enable an individual's accurate fluid status assessment. The cumulative balance is the 24-hour total, which is usually obtained at midnight. It is important that the healthcare facility's policy and procedure regarding recording of FBCs is adhered to.

NMBA Decision-making Framework considerations (refer to NMBA Decision-making framework for nursing and midwifery 2020):	Equipment:
1. Am I educated? 2. Am I authorised? 3. Am I competent? If you answer 'no' to any of these, do not perform that activity. Seek guidance and support from your teacher/a nurse team leader/clinical facilitator/educator.	Fluid balance chart (either in EMR or physical form) Weigh scale (calibrated) Calculator Bedpan and/or urinal if the person does not have an IDC Measuring jug/containers for each type of output Appropriate PPE

 PREPARE FOR THE SKILL

(Please refer to the Standard Steps on p. xii for related rationales.)
Mentally review the steps of the skill.
Discuss the skill with your instructor/supervisor/team leader, if required.
Confirm correct facility/organisation policy/safe operating procedures.
Validate the order in the individual's record.
Identify indication and rationale for performing the activity.
Assess for any contraindications.
Locate and gather equipment.
Perform hand hygiene.
Ensure therapeutic interaction.
Identify the individual using three individual identifiers.
Gain the individual's consent.
Assess for pain relief.
Prepare the environment.
Provide and maintain privacy.
Assist the individual to assume an appropriate position of comfort.

Skill activity	Rationale
Establish the reason for the commencement of a fluid balance chart (FBC): • Fluid restriction • IV fluid administration • Critically ill/haemodynamically unstable • Prevention of fluid overload • Actual or potential fluid imbalance • Dehydration • Electrolyte replacement • Multiple infusions • Blood product administration • Indwelling catheter (IDC)/urinary retention • IV medication administration	Ensures correct use of FBC.

CLINICAL SKILL 26.1 Fluid balance charting—cont'd

 PERFORM THE SKILL

(Please refer to the Standard Steps on p. xii for related rationales.)
Perform hand hygiene.
Apply PPE: gloves, eyewear, mask and gown as appropriate.
Ensure the individual's safety and comfort throughout skill.
Promote independence and involvement of the individual if possible and/or appropriate.
Assess the individual's tolerance to the skill throughout.
Dispose of used supplies, equipment, waste and sharps appropriately.
Remove PPE and discard or store appropriately.
Perform hand hygiene.

Skill activity	Rationale
Ensure a list of the correct amount of millilitres per container of fluid (intake) is available. Ensure all IV fluid administration is via an IV pump (where possible).	Ensures accuracy of individual's intake.
Ensure urinal, bedpan or plastic urinal female toilet available for the individual to urinate into, or that an IDC is in situ if haemodynamically unstable. Ensure all wound drainage, vomitus, loose bowel actions and gastric fluid is also recorded on the individual's output.	Ensures accuracy of individual's output.
Separate input and output routes in the columns on the FBC. Maintain and monitor hourly input and output over the 24-hour period. Calculate 6-hourly subtotals (or more frequently if indicated and as per organisation's guidelines). Obtain a cumulative 24-hour total at midnight (or as per healthcare organisation's guidelines). Subtract the difference between total input and output for the 24-hour period. Observe for any signs of under- or over-hydration.	Provides quantity or measurement via each input and output route/type. Establishes an accurate positive or negative balance to determine the individual's fluid status so that intervention may be prompt. Prevents circulatory overload and complications.

 AFTER THE SKILL

(Please refer to the Standard Steps on p. xii for related rationales.)
Communicate outcome to the individual, any ongoing care and to report any complications.
Restore the environment.
Report, record and document assessment findings, details of the skill performed and the individual's response.
Report, record and document any abnormalities and/or inability to perform the skill.
Reassess the individual to ensure there are no adverse effects/events from the skill.

(Berman et al 2020; Crisp et al 2021; Simpson & McIntosh 2021)

OBSERVATION CHECKLIST: FLUID BALANCE CHARTING

STUDENT NAME: _____

CLINICAL SKILL 26.1: Fluid balance charting

DEMONSTRATION OF: The ability to correctly and accurately complete a fluid balance chart

If the observation checklist is being used as an assessment tool, the student will need to obtain a scale of independence for each of the performance criteria/evidence.

Independent (I)
Supervised (S)
Assisted (A)
Marginal (M)
Dependent (D)

COMPETENCY ELEMENTS	PERFORMANCE CRITERIA/EVIDENCE	I	S	A	M	D
Preparation for the activity	Identifies indications and rationale for performing the activity Identifies the individual using three individual identifiers Ensures therapeutic interaction Gains the individual's consent Checks facility/organisation policy Validates the order in the individual's record Locates and gathers equipment					
Performs activity informed by evidence	Depending on the need for the FBC, records the total at least each shift to enable an accurate fluid status of the individual If the individual is on a fluid restriction, updates them on their progress for the day					
Applies critical thinking and reflective practice	Assesses the individual's ability to record their input Ensures all input and output recorded correctly including IV fluids and any IV medications, and all sensible losses that can be measured Is able to link theory to practice Demonstrates current best practice in the care provided Assesses own performance					
Practises within safety and quality assurance guidelines	Is aware of any fluid restrictions or any special fluid requirements when recording Reviews against facility/organisation policy Performs hand hygiene, dons appropriate PPE as per infection control protocols Cleans and disposes of equipment and waste appropriately					
Documentation and communication	Explains and communicates the activity clearly to the individual Communicates outcome and ongoing care to individual and significant others Communicates abnormal findings to appropriate personnel Reports and documents all relevant information and any complications correctly in the healthcare record Reports any complications and/or inability to perform the procedure to the RN and/or medical officer Asks the individual to report any complications during and post procedure					

Educator/Facilitator Feedback:

Educator/Facilitator Score: Competent   Needs further development

How would you rate your overall performance while undertaking this clinical activity? (use a ✓ & initial)

Unsatisfactory   Satisfactory   Good   Excellent

Student Reflection: (discuss how you would approach your practice differently or more effectively)

EDUCATOR/FACILITATOR NAME/SIGNATURE:

STUDENT NAME/SIGNATURE: **DATE:**

Evolve®

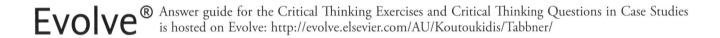 Answer guide for the Critical Thinking Exercises and Critical Thinking Questions in Case Studies is hosted on Evolve: http://evolve.elsevier.com/AU/Koutoukidis/Tabbner/

References

Berman, A., Frandsen, G., Snyder, S., et al., 2020. *Kozier and Erb's fundamentals of nursing*, 5th ed. Pearson, Melbourne.

Brown, D., Edwards, H., Buckley, T., et al., 2020. *Lewis's medical–surgical nursing: Assessment and management of clinical problems*, 5th ed. Elsevier, Sydney.

Crisp, J., Douglas, C., Rebeiro, G., et al. (eds.), 2021. *Potter & Perry's fundamentals of nursing*, 6th ed. Elsevier, Chatswood.

Nursing and Midwifery Board of Australia (NMBA), 2020. Decision-making framework for nursing and midwifery. Available at: <https://www.nursingmidwiferyboard.gov.au/Codes-Guidelines-Statements/Frameworks.aspx>.

Simpson, D., McIntosh, R., 2021. Measuring and monitoring fluid balance. *British Journal of Nursing* 20(12), 706–710.

Sivapuram, M., 2022. Fluid balance charts: Documentation. Evidence summaries. (JBI183.) The Joanna Briggs Institute. Available at: <http://ovidsp.ovid.com/ovidweb.cgi?T=JS&PAGE=reference&D=jbi&NEWS=N&AN=JBI183>.

MOVEMENT AND EXERCISE

Heather Wakefield

Overview

Movement and exercise are essential components for restoring, maintaining and enhancing physical and psychosocial health. The human body is ideally suited to movement. Regular exercise promotes health and feelings of wellbeing and prevents illness throughout the lifespan. Exercise is made possible by the muscular, skeletal and nervous systems. These interconnected systems work together to make movement possible; for most human movement they must function effectively for optimal physical performance. Disease processes that disable one or more of these systems may inhibit or restrict mobility.

This chapter includes how to position an individual in bed and assist with a transfer utilising the 'no lift technique', as well as how to assist with application of anti-embolic stockings.

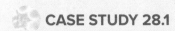

CASE STUDY 28.1

Lorenzo Durutto is an 87-year-old man with limited English. He has dense right hemiplegia and requires a shower after an incontinent episode. The care plan states he requires transferring using a hoist. You are an agency nurse, unfamiliar with the hoists used in this aged-care home; however, Lorenzo is becoming increasingly impatient and upset.

1. State what nursing care is priority at this time.
2. Outline how you will transfer this individual to a commode chair.
3. List other assessments you will make of Lorenzo while transferring and attending to his hygiene.

CRITICAL THINKING EXERCISE 28.4

You are caring for an individual who is recovering from a motor vehicle accident. The individual sustained a fractured left tibia and fibula and a fractured left humerus, both of which are in a full cast. Outline the strategies you will employ to ensure this individual mobilises comfortably and safely.

CLINICAL SKILL 28.1 Assisting with transfer

Please adhere to the policy and procedures of the facility/organisation prior to undertaking the skill. Ensure this skill is in your scope of practice.

NMBA Decision-making Framework considerations (refer to NMBA Decision-making framework for nursing and midwifery 2020):	Equipment (as needed):
1. Am I educated? 2. Am I authorised? 3. Am I competent? If you answer 'no' to any of these, do not perform that activity. Seek guidance and support from your teacher/a nurse team leader/clinical facilitator/educator.	Transfer belt Sling Lap board Slide sheet Mechanical/hydraulic lift

 PREPARE FOR THE SKILL

(Please refer to the Standard Steps on p. xii for related rationales.)
Mentally review the steps of the skill.
Discuss the skill with your instructor/supervisor/team leader, if required.
Confirm correct facility/organisation policy/safe operating procedures.
Validate the order in the individual's record.
Identify indication and rationale for performing the activity.
Assess for any contraindications.
Locate and gather equipment.
Perform hand hygiene.
Ensure therapeutic interaction.
Identify the individual using three individual identifiers.
Gain the individual's consent.
Assess for pain relief.
Prepare the environment.
Provide and maintain privacy.
Assist the individual to assume an appropriate position of comfort.

Skill activity	Rationale
Assess the individual for: • Joint mobility • Presence of paralysis or paresis • Activity tolerance • Orthostatic blood pressure • Level of consciousness • Pain level • Ability to follow instructions.	Provides information regarding the individual's ability to transfer and the number of people required to assist.

 PERFORM THE SKILL

(Please refer to the Standard Steps on p. xii for related rationales.)
Perform hand hygiene.
Apply PPE: gloves, eyewear, mask and gown as appropriate.
Ensure the individual's safety and comfort throughout skill.
Promote independence and involvement of the individual if possible and/or appropriate.
Assess the individual's tolerance to the skill throughout.
Dispose of used supplies, equipment, waste and sharps appropriately.
Remove PPE and discard or store appropriately.
Perform hand hygiene.

Skill activity	Rationale
Assisting individual into sitting position on side of bed	
With the individual in a supine position, raise the head of bed to 30 degrees.	Decreases amount of work required by the individual and nurse to raise person to a sitting position.

CLINICAL SKILL 28.1 Assisting with transfer—cont'd

Where possible, the individual should be encouraged to move into the position themselves.	Decreases amount of work needed by individual and nurse to raise person to a sitting position.
Turn the individual to the side, facing nurse on the side of bed on which the individual will be sitting.	Prepares the individual to move to the side of bed and protects the individual from falling.
Stand opposite to the individual's hips and turn diagonally to face the individual and the far corner of foot of bed.	Places nurse's centre of gravity near to individual. Reduces twisting.
Place feet apart with foot closer to head of bed in front of other foot.	Increases balance and allows nurse to transfer weight as individual is brought to sitting position on side of bed.
Place arm nearer head of bed under individual's shoulder, supporting head and neck.	Maintains alignment of head and neck as nurse brings individual to sitting position.
Place other arm over individual's thighs.	Supports hip and prevents individual from falling backwards during procedure.
Move individual's lower legs and feet over side of bed. Pivot towards rear leg, allowing the individual's upper legs to swing downwards.	Decreases friction and resistance. Weight of individual's legs when off bed provides gravity to lower legs, and weight of leg helps pull upper body into a sitting position.
At same time, shift weight to rear leg and elevate individual.	Allows nurse to transfer weight in direction of motion.
Remain in front of the individual until they regain balance.	Reduces risk of falling.
Transfer individual from bed to chair:	
Adjust the bed so that it is slightly higher than the chair. Assist the individual to a sitting position on side of the bed. Have chair in position at 45-degree angle to the bed and ensure the brakes are on.	Positions chair within easy access for transfer.
Apply transfer belt or other transfer aids if required.	Reduces risk of falling.
Ensure individual has stable, non-skid shoes. Weight-bearing or stronger leg is placed forwards with weaker foot back.	Decreases risk of slipping. Bare feet increases risk of falls.
Spread feet apart.	Ensures balance with wide base of support.
Flex hips and knees, aligning feet and knees with individual's feet.	Flexion of knees and hips lowers nurse's centre of gravity to object to be raised; aligning knees with individual allows for stabilisation of knees when individual stands.
Grasp transfer belt from underneath, if used, or reach through individual's axillae and place hands on individual's scapulae.	Transferring individual with hands on scapulae reduces pressure on axillae and maintains the individual's stability. Transfer belt is grasped at each side to provide movement of individual at centre of gravity.
Rock individual up to standing position on count of three while straightening hips and legs and keeping knees slightly flexed. Individual is instructed to use hands to push up if possible.	Rocking motion gives individual body momentum and requires less muscular effort to transfer individual.
Maintain stability of individual's weak or paralysed leg with knee.	Ability to stand can often be maintained in paralysed or weak limb with support of knee to stabilise.
Pivot on foot further from chair.	Maintains support of individual while allowing adequate space for individual to move.
Instruct the individual to use armrests on chair for support and ease themselves into chair.	Increases individual's stability.
Flex hips and knees while lowering individual into chair.	Prevents injury to nurse from poor body mechanics.

Continued

CLINICAL SKILL 28.1 Assisting with transfer—cont'd

Assess the individual for proper alignment for sitting position. Provide support for paralysed extremities. Lap board or sling will support flaccid arm. Stabilise leg with bath blanket or pillow.	Prevents injury to individual from poor body alignment.
Praise individual's progress, effort and performance.	Continued support and encouragement provides incentive for individuals.

Use mechanical/hydraulic lift to transfer individual from bed to chair (two nurses):

Assess the individual's mobility and strength.	To determine whether the individual can offer help during transfer.
Bring lift to bedside. Before using lift, be familiar with its operation. Check hoist sling, straps, hooks and chains in safe working order.	Prepares environment for safe use of lift and subsequent transfer.
Position chair near bed and allow adequate space to manoeuvre hoist.	Prepares environment for safe use of lift and subsequent transfer.
Raise bed to safe working height with mattress flat. Lower side rails.	Allows nurse to use proper body mechanics.
Roll the individual towards one nurse.	Positions individual for use of lift sling.
Place sling evenly under individual's back (follow manufacturer's guidelines) and roll individual to opposite side to position sling.	Places sling under individual's centre of gravity and greatest portion of body weight.
Roll individual supine on sling and position hoist over individual. Lower boom and attach sling to frame with the head end attached first. Raise individual's knees and feed the leg sections of the sling under the thighs and attach to frame.	Sling should extend from shoulders to knees to support individual's body weight equally.
Elevate head of bed.	Positions individual in sitting position.
Ask or assist the individual to fold arms over the chest.	To prevent injury during transfer.
Pump hydraulic handle using long, slow, even strokes, or activate electronic hoist until individual is raised off bed ensuring the head is supported.	
Using steering handle to move, lift from bed and manoeuvre to the chair. Slowly lower the individual onto chair.	Moves individual from bed to chair.
Detach sling from frame and remove hoist. Pull leg straps to the side, tilt the individual forwards to slide out of the sling.	Safely guides individual into back of chair as seat descends.
Reposition the individual to a comfortable and safe position.	

AFTER THE SKILL

(Please refer to the Standard Steps on p. xii for related rationales.)
Communicate outcome to the individual, any ongoing care and to report any complications .
Restore the environment.
Report, record and document assessment findings, details of the skill performed and the individual's response.
Report, record and document any abnormalities and/or inability to perform the skill.
Reassess the individual to ensure there are no adverse effects/events from the skill.

(Crisp et al 2021; Rebeiro et al 2021; Tollefson & Hillman 2022)

OBSERVATION CHECKLIST: ASSISTING WITH TRANSFER

STUDENT NAME: _____

CLINICAL SKILL 28.1: Assisting with transfer

DEMONSTRATION OF: The ability to assist with transferring individuals

If the observation checklist is being used as an assessment tool, the student will need to obtain a scale of independence for each of the performance criteria/evidence.

Independent (I)		
Supervised (S)		
Assisted (A)		
Marginal (M)		
Dependent (D)		

COMPETENCY ELEMENTS	PERFORMANCE CRITERIA/EVIDENCE	I	S	A	M	D
Preparation for the activity	Identifies indications and rationale for performing the activity Identifies the individual using three individual identifiers Ensures therapeutic interaction Gains the individual's consent Checks facility/organisation policy Validates the order in the individual's record Locates and gathers equipment Assists the individual into an appropriate position Asks the individual to report any feelings of dizziness, weakness or shortness of breath while mobilising					
Performs activity informed by evidence	Undertakes a risk assessment to identify any movement limitations and identifies pain Assesses for IV lines, incisions or equipment that may alter the procedure **Bed to chair** Encourages the individual to assist Positions chair at 45-degree angle to bed Assists individual to move their legs over side of bed Assesses the individual's footwear, balance and leg strength Rocks individual into standing position on count of three and supports individual to stand Encourages individual to pivot using foot furthest from the chair Instructs individual to use chair arms for stability and ease themselves down into chair Ensures individual is in a comfortable position with call bell within easy reach **Bed to chair using lifting machine** Positions lifting machine at side of bed Positions chair close to the bed Places sling evenly under individual's back by rolling individual laterally Lowers horizontal bar of lifting machine and attaches sling to bar Asks or assists individual to cross their arms or hold onto the straps Slowly elevates individual and provides reassurance Using the steering handle, moves lifting machine and individual over chair Slowly lowers individual and positions individual in chair Ensures individual is in a comfortable position with call bell within easy reach					

Continued

COMPETENCY ELEMENTS	PERFORMANCE CRITERIA/EVIDENCE	I	S	A	M	D
Applies critical thinking and reflective practice	Demonstrates critical thinking and problem-solving (e.g. privacy, correct positioning of individual, assesses for signs of pain or discomfort) Is able to link theory to practice Demonstrates current best practice in the care provided Assesses own performance					
Practises within safety and quality assurance guidelines	Reviews against facility/organisation policy Performs hand hygiene Adjusts the bed to the appropriate working position and re-adjusts at completion of activity Cleans equipment appropriately					
Documentation and communication	Explains and communicates the activity clearly to the individual Communicates outcome and ongoing care to individual and significant others Communicates abnormal findings to appropriate personnel Reports and documents all relevant information and any complications correctly in the healthcare record Reports any complications and/or inability to perform the procedure to the RN and/or medical officer Asks the individual to report any complications during and post procedure					

Educator/Facilitator Feedback:

Educator/Facilitator Score: Competent   Needs further development

How would you rate your overall performance while undertaking this clinical activity? (use a ✓ & initial)

Unsatisfactory   Satisfactory   Good   Excellent

Student Reflection: (discuss how you would approach your practice differently or more effectively)

EDUCATOR/FACILITATOR NAME/SIGNATURE:

STUDENT NAME/SIGNATURE: **DATE:**

CLINICAL SKILL 28.2 Positioning individuals in bed

Please adhere to the policy and procedures of the facility/organisation prior to undertaking the skill. Ensure this skill is in your scope of practice.

NMBA Decision-making Framework considerations (refer to NMBA Decision-making framework for nursing and midwifery 2020):	Equipment:
1. Am I educated? 2. Am I authorised? 3. Am I competent? If you answer 'no' to any of these, do not perform that activity. Seek guidance and support from your teacher/a nurse team leader/clinical facilitator/educator.	Slide sheet/slip sheet Pillows Lifting device, if required

 PREPARE FOR THE SKILL

(Please refer to the Standard Steps on p. xii for related rationales.)
Mentally review the steps of the skill.
Discuss the skill with your instructor/supervisor/team leader, if required.
Confirm correct facility/organisation policy/safe operating procedures.
Validate the order in the individual's record.
Identify indication and rationale for performing the activity.
Assess for any contraindications.
Locate and gather equipment.
Perform hand hygiene.
Ensure therapeutic interaction.
Identify the individual using three individual identifiers.
Gain the individual's consent.
Assess for pain relief.
Prepare the environment.
Provide and maintain privacy.
Assist the individual to assume an appropriate position of comfort.

Skill activity	Rationale
Assess the individual's physical ability to help with moving and positioning. Assess the individual's physical ability to help with moving and positioning.	Ensures individual's independence is maintained. Determines need for additional assistance. Ensures safety.
Account for all tubing, drains and attached equipment.	Prevents spillage and dislodgement if equipment catches on bedframe or mattress.
Place the individual in supine position with head of the bed flat and remove the pillows, place pillow at the head of the bed.	Enables nurse to assess body alignment. Reduces gravity's pull on individual's upper body. Prevents striking the individual's head against head of the bed.
Assess the need for extra help.	Ensures the individual's and nurse's safety.

 PERFORM THE SKILL

(Please refer to the Standard Steps on p. xii for related rationales.)
Perform hand hygiene.
Apply PPE: gloves, eyewear, mask and gown as appropriate.
Ensure the individual's safety and comfort throughout skill.
Promote independence and involvement of the individual if possible and/or appropriate.
Assess the individual's tolerance to the skill throughout.
Dispose of used supplies, equipment, waste and sharps appropriately.
Remove PPE and discard or store appropriately.
Perform hand hygiene.

CLINICAL SKILL 28.2 Positioning individuals in bed—cont'd

Skill activity	Rationale
Determine the most appropriate position for the individual.	Various conditions and diseases preclude moving individuals into some positions.
Utilise principles of efficient body mechanics.	To protect the nurse's back.
Perform pressure area care. Wash and dry area. Apply moisturiser, if appropriate. Change linen.	Prevents skin breakdown. Maintains skin integrity.
Move and position individual appropriately using appropriate friction-reducing device (such as slide sheet). Ensure pressure is relieved by positioning in a different position. Pressure-relieving devices may be utilised.	Promotes individual's comfort.
The body must be supported to maintain its natural contours, symmetry and alignment.	Maintains and helps to restore body functioning and helps to prevent the complications with bed rest and immobility.
Assess the skin.	Ongoing assessment of the skin is necessary to detect early signs of pressure damage.

 AFTER THE SKILL

(Please refer to the Standard Steps on p. xii for related rationales.)
Communicate outcome to the individual, any ongoing care and to report any complications.
Restore the environment.
Report, record and document assessment findings, details of the skill performed and the individual's response.
Report, record and document any abnormalities and/or inability to perform the skill.
Reassess the individual to ensure there are no adverse effects/events from the skill.

(Perry et al 2019; Rebeiro et al 2021; Tollefson & Hillman 2022)

OBSERVATION CHECKLIST: POSITIONING INDIVIDUALS IN BED

STUDENT NAME: _____

CLINICAL SKILL 28.2: Positioning individuals in bed

DEMONSTRATION OF: The ability to position an individual in bed

If the observation checklist is being used as an assessment tool, the student will need to obtain a scale of independence for each of the performance criteria/evidence.

Independent (I)

Supervised (S)

Assisted (A)

Marginal (M)

Dependent (D)

COMPETENCY ELEMENTS	PERFORMANCE CRITERIA/EVIDENCE	I	S	A	M	D
Preparation for the activity	Identifies indications and rationale for performing the activity Identifies the individual using three individual identifiers Ensures therapeutic interaction Gains the individual's consent Checks facility/organisation policy Validates the order in the individual's record Locates and gathers equipment Assists the individual into an appropriate position					
Performs activity informed by evidence	Undertakes a risk assessment to identify individual's capability, movement limitations and any movement that may be contraindicated Removes clutter from area Assists the individual to a comfortable position and positions in correct alignment Uses equipment as required (e.g. slide sheet) Uses pillows or other supports under the legs and arms as needed Readjusts the pillow under the individual's head Elevates the head of the bed as needed for comfort					
Applies critical thinking and reflective practice	Demonstrates critical thinking and problem-solving (e.g. privacy, correct position of individual, abnormalities and pain noted) Is able to link theory to practice Demonstrates current best practice in the care provided Assesses own performance					
Practises within safety and quality assurance guidelines	Reviews against facility/organisation policy Performs hand hygiene Lowers the bed to the appropriate working position and raises at completion of activity Cleans equipment appropriately					
Documentation and communication	Explains and communicates the activity clearly to the individual Communicates outcome and ongoing care to individual and significant others Communicates abnormal findings to appropriate personnel Reports and documents all relevant information and any complications correctly in the healthcare record Reports any complications and/or inability to perform the procedure to the RN and/or medical officer Asks the individual to report any complications during and post procedure					

Educator/Facilitator Feedback:

Educator/Facilitator Score: Competent   Needs further development

How would you rate your overall performance while undertaking this clinical activity? (use a ✓ & initial)

Unsatisfactory   Satisfactory   Good   Excellent

Student Reflection: (discuss how you would approach your practice differently or more effectively)

EDUCATOR/FACILITATOR NAME/SIGNATURE:

STUDENT NAME/SIGNATURE: **DATE:**

CLINICAL SKILL 28.3 Application of anti-embolic stockings

Please adhere to the policy and procedures of the facility/organisation prior to undertaking the skill. Ensure this skill is in your scope of practice.

NMBA Decision-making Framework considerations (refer to NMBA Decision-making framework for nursing and midwifery 2020):	Equipment:
1. Am I educated? 2. Am I authorised? 3. Am I competent? If you answer 'no' to any of these, do not perform that activity. Seek guidance and support from your teacher/a nurse team leader/clinical facilitator/educator.	Tape measure Correct size of anti-embolic elastic stockings Talcum powder (optional)

 PREPARE FOR THE SKILL

(Please refer to the Standard Steps on p. xii for related rationales.)
Mentally review the steps of the skill.
Discuss the skill with your instructor/supervisor/team leader, if required.
Confirm correct facility/organisation policy/safe operating procedures.
Validate the order in the individual's record.
Identify indication and rationale for performing the activity.
Assess for any contraindications.
Locate and gather equipment.
Perform hand hygiene.
Ensure therapeutic interaction.
Identify the individual using three individual identifiers.
Gain the individual's consent.
Assess for pain relief.
Prepare the environment.
Provide and maintain privacy.
Assist the individual to assume an appropriate position of comfort.

Skill activity	Rationale
Observe for signs and symptoms and conditions that might contraindicate the use of anti-embolic elastic stockings.	Anti-embolic elastic stockings may aggravate skin conditions. Continuous pressure is necessary to keep graft adherent to recipient bed, but pressure should not be firm as to cause death of the graft. Anti-embolic elastic stockings that do not fit correctly due to larger thighs may cause excessive pressure and constriction around the thighs, which could then lead to reduced venous return. Circulation may be further reduced in conditions of altered circulation.

 PERFORM THE SKILL

(Please refer to the Standard Steps on p. xii for related rationales.)
Perform hand hygiene.
Apply PPE: gloves, eyewear, mask and gown as appropriate.
Ensure the individual's safety and comfort throughout skill.
Promote independence and involvement of the individual if possible and/or appropriate.
Assess the individual's tolerance to the skill throughout.
Dispose of used supplies, equipment, waste and sharps appropriately.
Remove PPE and discard or store appropriately.
Perform hand hygiene.

CLINICAL SKILL 28.3 Application of anti-embolic stockings—cont'd

Skill activity	Rationale
Assess individual's skin, colouration and circulation of legs.	Identifies a baseline of skin condition and quality of pedal pulses.
Use tape measure to measure individual's legs to determine correct stocking size.	Stockings must be measured as per the instructions on the packaging. The length of the stockings will be determined by the medical orders and the individual's condition. If stockings are too large, they will not support the extremities adequately. If stockings are too small, circulation may be impeded.
Position individual in supine position.	Ensures good body mechanics for the nurse and enables ease of application. Stockings should be applied before standing to prevent stagnation of blood in lower extremities.
Ensure the individual's legs are clean and dry and apply a small amount of talcum powder.	Allows for easier application and reduces friction.
Stockings are applied by rolling them slowly from the foot up the leg. Ensure the foot fits into toe and heel position of the stocking. Ensure the stocking is completely extended up the leg. Ensure it is smooth and no creases are present. Ensure toes are able to be exposed to check they remain warm and pink and blood supply is not impeded by the stockings.	Creases in stockings can impede circulation to lower region of extremities.
Inspect stockings to make sure there are no creases or binding at the top.	Can lead to increased pressure and alter circulation.
Ensure individual is aware not to adjust stockings or roll them down. Note individual's reaction to stockings.	Rolling down of stockings can have a constricting effect and impede venous return. Ensure the individual is adapting to stockings and is not experiencing discomfort.
Ensure individual wears shoes/slippers over stockings to ambulate.	Slip/fall prevention strategy.
Remove stockings once per shift.	Ensures they remain in the correct position. Ensures skin intact. Ensures adequate circulation. Identifies any complications.

 AFTER THE SKILL

(Please refer to the Standard Steps on p. xii for related rationales.)
Communicate outcome to the individual, any ongoing care and to report any complications.
Restore the environment.
Report, record and document assessment findings, details of the skill performed and the individual's response.
Report, record and document any abnormalities and/or inability to perform the skill.
Reassess the individual to ensure there are no adverse effects/events from the skill.

Skill activity	Rationale
Document size and length of stockings that were applied. Record skin condition and circulatory assessment.	Informs healthcare professionals and assists with planning and implementing care.

(Crisp et al 2021; Rebeiro et al 2021)

OBSERVATION CHECKLIST: APPLICATION OF ANTI-EMBOLIC STOCKINGS

STUDENT NAME: _____

CLINICAL SKILL 28.3: Application of anti-embolic stockings

DEMONSTRATION OF: The ability to apply anti-embolic stockings

If the observation checklist is being used as an assessment tool, the student will need to obtain a scale of independence for each of the performance criteria/evidence.

Independent (I)
Supervised (S)
Assisted (A)
Marginal (M)
Dependent (D)

COMPETENCY ELEMENTS	PERFORMANCE CRITERIA/EVIDENCE	I	S	A	M	D
Preparation for the activity	Identifies indications and rationale for performing the activity Identifies the individual using three individual identifiers Ensures therapeutic interaction Gains the individual's consent Checks facility/organisation policy Validates the order in the individual's record Locates and gathers equipment					
Performs activity informed by evidence	Assists individual into a supine position Exposes one leg at a time Powders the leg if appropriate Turns stockings inside out, places over individual's toes Slides stocking over individual's foot Slides stocking up over individual's calf and ensures stocking is smooth with no creases Repositions individual Ensures call bell is within reach Ensures shoes are available to avoid slipping					
Applies critical thinking and reflective practice	Demonstrates critical thinking and problem-solving (e.g. correctly measures legs and obtains correct-size stockings) Assesses individual for any abnormalities or pain Is able to link theory to practice Demonstrates current best practice in the care provided Assesses own performance					
Practises within safety and quality assurance guidelines	Reviews against facility/organisation policy Performs hand hygiene Raises the bed to the appropriate working position based on nurse's height and lowers at completion of activity Correctly measures according to manufacturer's instructions					
Documentation and communication	Explains and communicates the activity clearly to the individual Communicates outcome and ongoing care to individual and significant others Communicates abnormal findings to appropriate personnel Reports and documents all relevant information and any complications correctly in the healthcare record Reports any complications and/or inability to perform the procedure to the RN and/or medical officer Asks the individual to report any complications during and post procedure					

Educator/Facilitator Feedback:

Educator/Facilitator Score: Competent   Needs further development

How would you rate your overall performance while undertaking this clinical activity? (use a ✓ & initial)

Unsatisfactory   Satisfactory   Good   Excellent

Student Reflection: (discuss how you would approach your practice differently or more effectively)

EDUCATOR/FACILITATOR NAME/SIGNATURE:

STUDENT NAME/SIGNATURE: **DATE:**

Evolve®

Answer guide for the Critical Thinking Exercises and Critical Thinking Questions in Case Studies is hosted on Evolve: http://evolve.elsevier.com/AU/Koutoukidis/Tabbner/

References

Crisp, J., Douglas, C., Rebeiro, G., Waters, D., 2021. *Potter & Perry's fundamentals of nursing*, 6th ed. Elsevier, Sydney.

Nursing and Midwifery Board of Australia (NMBA), 2020. Decision-making framework for nursing and midwifery. Available at: <https://www.nursingmidwiferyboard.gov.au/codes-guidelines-statements/frameworks.aspx>.

Perry, A.G., Potter, P.A., Ostendorf, W.R., 2019. *Nursing interventions & clinical skills*, 7th ed. Elsevier, St Louis.

Rebeiro, G., Wilson, D., Fuller, S., 2021. *Potter and Perry's fundamentals of nursing workbook*, 4th ed. Elsevier, Chatswood.

Tollefson, J., Hillman, E., 2022. *Clinical psychomotor skills: Assessment tools for nursing students*, 8th ed. Cengage Learning Australia, South Melbourne.

SKIN INTEGRITY AND WOUND CARE

Jing Wan (Persephone Wan)

Overview

The integumentary system is the largest organ of the body. As the skin is exposed to infection and trauma, promotion of skin integrity is important to maintain and protect underlying organs and structures. The skin also provides the first line of defence for microorganisms to prevent entry into the body. Not only is it important to promote wound healing—understanding wound healing and measures to promote optimal conditions for healing are also required.

The skin has several functions that are largely concerned with protection of the body against infection, physical trauma and ultraviolet radiation. Any disorder that disrupts normal skin function will affect the efficiency with which it carries out its functions and may place the physiological integrity of the individual at risk. Maintenance of skin integrity and wound management are major roles of the nurse. It is important that all nurses understand normal wound healing and the variances that can occur with ageing and disease processes.

Aseptic non-touch technique (ANTT) is a framework used in conjunction with standard precautions and the 5 Moments for Hand Hygiene to protect Key-Parts and Key-Sites when performing clinical procedures and utilising a surgical or standard ANTT. The introduction of ANTT has been based on the resources provided by The Association for Safe Aseptic Practice (The-ASAP) UK and the ANTT project (see www.antt.org).

Asepsis is maintained and/or ensured by the use of six core infection prevention and control components:

1. Key-Part and Key-Site identification and protection
2. Hand hygiene
3. Glove use and a non-touch technique
4. Aseptic fields to promote and ensure asepsis
5. Environmental controls
6. Sequencing of procedures.

A *Key-Part* is the part of the equipment that must remain sterile or aseptic, such as the forceps tips and scissor tips; it must only make contact with other Key-Parts or Key-Sites.

A *Key-Site* is the area on the person, such as a wound, that must be protected from microorganisms. Key-Sites are protected by non-touch techniques and aseptic fields.

Hand hygiene involves using alcohol-based hand rub or soap and water using correct technique and performed at the correct time in the sequence for the procedure. Glove use and non-touch technique reduce the risk of contamination for the individual and carer during contact with the procedural equipment. Non-sterile gloves are used to minimise the risk of contamination and body fluid exposure during the procedure and for basic dressings. Sterile gloves are used if it is necessary to touch Key-Parts or Key-Sites directly.

Standard aseptic technique can be used when procedures:
- Involve a small number of Key-Parts and Key-Sites
- Involve small Key-Parts and Key-Sites
- Are technically simple
- Are short in duration (e.g. less than 20 minutes).

Standard aseptic technique requires the clinician to:
- Identify Key-Parts and Key-Sites
- Protect those Key-Parts and Key-Sites from contamination during the procedure
- Decontaminate non-aseptic Key-Parts as required
- Create and maintain aseptic fields
- Perform hand hygiene
- Wear gloves
- Use a non-touch technique
- Control environmental risks.

Surgical aseptic technique is required when procedures:
- Involve a large number of Key-Parts or Key-Sites
- Involve large-sized Key-Parts or Key-Sites
- Are technically complex
- Are long in duration (e.g. more than 20 minutes).

Surgical aseptic technique requires the clinician to:
- Identify Key-Parts and Key-Sites
- Protect those Key-Parts and Key-Sites from contamination during the procedure
- Decontaminate non-aseptic Key-Parts as required
- Maintain aseptic fields
- Perform hand hygiene
- Wear sterile gloves
- Use a non-touch technique whenever possible
- Control environmental risks.

This chapter contains skills related to wounds including collecting a wound swab, assessment and management of skin tears, dressing a wound, packing a wound, shortening a drain tube and removal of sutures or staples. The standard steps for all clinical skills/interventions should be reviewed before undertaking the skill. The dressing trolley should be cleaned before and after use, with equipment to be used placed on the bottom shelf. This leaves the top surface as clean as possible. Confirm the sterility/use-by dates of equipment to be used. Ensure adequate lighting to facilitate observation of the wound and adjust the bed height to an appropriate working position based on your height to promote comfort and facilitate performance of the procedure. After the procedure readjust the bed to an appropriate height for the individual to promote comfort and independence of the individual and reduce the risk of falls. Clean dressing trolley as per organisational policy.

 CASE STUDY 29.2

Skin tears

Eleanor Parker is a frail 89-year-old who has been admitted to hospital for functional decline and increased confusion. Her medical history includes hypertension (on twice daily furosemide), COPD (on a regular inhaler) and rheumatoid arthritis (on disease-modifying anti-rheumatic drugs). She walks with a four-wheelie walker, and her gait has become increasingly unsteady over the past 6 months. She used to cook for herself, but recently has been living on sandwiches and only weighs 42 kg for her 158 cm height. Upon arrival to the clinical area, a bleeding skin tear is noted on her left leg (pre-tibial region). Eleanor cannot recall how it was sustained. Upon skin assessment, the skin tear is classified as type 2 with partial flap loss according to the ISTAP skin tear classification.

1. In addition to the skin tear classification, what other assessments are required prior to the wound management?
2. What is the required wound care/management for Mrs Parker's skin tear?
3. What preventative measures can be taken for Mrs Parker?

CRITICAL THINKING EXERCISE 29.1

What factors do you consider in terms of selecting an appropriate dressing product for a given wound type?

CLINICAL SKILL 29.1 Wound swab

Please adhere to the policy and procedures of the facility/organisation prior to undertaking the skill. Ensure this skill is in your scope of practice.

NMBA Decision-making Framework considerations (refer to NMBA Decision-making framework for nursing and midwifery 2020):	Equipment:
1. Am I educated? 2. Am I authorised? 3. Am I competent? If you answer 'no' to any of these, do not perform that activity. Seek guidance and support from your teacher/a nurse team leader/clinical facilitator/educator.	Disposable gloves Wound swab kit Sterile dressing pack Sterile normal saline 0.9% Biohazard specimen transport bag Laboratory request form (signed by a medical practitioner or Nurse Practitioner—may be an electronic document) Dressing trolley Disinfectant wipes/solution Waste receptacle

 ### PREPARE FOR THE SKILL

(Please refer to the Standard Steps on p. xii for related rationales.)
Mentally review the steps of the skill.
Discuss the skill with your instructor/supervisor/team leader, if required.
Confirm correct facility/organisation policy/safe operating procedures.
Validate the order in the individual's record.
Identify indication and rationale for performing the activity.
Assess for any contraindications.
Locate and gather equipment.
Perform hand hygiene.
Ensure therapeutic interaction.
Identify the individual using three individual identifiers.
Gain the individual's consent.
Assess for pain relief.
Prepare the environment.
Provide and maintain privacy.
Assist the individual to assume an appropriate position of comfort.

Skill activity	Rationale
Wound swabs are often taken at the time of wound dressing changes. These are taken when the wound is suspected of containing microorganisms. Identification of the microorganism will enable correct treatment regimens to be implemented.	
Assess the individual's record to determine previous appearance of wound and any previous dressings.	Determines requirements for equipment and dressing requirements.

 ### PERFORM THE SKILL

(Please refer to the Standard Steps on p. xii for related rationales.)
Perform hand hygiene.
Apply PPE: gloves, eyewear, mask and gown as appropriate.
Ensure the individual's safety and comfort throughout skill.
Promote independence and involvement of the individual if possible and/or appropriate.
Assess the individual's tolerance to the skill throughout.
Dispose of used supplies, equipment, waste and sharps appropriately.
Remove PPE and discard or store appropriately.
Perform hand hygiene.

Skill activity	Rationale
Create the aseptic field by using the sterile dressing pack and adding sterile equipment including 0.9% sodium chloride to the field. Open sterile dressing pack by using corners. Open the sterile dressing products away from the aseptic field and add into the field.	Prevents contamination of sterile items and Key-Parts.

Continued

CLINICAL SKILL 29.1 Wound swab—cont'd

Loosen and remove the existing wound dressing and assess wound for suspected clinical signs and symptoms of infection, including the type and amount of exudate on the removed dressing and peri-wound condition. Dispose of wound dressing and the used gloves.	Assesses for signs and symptoms of wound infection (e.g. redness, swelling, warmth, exudate amount and type). Prevents spread of microorganisms.
Position sterile dressing drape below or near the wound.	Protects wound from environmental contamination.
Cleanse the wound with sterile 0.9% sodium chloride.	Removes excessive debris and any dressing residue. Prevents swab from becoming contaminated, which could lead to false positive swab results. If the wound is dry, the swab may be moistened with sterile normal saline; if the wound is moist, the dry swab can be used dry.
Remove wound swab from the swab container and perform Levine technique (rotate swab over a 1 cm² area with sufficient pressure to express fluid from tissue) from the cleanest part of the wound bed. Return the wound swab back to the transport medium. Place used wound swab kit(s) on the lower shelf of the dressing trolley or a clean surface. Repeat with another wound swab if required.	Obtains causative pathogen from both superficial and deep in the wound bed (aerobic and anaerobic bacteria from the wound fluid). Do not swab pus or exudate since these surface organisms may contain contaminants that are different from those causing the wound infection. Minimises the risk of obtaining contaminated wound swab leading to false positive result.
Apply an appropriate sterile wound dressing (if required) using ANTT and secure. (See Clinical Skill 29.2 for dressing a wound.)	Covers wound and prevents spread of microorganisms.
Label specimen container with the person's name, date of birth, hospital or patient number and the date, time and site of the specimen collection. Add collector's signature/initial.	Ensures that the correct specimen is sent for testing and that it is for the correct person.
Specimen is placed in the zip lock section of the plastic biohazard bag.	Standard infection control precaution.
Pathology request form is checked for the person's details. The pathology request form is placed in the other section of the bag.	Ensures correct form and specimen are sent to pathology department and correct test will be undertaken in the pathology department.

AFTER THE SKILL

(Please refer to the Standard Steps on p. xii for related rationales.)
Communicate outcome to the individual, any ongoing care and report any complications.
Restore the environment.
Report, record and document assessment findings, details of the skill performed and the individual's response.
Report, record and document any abnormalities and/or inability to perform the skill.
Reassess the individual to ensure there are no adverse effects/events from the skill.

Skill activity	Rationale
The specimen should be transported to the laboratory as soon as possible, or stored in a refrigerator until transport can be arranged.	Decomposition and cell growth occur if the specimen is left standing, and may provide an inaccurate result.

(Adapted from ACIPC 2015; LeMone et al 2020; Berman et al 2020; IWII 2022; Lynn 2022; The-ASAP 2019)

OBSERVATION CHECKLIST: WOUND SWAB

STUDENT NAME: _____

CLINICAL SKILL 29.1: Wound swab

DEMONSTRATION OF: The ability to obtain a wound swab

If the observation checklist is being used as an assessment tool, the student will need to obtain a scale of independence for each of the performance criteria/evidence.

Independent (I)
Supervised (S)
Assisted (A)
Marginal (M)
Dependent (D)

COMPETENCY ELEMENTS	PERFORMANCE CRITERIA/EVIDENCE	I	S	A	M	D
Preparation for the activity	Identifies indications and rationale for performing the activity Identifies the individual using three individual identifiers Ensures therapeutic interaction Gains the individual's consent Checks facility/organisational policy Visually assesses the wound and any dressing Assesses pain, provides analgesia if required Validates the order in the individual's record Locates and gathers equipment Assists the individual into an appropriate position Ensures privacy and dignity					
Performs activity informed by evidence	Prepares and maintains aseptic field Removes and appropriately discards existing dressing Correctly positions dressing towels around the wound Cleanses the wound from a clean area towards a less clean area Performs wound swab using Levine technique (rotating the wound swab over a 1 cm² area of the wound by using gentle pressure) Repeats with another swab if required Applies and secures wound dressing as required Labels specimen according to organisational policies and procedures Places in specimen bag Dispatches specimen to laboratory with request form					
Applies critical thinking and reflective practice	Is able to link theory to practice Demonstrates current best practice in the care provided Obtains assistance as required Selects appropriate dressing (if required) Stores specimen in refrigerator if a delay of more than 24 hours between collection and transport to the laboratory is expected Assesses own performance					
Practises within safety and quality assurance guidelines	Reviews against facility/organisational policy Performs hand hygiene, dons and doffs PPE as per infection control protocols Raises the bed to the appropriate working position based on nurse's height and lowers at completion of activity Adheres to infection control/ANTT principles Labels specimen correctly Cleans and disposes of equipment and waste appropriately					

Continued

COMPETENCY ELEMENTS	PERFORMANCE CRITERIA/EVIDENCE	I	S	A	M	D
Documentation and communication	Explains and communicates the activity clearly to the individual Communicates outcome and ongoing care to individual and significant others Communicates abnormal findings to appropriate personnel Reports and documents all relevant information and any complications correctly in the healthcare record Reports any complications and/or inability to perform the procedure to the RN and/or medical officer Asks the individual to report any complications during and post procedure					

Educator/Facilitator Feedback:

Educator/Facilitator Score: Competent   Needs further development

How would you rate your overall performance while undertaking this clinical activity? (use a ✓ & initial)

Unsatisfactory ☐   Satisfactory ☐   Good ☐   Excellent ☐

Student Reflection: (discuss how you would approach your practice differently or more effectively)

EDUCATOR/FACILITATOR NAME/SIGNATURE:

STUDENT NAME/SIGNATURE: **DATE:**

CLINICAL SKILL 29.2 Dressing a wound

Please adhere to the policy and procedures of the facility/organisation prior to undertaking the skill. Ensure this skill is in your scope of practice.

NMBA Decision-making Framework considerations (refer to NMBA Decision-making framework for nursing and midwifery 2020):	Equipment:
1. Am I educated? 2. Am I authorised? 3. Am I competent? If you answer 'no' to any of these, do not perform that activity. Seek guidance and support from your teacher/a nurse team leader/clinical facilitator/educator.	Sterile dressing pack Sterile dressing materials Sterile 0.9% sodium chloride Additional light source (if required) Disposable gloves Waste receptacle Dressing trolley Disinfectant wipes/solution

 PREPARE FOR THE SKILL

(Please refer to the Standard Steps on p. xii for related rationales.)
Mentally review the steps of the skill.
Discuss the skill with your instructor/supervisor/team leader, if required.
Confirm correct facility/organisation policy/safe operating procedures.
Validate the order in the individual's record.
Identify indication and rationale for performing the activity.
Assess for any contraindications.
Locate and gather equipment.
Perform hand hygiene.
Ensure therapeutic interaction.
Identify the individual using three individual identifiers.
Gain the individual's consent.
Assess for pain relief.
Prepare the environment.
Provide and maintain privacy.
Assist the individual to assume an appropriate position of comfort.

Skill activity	Rationale
Wound dressings are undertaken to provide a moist cover for the wound to prevent the introduction of microorganisms and to promote healing. They also absorb exudate.	
Assess the individual's record to determine previous appearance of wound and any previous dressings.	Determines requirements for equipment and dressing requirements.

 PERFORM THE SKILL

(Please refer to the Standard Steps on p. xii for related rationales.)
Perform hand hygiene.
Apply PPE: gloves, eyewear, mask and gown as appropriate.
Ensure the individual's safety and comfort throughout skill.
Promote independence and involvement of the individual if possible and/or appropriate.
Assess the individual's tolerance to the skill throughout.
Dispose of used supplies, equipment, waste and sharps appropriately.
Remove PPE and discard or store appropriately.
Perform hand hygiene.

Skill activity	Rationale
Create the aseptic field by using the sterile dressing pack and adding sterile equipment including 0.9% sodium chloride to the field. Open sterile dressing pack by using corners. Open the sterile dressing products away from the aseptic field and add into the field.	Prevents contamination of sterile items and Key-Parts.

CLINICAL SKILL 29.2 Dressing a wound—cont'd

Loosen and remove the existing wound dressing and assess wound for suspected clinical signs and symptoms of infection, including the type and amount of exudate on the removed dressing and peri-wound condition. Dispose of wound dressing and the used gloves.	Assesses for signs and symptoms of wound infection (e.g. redness, swelling, warmth, exudate amount and type). Prevents spread of microorganisms.
Rearrange and assemble the required sterile dressing and equipment in the aseptic field using ANTT without contaminating the Key-Parts.	Maintains ANTT to protect the wound from environmental contamination. Prevents contamination of the Key-Parts.
Position sterile dressing drape below or near the wound.	Protects wound from environmental contamination.
Cleanse the wound with sterile 0.9% sodium chloride. Clean from top to bottom and from a clean area towards a less clean area, usually an outward direction.	Removes debris from the wound bed. Avoids transferring wound exudate and normal flora from the surrounding skin into the wound. Prevents wound contamination.
Assess the wound size, type(s) of tissue in the wound bed and the quantity of each tissue type in percentage (%), signs of infection, type and amount of exudate, odour, inflammation and healing. Assess for pain.	Evaluates condition of the wound, the peri-wound condition, and the stage of healing.
Apply sterile wound dressing using ANTT and secure. If ordered, wound may be left exposed to the air.	Provides a moist wound environment. Facilitates healing, absorbs exudate, protects the wound from infection and irritation (e.g. from clothing).

 AFTER THE SKILL

(Please refer to the Standard Steps on p. xii for related rationales.)
Communicate outcome to the individual, any ongoing care and report any complications.
Restore the environment.
Report, record and document assessment findings, details of the skill performed and the individual's response.
Report, record and document any abnormalities and/or inability to perform the skill.
Reassess the individual to ensure there are no adverse effects/events from the skill.

(Adapted from ACIPC 2015; LeMone et al 2020; Berman et al 2020; IWWII 2022; Lynn 2022; The-ASAP-2019)

OBSERVATION CHECKLIST: DRESSING A WOUND

STUDENT NAME: _____

CLINICAL SKILL 29.2: Dressing a wound

DEMONSTRATION OF: The ability to clean and dress a wound

If the observation checklist is being used as an assessment tool, the student will need to obtain a scale of independence for each of the performance criteria/evidence.

Independent (I)
Supervised (S)
Assisted (A)
Marginal (M)
Dependent (D)

COMPETENCY ELEMENTS	PERFORMANCE CRITERIA/EVIDENCE	I	S	A	M	D
Preparation for the activity	Identifies indications and rationale for performing the activity Identifies the individual using three individual identifiers Ensures therapeutic interaction Gains the individual's consent Checks facility/organisational policy Visually assesses the wound and dressing Assesses pain, provides analgesia if required Validates the order in the individual's record Locates and gathers equipment Assists the individual into an appropriate position Ensures privacy and dignity					
Performs activity informed by evidence	Prepares and maintains aseptic field Removes and appropriately discards existing dressing Correctly positions dressing towels around the wound Cleanses the wound from a clean area towards a less clean area Observes the wound for size, union, signs of infection, exudate, odour, inflammation and healing Applies and secures wound dressing as required					
Applies critical thinking and reflective practice	Is able to link theory to practice Demonstrates current best practice in the care provided Offers and provides pain relief as required Obtains assistance as required Selects appropriate dressing Assesses own performance					
Practises within safety and quality assurance guidelines	Reviews against facility/organisational policy Performs hand hygiene, dons and doffs PPE as per infection control protocols Adheres to infection control/ANTT principles Raises the bed to the appropriate working position based on nurse's height and lowers at completion of activity Cleans and disposes of equipment and waste appropriately					
Documentation and communication	Explains and communicates the activity clearly to the individual Communicates outcome and ongoing care to individual and significant others Communicates abnormal findings to appropriate personnel Reports and documents all relevant information and any complications correctly in the healthcare record Reports any complications and/or inability to perform the procedure to the RN and/or medical officer Asks the individual to report any complications during and post procedure					

Educator/Facilitator Feedback:

Educator/Facilitator Score: Competent   Needs further development

How would you rate your overall performance while undertaking this clinical activity? (use a ✓ & initial)

Unsatisfactory ☐   Satisfactory ☐   Good ☐   Excellent ☐

Student Reflection: (discuss how you would approach your practice differently or more effectively)

EDUCATOR/FACILITATOR NAME/SIGNATURE:

STUDENT NAME/SIGNATURE: **DATE:**

CLINICAL SKILL 29.3 Assessment and management of skin tears

Please adhere to the policy and procedures of the facility/organisation prior to undertaking the skill. Ensure this skill is in your scope of practice.

NMBA Decision-making Framework considerations (refer to NMBA Decision-making framework for nursing and midwifery 2020):	Equipment:
1. Am I educated? 2. Am I authorised? 3. Am I competent? If you answer 'no' to any of these, do not perform that activity. Seek guidance and support from your teacher/a nurse team leader/clinical facilitator/educator.	Sterile dressing pack Sterile dressing materials Additional light source (if required) Additional sterile gauze Disposable gloves Sterile 0.9% sodium chloride Waste receptacle Dressing trolley Disinfectant wipes/solution

 PREPARE FOR THE SKILL

(Please refer to the Standard Steps on p. xii for related rationales.)
Mentally review the steps of the skill.
Discuss the skill with your instructor/supervisor/team leader, if required.
Confirm correct facility/organisation policy/safe operating procedures.
Validate the order in the individual's record.
Identify indication and rationale for performing the activity.
Assess for any contraindications.
Locate and gather equipment.
Perform hand hygiene.
Ensure therapeutic interaction.
Identify the individual using three individual identifiers.
Gain the individual's consent.
Assess for pain relief.
Prepare the environment.
Provide and maintain privacy.
Assist the individual to assume an appropriate position of comfort.

Skill activity	Rationale
Skin tears can result in partial or full separation of the layers of the skin. They may be caused by friction and/or shearing forces and require treatment to prevent wound contamination and infections.	
Assess the skin tear to determine the severity: assess degree of tissue loss and skin or flap colour using ISTAP or STAR classification system. Assess the size of the wound and surrounding skin for swelling, discolouration or bruising, fragility. Choose appropriate dressing according to skin tear assessment.	Severity will depend on the treatment and the type of dressing required. Dressing choice will maintain a moist wound-healing environment, control or manage exudate, reduce the risk of infection, and atraumatic removal during dressing change.

 PERFORM THE SKILL

(Please refer to the Standard Steps on p. xii for related rationales.)
Perform hand hygiene.
Apply PPE: gloves, eyewear, mask and gown as appropriate.
Ensure the individual's safety and comfort throughout skill.
Promote independence and involvement of the individual if possible and/or appropriate.
Assess the individual's tolerance to the skill throughout.
Dispose of used supplies, equipment, waste and sharps appropriately.

CLINICAL SKILL 29.3 Assessment and management of skin tears—cont'd

Skill activity	Rationale
Create the aseptic field by using the sterile dressing pack and add sterile equipment including 0.9% sodium chloride to the field. Open sterile dressing pack by using corners. Open the sterile dressing products away from the aseptic field and add into the field.	Prevents contamination of sterile items and Key-Parts.
Rearrange and assemble the required sterile dressing and equipment in the aseptic field using ANTT without contaminating the Key-Parts.	Maintains ANTT to protect the wound from environmental contamination. Prevents contamination of the Key-Parts.
Position sterile dressing drape below or near the wound.	Protects wound from environmental contamination.
Control bleeding (if required). Cleanse wound with warm 0.9% sodium chloride solution, and remove debris (if required).	Cleans wound, removes debris and prepares for flap realignment. Allows for more accurate wound assessment.
Gently roll out (realign) the skin flap. Avoid stretching and pulling the flap.	Replaces the skin flap into anatomical position. Stretching and pulling may cause the skin flap to be damaged and devitalised or shrink back on itself or it may tear off completely.
Apply an appropriate sterile wound dressing using ANTT and secure. Ensure dressing extends over the wound edge by at least 1.5–2 cm. Date and draw arrow on the dressing in direction of skin flap.	Covers wound and prevents spread of microorganisms. Indicates the direction of dressing removal to reduce the risk of re-trauma to the flap upon removal of dressing as scheduled.

 AFTER THE SKILL

(Please refer to the Standard Steps on p. xii for related rationales.)
Communicate outcome to the individual, any ongoing care and report any complications.
Restore the environment.
Report, record and document assessment findings, details of the skill performed and the individual's response.
Report, record and document any abnormalities and/or inability to perform the skill.
Reassess the individual to ensure there are no adverse effects/events from the skill.

(Adapted from ACIPC 2015; LeMone et al 2020; Berman et al 2020; IWII 2022; LeBlanc et al 2018; Lynn 2022; The-ASAP 2019)

OBSERVATION CHECKLIST: ASSESSMENT AND MANAGEMENT OF SKIN TEARS

STUDENT NAME: _____

CLINICAL SKILL 29.3: Assessment and management of skin tears

DEMONSTRATION OF: The ability to assess and dress a skin tear

If the observation checklist is being used as an assessment tool, the student will need to obtain a scale of independence for each of the performance criteria/evidence.

Independent (I)
Supervised (S)
Assisted (A)
Marginal (M)
Dependent (D)

COMPETENCY ELEMENTS	PERFORMANCE CRITERIA/EVIDENCE	I	S	A	M	D
Preparation for the activity	Identifies indications and rationale for performing the activity Identifies the individual using three individual identifiers Ensures therapeutic interaction Gains the individual's consent Checks facility/organisational policy Validates the order in the individual's record Assesses the skin tear to determine the severity, need for analgesia Chooses appropriate dressing according to skin tear assessment Locates and gathers equipment Assists the individual into an appropriate position Ensures privacy and dignity					
Performs activity informed by evidence	Prepares and maintains aseptic field Removes and appropriately discards existing dressing Correctly positions dressing towels around the wound Controls bleeding (if present), cleanses wound with warmed sterile 0.9% sodium chloride solution, removes debris (if required), reassesses severity of tear, realigns skin tear Applies and secures wound dressing as required					
Applies critical thinking and reflective practice	Is able to link theory to practice Demonstrates current best practice in the care provided Obtains assistance as required Offers and provides pain relief as required Selects appropriate dressing Assesses own performance					
Practises within safety and quality assurance guidelines	Reviews against facility/organisational policy Performs hand hygiene, dons and doffs PPE as per infection control protocols Adheres to infection control/ANTT principles Raises the bed to the appropriate working position based on nurse's height and lowers at completion of activity Cleans and disposes of equipment and waste appropriately					
Documentation and communication	Explains and communicates the activity clearly to the individual Communicates outcome and ongoing care to individual and significant others Communicates abnormal findings to appropriate personnel Reports and documents all relevant information and any complications correctly in the healthcare record Reports any complications and/or inability to perform the procedure to the RN and/or medical officer Asks the individual to report any complications during and post procedure					

Educator/Facilitator Feedback:

Educator/Facilitator Score: Competent   Needs further development

How would you rate your overall performance while undertaking this clinical activity? (use a ✓ & initial)

Unsatisfactory ☐   Satisfactory ☐   Good ☐   Excellent ☐

Student Reflection: (discuss how you would approach your practice differently or more effectively)

EDUCATOR/FACILITATOR NAME/SIGNATURE:

STUDENT NAME/SIGNATURE: **DATE:**

CLINICAL SKILL 29.4 Packing a wound

Please adhere to the policy and procedures of the facility/organisation prior to undertaking the skill. Ensure this skill is in your scope of practice.

NMBA Decision-making Framework considerations (refer to NMBA Decision-making framework for nursing and midwifery 2020):

1. Am I educated?
2. Am I authorised?
3. Am I competent?

If you answer 'no' to any of these, do not perform that activity. Seek guidance and support from your teacher/a nurse team leader/clinical facilitator/educator.

Equipment:
Sterile dressing pack
Sterile dressing materials
Additional light source (if required)
Sterile 0.9% sodium chloride
Additional gauze
Sterile scissors
Sterile gloves
Disposable gloves
Waste receptacle
Dressing trolley
Disinfectant wipes/solution

 PREPARE FOR THE SKILL

(Please refer to the Standard Steps on p. xii for related rationales.)
Mentally review the steps of the skill.
Discuss the skill with your instructor/supervisor/team leader, if required.
Confirm correct facility/organisation policy/safe operating procedures.
Validate the order in the individual's record.
Identify indication and rationale for performing the activity.
Assess for any contraindications.
Locate and gather equipment.
Perform hand hygiene.
Ensure therapeutic interaction.
Identify the individual using three individual identifiers.
Gain the individual's consent.
Assess for pain relief.
Prepare the environment.
Provide and maintain privacy.
Assist the individual to assume an appropriate position of comfort.

Skill activity	Rationale
Wound packing is undertaken to provide a moist cover for the wound to prevent the introduction of microorganisms and to promote healing. Wounds requiring packing heal by secondary intent. The wound packing promotes healing for this type of wound, facilitates mechanical debridement, and minimises dead space. The type of dressing used also absorbs exudate.	
Assess the individual's record to determine previous appearance of wound and previous dressing.	Determines requirements for equipment and dressing requirements.

 PERFORM THE SKILL

(Please refer to the Standard Steps on p. xii for related rationales.)
Perform hand hygiene.
Apply PPE: gloves, eyewear, mask and gown as appropriate.
Ensure the individual's safety and comfort throughout skill.
Promote independence and involvement of the individual if possible and/or appropriate.
Assess the individual's tolerance to the skill throughout.
Dispose of used supplies, equipment, waste and sharps appropriately.
Remove PPE and discard or store appropriately.
Perform hand hygiene.

CLINICAL SKILL 29.4 Packing a wound—cont'd

Skill activity	Rationale
Create the aseptic field by using the sterile dressing pack and add sterile equipment including 0.9% sodium chloride to the field. Open sterile dressing pack by using corners. Open the sterile dressing products away from the aseptic field and add into the field.	Prevents contamination of sterile items and Key-Parts.
Loosen and remove the existing wound dressing for the visual wound assessment including the type and amount of exudate on the removed dressing and peri-wound condition. Dispose of wound dressing and the used gloves.	Assesses the signs and symptoms of wound infection (e.g. redness, swelling, warmth, exudate amount and type on the dressing). Prevents spread of microorganisms.
Rearrange and assemble the required sterile dressing and equipment in the aseptic field using ANTT without contaminating the Key-Parts.	Maintains ANTT to protect the wound from environmental contamination. Prevents contamination of the Key-Parts.
Position sterile dressing drape below or near the wound.	Protects the wound from environmental contamination.
Remove all existing packing/dressings (irrigate packing if required).	Provides the view for assessing wound bed. Irrigates the existing packing further to minimise pain/discomfort upon removal.
Cleanse the wound with sterile 0.9% sodium chloride. Clean from a clean area towards a less clean area, usually an outward direction.	Removes debris from the wound bed. Avoids transferring wound exudate and normal flora from the surrounding skin into the wound. Prevents wound contamination.
Assess the wound size (including depth), type(s) of tissue in the wound bed and the quantity of each tissue type in percentage (%), signs of infection, type and amount of exudate, odour, and direction and depth of tunnelling (if present). Assess for pain.	Evaluates condition of the wound and the stage of healing.
Gently pack the wound with the required packing materials. (See medical officer's or wound management consultant's orders.) Ribbon or packing gauze is gently placed into the wound cavity.	Do not tightly pack the wound cavity since the dressing will expand as it absorbs exudate and may cause discomfort and pressure to the wound bed. Packing allows for secondary wound healing.
Apply an appropriate sterile wound dressing using ANTT, and secure.	Provides a moist wound environment. Facilitates healing, absorbs exudate, protects the wound from infection and irritation (e.g. from clothing).

 ### AFTER THE SKILL

(Please refer to the Standard Steps on p. xii for related rationales.)
Communicate outcome to the individual, any ongoing care and report any complications.
Restore the environment.
Report, record and document assessment findings, details of the skill performed and the individual's response.
Report, record and document any abnormalities and/or inability to perform the skill.
Reassess the individual to ensure there are no adverse effects/events from the skill.

(Adapted from ACIPC 2015; LeMone et al 2020; Berman et al 2020; IWII 2022; Lynn 2022; The-ASAP 2019)

OBSERVATION CHECKLIST: PACKING A WOUND

STUDENT NAME: _____

CLINICAL SKILL 29.4: Packing a wound

DEMONSTRATION OF: The ability to pack a wound

If the observation checklist is being used as an assessment tool, the student will need to obtain a scale of independence for each of the performance criteria/evidence.

Independent (I)
Supervised (S)
Assisted (A)
Marginal (M)
Dependent (D)

COMPETENCY ELEMENTS	PERFORMANCE CRITERIA/EVIDENCE	I	S	A	M	D
Preparation for the activity	Identifies indications and rationale for performing the activity Identifies the individual using three individual identifiers Ensures therapeutic interaction Gains the individual's consent Visually assesses the wound and dressing Assesses pain, provides analgesia if required Checks facility/organisational policy Validates the order in the individual's record Locates and gathers equipment Assists the individual into an appropriate position Ensures privacy and dignity					
Performs activity informed by evidence	Prepares and maintains aseptic field Removes and appropriately discards existing dressing Correctly positions dressing towels around the wound Irrigates wound packing with sterile 0.9% sodium chloride (if required) Removes packing material from the wound Observes the wound for size, union, signs of infection, exudate, odour, inflammation and healing Cleanses the wound from a clean area towards a less clean area Packs wound with appropriate packing material Applies and secures dressing over the wound					
Applies critical thinking and reflective practice	Is able to link theory to practice Demonstrates current best practice in the care provided Obtains assistance as required Offers and provides pain relief as required Selects appropriate dressing Assesses own performance					
Practises within safety and quality assurance guidelines	Reviews against facility/organisational policy Performs hand hygiene, dons and doffs PPE as per infection control protocols Adheres to infection control/ANTT principles Raises the bed to the appropriate working position based on nurse's height and lowers at completion of activity Cleans and disposes of equipment and waste appropriately					
Documentation and communication	Explains and communicates the activity clearly to the individual Communicates outcome and ongoing care to individual and significant others Communicates abnormal findings to appropriate personnel Reports and documents all relevant information and any complications correctly in the healthcare record Reports any complications and/or inability to perform the procedure to the RN and/or medical officer Asks the individual to report any complications during and post procedure					

Educator/Facilitator Feedback:

Educator/Facilitator Score: Competent   Needs further development

How would you rate your overall performance while undertaking this clinical activity? (use a ✓ & initial)

Unsatisfactory ☐   Satisfactory ☐   Good ☐   Excellent ☐

Student Reflection: (discuss how you would approach your practice differently or more effectively)

EDUCATOR/FACILITATOR NAME/SIGNATURE:

STUDENT NAME/SIGNATURE: **DATE:**

CLINICAL SKILL 29.5 Removal of sutures and staples

Please adhere to the policy and procedures of the facility/organisation prior to undertaking the skill. Ensure this skill is in your scope of practice.

NMBA Decision-making Framework considerations (refer to NMBA Decision-making framework for nursing and midwifery 2020):	Equipment:
1. Am I educated? 2. Am I authorised? 3. Am I competent? If you answer 'no' to any of these, do not perform that activity. Seek guidance and support from your teacher/a nurse team leader/clinical facilitator/educator.	Sterile dressing pack Sterile dressing materials including sterile wound closure strips Sterile 0.9% sodium chloride Additional sterile gauze Sterile staple remover Sterile suture cutter Additional light source (if required) Disposable gloves Waste receptacle Sharps bin Dressing trolley Disinfectant wipes/solution

 PREPARE FOR THE SKILL

(Please refer to the Standard Steps on p. xii for related rationales.)
Mentally review the steps of the skill.
Discuss the skill with your instructor/supervisor/team leader, if required.
Confirm correct facility/organisation policy/safe operating procedures.
Validate the order in the individual's record.
Identify indication and rationale for performing the activity.
Assess for any contraindications.
Locate and gather equipment.
Perform hand hygiene.
Ensure therapeutic interaction.
Identify the individual using three individual identifiers.
Gain the individual's consent.
Assess for pain relief.
Prepare the environment.
Provide and maintain privacy.
Assist the individual to assume an appropriate position of comfort.

Skill activity	Rationale
Sutures and staples are removed once wound healing has occurred. Alternate sutures and staples may be removed with the remainder the following day.	
Assess the individual's record to determine previous appearance of wound and previous dressing.	Determines requirements for equipment and dressing requirements.

 PERFORM THE SKILL

(Please refer to the Standard Steps on p. xii for related rationales.)
Perform hand hygiene.
Apply PPE: gloves, eyewear, mask and gown as appropriate.
Ensure the individual's safety and comfort throughout skill.
Promote independence and involvement of the individual if possible and/or appropriate.
Assess the individual's tolerance to the skill throughout.
Dispose of used supplies, equipment, waste and sharps appropriately.
Remove PPE and discard or store appropriately.
Perform hand hygiene.

CLINICAL SKILL 29.5 Removal of sutures and staples—cont'd

Skill activity	Rationale
Create the aseptic field by using the sterile dressing pack and add sterile equipment including 0.9% sodium chloride to the field. Open sterile dressing pack by using corners. Open the sterile dressing products away from the aseptic field and add into the field.	Prevents contamination of sterile items and Key-Parts.
Loosen and remove the existing wound dressing for the visual wound assessment including the type and amount of exudate on the removed dressing and peri-wound condition, and count the number of sutures or staples. Dispose of wound dressing and used gloves.	Assesses the signs and symptoms of wound infection (e.g. redness, swelling, warmth, exudate amount and type). Prevents spread of microorganisms.
Rearrange and assemble the required sterile dressing and equipment in the aseptic field using ANTT without contaminating the Key-Parts.	Maintains ANTT to protect the wound from environmental contamination. Prevents contamination of the Key-Parts.
Position sterile dressing drape below or near the wound.	Protects the wound from environmental contamination.
Cleanse the wound with sterile 0.9% sodium chloride Clean from top to bottom and from a clean area towards a less clean area, usually an outward direction.	Removes debris from the wound bed. Avoids transferring wound exudate and normal flora from the surrounding skin into the wound. Prevents wound contamination.
Reassess the suture wound for any signs of infection or dehiscence.	Assesses for any signs of infection and wound dehiscence.
Removal of sutures: • Start with the second suture, using forceps to grasp the knot and gently raise it off the skin. • Cut the suture as close to the skin as possible, away from the knot. • Pull the cut suture up and out of the skin, ensuring that the exposed portion of the suture is not pulled through the tissues. • Remove alternating sutures by using the same technique leaving the first and last sutures till last to remove.	Allows for assessment of union. Avoids risk of pulling exposed suture through the tissues, which prevents infection.
Removal of staples: • Place the staple remover's lower jaw under the centre of the staple. • Squeeze the handles of the staple remover until the jaws are completely closed. • Slightly tilt the staple remover from side to side to facilitate removal. • Gently lift the staple remover to remove the staple from the skin. • Place the staple(s) onto the extended sterile field for counting later. • Repeat the same process for alternating staples leaving first and last staple till last to remove.	The extractor reforms the shape of the staple and pulls the prongs out of the intradermal tissue. Ensures that the incision has healed before removing all staples.
Apply an appropriate sterile wound dressing using ANTT and secure.	If necessary, apply sterile wound closure strips to provide additional support in wound edge closure. Provides protection from infection and irritation if required.
Count and dispose of staples.	Ensures required number of staples were removed and disposed.

Continued

CLINICAL SKILL 29.5 Removal of sutures and staples—cont'd

 AFTER THE SKILL

(Please refer to the Standard Steps on p. xii for related rationales.)

Communicate outcome to the individual, any ongoing care and report any complications.

Restore the environment.

Report, record and document assessment findings, details of the skill performed and the individual's response.

Report, record and document any abnormalities and/or inability to perform the skill.

Reassess the individual to ensure there are no adverse effects/events from the skill.

(Adapted from ACIPC 2015; LeMone et al 2020; Berman et al 2020; Lynn 2022; The-ASAP 2019)

OBSERVATION CHECKLIST: REMOVAL OF SUTURES AND STAPLES

STUDENT NAME: _____

CLINICAL SKILL 29.5: Removal of sutures and staples

DEMONSTRATION OF: The ability to remove sutures and staples

If the observation checklist is being used as an assessment tool, the student will need to obtain a scale of independence for each of the performance criteria/evidence.

Independent (I)

Supervised (S)

Assisted (A)

Marginal (M)

Dependent (D)

COMPETENCY ELEMENTS	PERFORMANCE CRITERIA/EVIDENCE	I	S	A	M	D
Preparation for the activity	Identifies indications and rationale for performing the activity Identifies the individual using three individual identifiers Ensures therapeutic interaction Gains the individual's consent Visually assesses the wound and dressing Assesses pain, provides analgesia if required Checks facility/organisational policy Validates the order in the individual's record Locates and gathers equipment Assists the individual into an appropriate position Ensures privacy and dignity					
Performs activity informed by evidence	Prepares and maintains aseptic field Removes and appropriately discards existing dressing Correctly positions dressing towels around the wound Cleanses the wound from a clean area towards a less clean area Examines the incision to determine the amount of healing and type of suture/clip used Removes suture or staple as ordered Applies and secures wound dressing as required					
Applies critical thinking and reflective practice	Is able to link theory to practice Demonstrates current best practice in the care provided Obtains assistance as required Offers and provides pain relief as required Selects appropriate dressing (if required) Assesses own performance					
Practises within safety and quality assurance guidelines	Reviews against facility/organisational policy Performs hand hygiene, dons and doffs PPE as per infection control protocols Adheres to infection control/ANTT principles Raises the bed to the appropriate working position based on nurse's height and lowers at completion of activity Cleans and disposes of equipment and waste appropriately					
Documentation and communication	Explains and communicates the activity clearly to the individual Communicates outcome and ongoing care to individual and significant others Communicates abnormal findings to appropriate personnel Reports and documents all relevant information and any complications correctly in the healthcare record Reports any complications and/or inability to perform the procedure to the RN and/or medical officer Asks the individual to report any complications during and post procedure					

Educator/Facilitator Feedback:

Educator/Facilitator Score: Competent   Needs further development

How would you rate your overall performance while undertaking this clinical activity? (use a ✓ & initial)

Unsatisfactory ☐   Satisfactory ☐   Good ☐   Excellent ☐

Student Reflection: (discuss how you would approach your practice differently or more effectively)

EDUCATOR/FACILITATOR NAME/SIGNATURE:

STUDENT NAME/SIGNATURE: **DATE:**

CLINICAL SKILL 29.6 Shortening a drain tube

Please adhere to the policy and procedures of the facility/organisation prior to undertaking the skill. Ensure this skill is in your scope of practice.

NMBA Decision-making Framework considerations (refer to NMBA Decision-making framework for nursing and midwifery 2020):	Equipment:
1. Am I educated? 2. Am I authorised? 3. Am I competent? If you answer 'no' to any of these, do not perform that activity. Seek guidance and support from your teacher/a nurse team leader/clinical facilitator/educator.	Sterile dressing pack Sterile dressing materials Sterile gloves Disposable gloves Additional light source (if required) Sterile 0.9% sodium chloride Additional gauze Sterile scissors Sterile suture cutter Sterile safety pin Ostomy/appliance bag (if required) Protective eyewear Waste receptacle Sharps bin Dressing trolley Disinfectant wipes/solution

 PREPARE FOR THE SKILL

(Please refer to the Standard Steps on p. xii for related rationales.)
Mentally review the steps of the skill.
Discuss the skill with your instructor/supervisor/team leader, if required.
Confirm correct facility/organisation policy/safe operating procedures.
Validate the order in the individual's record.
Identify indication and rationale for performing the activity.
Assess for any contraindications.
Locate and gather equipment.
Perform hand hygiene.
Ensure therapeutic interaction.
Identify the individual using three individual identifiers.
Gain the individual's consent.
Assess for pain relief.
Prepare the environment.
Provide and maintain privacy.
Assist the individual to assume an appropriate position of comfort.

Skill activity	Rationale
Drain tubes are shortened to reduce irritation to the bottom of the wound and promote healing.	
Assess the individual's record to determine previous appearance of wound and previous dressing.	Determines requirements for equipment and dressing requirements.

 PERFORM THE SKILL

(Please refer to the Standard Steps on p. xii for related rationales.)
Perform hand hygiene.
Apply PPE: gloves, eyewear, mask and gown as appropriate.
Ensure the individual's safety and comfort throughout skill.
Promote independence and involvement of the individual if possible and/or appropriate.
Assess the individual's tolerance to the skill throughout.
Dispose of used supplies, equipment, waste and sharps appropriately.
Remove PPE and discard or store appropriately.
Perform hand hygiene.

Continued

CLINICAL SKILL 29.6 Shortening a drain tube—cont'd

Skill activity	Rationale
Create the aseptic field by using the sterile dressing pack and add sterile equipment including 0.9% sodium chloride to the field. Open sterile dressing pack by using corners. Open the sterile dressing products away from the aseptic field and add into the field.	Prevents contamination of sterile items and Key-Parts.
Loosen and remove the existing wound dressing for the visual wound assessment including the type and amount of exudate on the removed dressing and peri-wound condition. Dispose of wound dressing and used gloves.	Assesses the signs and symptoms of wound infection (e.g. redness, swelling, warmth, exudate amount and type). Prevents spread of microorganisms.
Rearrange and assemble the required sterile dressing and equipment in the aseptic field using ANTT without contaminating the Key-Parts.	Maintains ANTT to protect the wound from environmental contamination. Prevents contamination of the Key-Parts.
Position sterile dressing drape below or near the wound.	Protects the wound from environmental contamination.
Cleanse the drain tube site at the point where the tubing enters/exits with sterile 0.9% sodium chloride. Assess drain tube site. Allow to dry.	Removes debris from the wound bed. Avoids transferring wound exudate and normal flora from the surrounding skin into the wound. Observes for any signs of infection (e.g. warmth, redness, increasing amount of exudate, odour) and peri-wound condition. Prevents wound contamination.
Cut and remove the drain tube securing suture with suture cutter and remove (if present).	Enables the tube to be free for retraction and/or rotation.
Hold onto the drain tube close to the exit point. Gently rotate the drain tube before using smooth and gentle traction to withdraw/shorten the drain tube by the specified amount (cease procedure immediately if excessive force is required to withdraw drain tube).	Rotates the tube free from any adherent granulation tissue.
Place the sterile safety pin through the drain tube after shortening (open drains only). Trim excess length below the sterile safety pin.	Prevents drain tube retraction or extrusion. Prevents it pressing on the wound.
Apply an appropriate sterile wound dressing or appliance bag (e.g. ostomy bag) using ANTT and secure.	Collects exudate to facilitate moist healing environment. Covers wound and prevents spread of microorganisms.

 AFTER THE SKILL

(Please refer to the Standard Steps on p. xii for related rationales.)
Communicate outcome to the individual, any ongoing care and report any complications.
Restore the environment.
Report, record and document assessment findings, details of the skill performed and the individual's response.
Report, record and document any abnormalities and/or inability to perform the skill.
Reassess the individual to ensure there are no adverse effects/events from the skill.

(Adapted from ACIPC 2015; LeMone et al 2020; Berman et al 2020; IWII 2022; Lynn 2022; The-ASAP 2019)

OBSERVATION CHECKLIST: SHORTENING A DRAIN TUBE

STUDENT NAME: _____

CLINICAL SKILL 29.6: Shortening a drain tube

DEMONSTRATION OF: The ability to shorten a drain tube

If the observation checklist is being used as an assessment tool, the student will need to obtain a scale of independence for each of the performance criteria/evidence.

Independent (I)
Supervised (S)
Assisted (A)
Marginal (M)
Dependent (D)

COMPETENCY ELEMENTS	PERFORMANCE CRITERIA/EVIDENCE	I	S	A	M	D
Preparation for the activity	Identifies indications and rationale for performing the activity Identifies the individual using three individual identifiers Ensures therapeutic interaction Gains the individual's consent Checks facility/organisation policy Visually assesses the wound and dressing Assesses pain, provides analgesia if required Validates the order in the individual's record Locates and gathers equipment Assists the individual into an appropriate position Ensures privacy and dignity					
Performs activity informed by evidence	Prepares and maintains aseptic field Removes and appropriately discards existing dressing Correctly positions dressing towels around the wound Cleanses the wound from a clean area towards a less clean area Observes the wound for size, union, signs of infection, exudate, odour, inflammation and healing Removes any suture securing the tube in the wound Gently rotates tube (if round) Withdraws tube to the prescribed length Replaces the sterile safety pin on the tube Cuts off excess tube below the safety pin Applies and secures wound dressing or appliance bag over the wound					
Applies critical thinking and reflective practice	Is able to link theory to practice Demonstrates current best practice in the care provided Offers and provides pain relief as required Obtains assistance as required Selects appropriate dressing Assesses own performance					
Practises within safety and quality assurance guidelines	Reviews against facility/organisational policy Performs hand hygiene, dons and doffs PPE as per infection control protocols Adheres to infection control/ANTT principles Raises the bed to the appropriate working position based on nurse's height and lowers at completion of activity Cleans and disposes of equipment and waste appropriately					
Documentation and communication	Explains and communicates the activity clearly to the individual Communicates outcome and ongoing care to individual and significant others Communicates abnormal findings to appropriate personnel Reports and documents all relevant information and any complications correctly in the healthcare record Reports any complications and/or inability to perform the procedure to the RN and/or medical officer Asks the individual to report any complications during and post procedure					

Educator/Facilitator Feedback:

Educator/Facilitator Score: Competent Needs further development

How would you rate your overall performance while undertaking this clinical activity? (use a ✓ & initial)

Unsatisfactory ☐ Satisfactory ☐ Good ☐ Excellent ☐

Student Reflection: (discuss how you would approach your practice differently or more effectively)

EDUCATOR/FACILITATOR NAME/SIGNATURE:

CLINICAL SKILL 29.7 Removal of a drain tube

Please adhere to the policy and procedures of the facility/organisation prior to undertaking the skill. Ensure this skill is in your scope of practice.

NMBA Decision-making Framework considerations (refer to NMBA Decision-making framework for nursing and midwifery 2020):	Equipment:
1. Am I educated? 2. Am I authorised? 3. Am I competent? If you answer 'no' to any of these, do not perform that activity. Seek guidance and support from your teacher/a nurse team leader/clinical facilitator/educator.	Sterile dressing pack Sterile dressing materials Sterile gloves Disposable gloves Additional light source (if required) Sterile 0.9% sodium chloride Additional sterile gauze Sterile suture cutter Protective eyewear Waste receptacle Sharps bin Dressing trolley Disinfectant wipes/solution

 PREPARE FOR THE SKILL

(Please refer to the Standard Steps on p. xii for related rationales.)
Mentally review the steps of the skill.
Discuss the skill with your instructor/supervisor/team leader, if required.
Confirm correct facility/organisation policy/safe operating procedures.
Validate the order in the individual's record.
Identify indication and rationale for performing the activity.
Assess for any contraindications.
Locate and gather equipment.
Perform hand hygiene.
Ensure therapeutic interaction.
Identify the individual using three individual identifiers.
Gain the individual's consent.
Assess for pain relief.
Prepare the environment.
Provide and maintain privacy.
Assist the individual to assume an appropriate position of comfort.

Skill activity	Rationale
Drain tubes are removed to reduce irritation to the bottom of the wound and promote healing.	
Assess drain tube condition and output.	Inspects for signs of infection, bleeding, leakage, suction patency, the quantity and type of drain.
Dissipate suction.	Prevents trauma to tissue around the drain tube upon removal. Prevents pain associated with drain tube removal.

 PERFORM THE SKILL

(Please refer to the Standard Steps on p. xii for related rationales.)
Perform hand hygiene.
Apply PPE: gloves, eyewear, mask and gown as appropriate.
Ensure the individual's safety and comfort throughout skill.
Promote independence and involvement of the individual if possible and/or appropriate.
Assess the individual's tolerance to the skill throughout.
Dispose of used supplies, equipment, waste and sharps appropriately.
Remove PPE and discard or store appropriately.
Perform hand hygiene.

Continued

CLINICAL SKILL 29.7 Removal of a drain tube—cont'd

Skill activity	Rationale
Create the aseptic field by using the sterile dressing pack and add sterile equipment including 0.9% sodium chloride to the field. Open sterile dressing pack by using corners. Open the sterile dressing products away from the aseptic field and add into the field.	Prevents contamination of sterile items and Key-Parts.
Loosen and remove the existing wound dressing for the visual assessment of the drain tube site. Dispose of wound dressing and used gloves.	Assesses the signs and symptoms of wound infection at the drain tube site (e.g. redness, exudate amount and type). Prevents spread of microorganisms.
Rearrange and assemble the required sterile dressing and equipment in the aseptic field using ANTT without contaminating the Key-Parts.	Maintains ANTT to protect the wound from environmental contamination. Prevents contamination of the Key-Parts.
Position sterile dressing drape below or near the wound.	Protects the wound from environmental contamination.
Cleanse the drain tube site at the point where the tubing enters/exits with sterile 0.9% sodium chloride. Reassess drain tube site. Allow to dry.	Removes debris from the wound bed. Avoids transferring wound exudate and normal flora from the surrounding skin into the wound. Observes for any signs of infection (e.g. redness, exudate type and amount), and peri-wound condition. Prevents wound contamination.
Cut and remove the drain tube securing suture with suture cutter (if present).	Ensures the tube is free for retraction and/or rotation.
Hold onto the drain tube close to the exit point. Gently rotate the drain tube (if the drain tube is round), and apply smooth and gentle traction to fully remove the drain tube (avoid forceful pulling of the tube). Inspect the drain tube tip for its integrity.	Rotates the tube free from any adherent granulation tissue to facilitate removal and to minimise pain/discomfort upon drain tube removal. Gentle traction to prevent drain tube fracture from forceful pulling action. Checks for integrity of the drain tube tip and escalates concerns if tube fracture is suspected.
Apply an appropriate sterile wound dressing using ANTT and secure.	Collects exudate to facilitate moist healing environment. Covers wound and prevents spread of microorganisms.

 AFTER THE SKILL

(Please refer to the Standard Steps on p. xii for related rationales.)
Communicate outcome to the individual, any ongoing care and report any complications.
Restore the environment.
Report, record and document assessment findings, details of the skill performed and the individual's response.
Report, record and document any abnormalities and/or inability to perform the skill.
Reassess the individual to ensure there are no adverse effects/events from the skill.

(Adapted from LeMone et al 2020; Berman et al 2020; LeBlanc et al 2018; Lynn 2022; The-ASAP 2019)

OBSERVATION CHECKLIST: REMOVAL OF A DRAIN TUBE

STUDENT NAME: _____

CLINICAL SKILL 29.7: Removal of a drain tube

DEMONSTRATION OF: The ability to remove a drain tube

If the observation checklist is being used as an assessment tool, the student will need to obtain a scale of independence for each of the performance criteria/evidence.

Independent (I)
Supervised (S)
Assisted (A)
Marginal (M)
Dependent (D)

COMPETENCY ELEMENTS	PERFORMANCE CRITERIA/EVIDENCE	I	S	A	M	D
Preparation for the activity	Identifies indications and rationale for performing the activity Identifies the individual using three individual identifiers Ensures therapeutic interaction Gains the individual's consent Checks facility/organisation policy Visually assesses the wound and dressing Assesses pain, provides analgesia if required Validates the order in the individual's record Locates and gathers equipment Assists the individual into an appropriate position Ensures privacy and dignity					
Performs activity informed by evidence	Prepares and maintains aseptic field Removes and appropriately discards existing dressing Correctly positions dressing towels around the wound Cleanses the wound from a clean area towards a less clean area Observes the drain tube and drain site condition Removes any suture securing the tube in the wound Gently rotates tube (if round) Withdraws drain tube Applies sterile dressing or appliance bag over the wound Secures dressing in position					
Applies critical thinking and reflective practice	Is able to link theory to practice Demonstrates current best practice in the care provided Offers and provides pain relief as required Obtains assistance as required Selects appropriate dressing Assesses own performance					
Practises within safety and quality assurance guidelines	Reviews against facility/organisational policy Performs hand hygiene, dons and doffs PPE as per infection control protocols Adheres to infection control/ANTT principles Raises the bed to the appropriate working position based on nurse's height and lowers at completion of activity Cleans and disposes of equipment and waste appropriately					
Documentation and communication	Explains and communicates the activity clearly to the individual Communicates outcome and ongoing care to individual and significant others Communicates abnormal findings to appropriate personnel Reports and documents all relevant information and any complications correctly in the healthcare record Reports any complications and/or inability to perform the procedure to the RN and/or medical officer Asks the individual to report any complications during and post procedure					

Educator/Facilitator Feedback:

Educator/Facilitator Score: Competent Needs further development

How would you rate your overall performance while undertaking this clinical activity? (use a ✓ & initial)

Unsatisfactory ☐ Satisfactory ☐ Good ☐ Excellent ☐

Student Reflection: (discuss how you would approach your practice differently or more effectively)

EDUCATOR/FACILITATOR NAME/SIGNATURE:

STUDENT NAME/SIGNATURE: **DATE:**

Evolve®

Answer guide for the Critical Thinking Exercises and Critical Thinking Questions in Case Studies is hosted on Evolve: http://evolve.elsevier.com/AU/Koutoukidis/Tabbner/

References

Australian College for Infection Prevention and Control (ACIPC), 2015. Aseptic technique policy and practice guidelines. Available at: <https://www.acipc.org.au/aseptic-technique-resources/>.

Berman, A., Snyder, S., Levett-Jones, T., et al., 2020. *Kozier and Erb's fundamentals of nursing*, 5th ed. Pearson, Melbourne.

International Wound Infection Institute (IWII), 2022. Wound infection in clinical practice: Principles of best practice. Wounds International. Available at: <https://woundinfection-institute.com/wp-content/uploads/IWII-CD-2022-web-1.pdf>.

LeBlanc, K., Campbell, K., Beeckman, D., et al., 2018. Best practice recommendations for prevention and management of skin tears in aged skin: An overview. *Journal of Wound, Ostomy and Continence Nursing* 45(6), 540–542.

LeMone, P., Bauldoff, G., Gubrud-Howe, P., et al., 2020. *Medical–surgical nursing: Critical thinking in person-centred care*, 4th ed. Pearson, Melbourne.

Lynn, P., 2022. *Taylor's clinical nursing skills. A nursing process approach*, 6th ed. Wolters Kluwer Lippincott Williams & Wilkins, Philadelphia.

Nursing and Midwifery Board of Australia (NMBA), 2020. Decision-making framework summary for nursing and midwifery. Available at: <https://www.nursingmidwiferyboard.gov.au/Codes-Guidelines-Statements/Frameworks.aspx>.

The Association for Safe Aseptic Practice (The-ASAP), 2019. Aseptic Non Touch Technique (ANTT), The ANTT clinical practice framework V4.0. Available at: <https://www.antt.org/antt-practice-framework.html>.

Online Sources and Recommended Reading

Aseptic Non-Touch Technique (ANTT) <https://www.antt.org>.

Australasian College for Infection Prevention and Control (ACIPC): <https://www.acipc.org.au/>.

Australian Commission on Safety and Quality in Health Care (ACSQHC): <https://www.safetyandquality.gov.au/>.

Australian Wound Management Association: <www.awma.com.au>.

Hand Hygiene Australia: <https://www.hha.org.au/>.

National Health and Medical Research Council (NHMRC), 2019. Australian guidelines for the prevention and control of infection in healthcare. Canberra. Available at: <https://www.nhmrc.gov.au/about-us/publications/australian-guidelines-prevention-and-control-infection-healthcare-2019>.

Prevention and Treatment of Pressure Ulcers/Injuries: Clinical Practice Guidelines: <www.internationalguideline.com>.

The Association for Safe Aseptic Practice (The-ASAP), 2019. Aseptic Non Touch Technique (ANTT), The ANTT clinical practice framework V4.0. Available at: <https://www.antt.org/antt-practice-framework.html>.

Wounds Australia: <https://woundsaustralia.org/ocd.aspx>.

NUTRITION

Ashleigh Djachenko

Overview

This chapter focuses on the nutritional nursing care required to assist an individual to meet and maintain their nutritional needs. Nurses are required to assess and educate individuals to maintain nutritional health status and provide information on how to undertake care related to nutrition. Nutritional practices and requirements may vary according to age, height, sex, religion, culture, socioeconomic factors and physical and psychological status. Nurses must be able to accommodate all these different factors when they plan, care and provide health education to individuals.

Nursing care skills and assessments included in this chapter are assisting with eating and drinking, inserting a nasogastric tube and enteral feeds. Provision of these nursing skills ensures the correct quantity and quality of absorbed nutrients to maintain efficient body function. Enteral nutrition refers to nutrition given via the gastrointestinal tract and is used in individuals who are not able to take adequate nutrition orally but who have a functional gastrointestinal tract.

CASE STUDY 30.2

Francis is a 73-year-old man with dementia who has recently been admitted into an aged-care home. Francis is from a remote community and his daughter and extended family are not able to visit regularly due to distance and lack of transport. You have noticed that since his admission one month ago Francis has become withdrawn and has lost 5 kg in weight. During his meals he eats very little and says he is not hungry.

1. What are some possible adverse effects of malnutrition on an older person?
2. What are some strategies that the nurse and the organisation can implement to improve Francis's mealtime experience?

CRITICAL THINKING EXERCISE 30.5

Ian is a 77-year-old male recently diagnosed with oesophageal cancer. He presented to hospital with a history of unintentional weight loss, difficulty swallowing, loss of appetite and a persistent cough. His medical officer has recommended that Ian be discharged home with enteral feeding while he waits to commence radiotherapy and surgical treatment. What education could you provide to Ian about enteral feeding?

CLINICAL SKILL 30.1 Assisting with eating and drinking

Please adhere to the policy and procedures of the facility/organisation prior to undertaking the skill. Ensure this skill is in your scope of practice.

NMBA Decision-making Framework considerations (refer to NMBA Decision-making framework for nursing and midwifery 2020):	Equipment:
1. Am I educated? 2. Am I authorised? 3. Am I competent? If you answer 'no' to any of these, do not perform that activity. Seek guidance and support from your teacher/a nurse team leader/clinical facilitator/educator.	Appropriate adaptive aids (e.g. plate guard) Dysphagia cup Cutlery Straw Clothes protector and/or serviette

 PREPARE FOR THE SKILL

(Please refer to the Standard Steps on p. xii for related rationales.)
Mentally review the steps of the skill.
Discuss the skill with your instructor/supervisor/team leader, if required.
Confirm correct facility/organisation policy/safe operating procedures.
Validate the order in the individual's record.
Identify indication and rationale for performing the activity.
Assess for any contraindications.
Locate and gather equipment.
Perform hand hygiene.
Ensure therapeutic interaction.
Identify the individual using three individual identifiers.
Gain the individual's consent.
Assess for pain relief.
Prepare the environment.
Provide and maintain privacy.
Assist the individual to assume an appropriate position of comfort.

Skill activity	Rationale
Critically think through the assessment data and problem-solving—level of consciousness, position of individual, dysphagia, chronic diseases that require dietary management, food allergies, appetite, assistance needed (personnel and equipment), social and psychological issues that may affect eating, appetite or food and drink choices, food texture, fluid viscosity, check if individual is wearing dentures if applicable.	Evaluate each aspect and its relationship to other data to help identify specific problems and modifications of the procedure that may be needed for the individual.
Assist the individual into the high Fowler's position or sit out of bed unless contraindicated. If contraindicated elevate head of bed >30 degrees. Individual to be centred in midline position, head flexed forwards and down.	Reduces risk of gastro-oesophageal reflux and aspiration by ensuring individual is safely positioned prior to commencement of feeding. Promotes comfort and reduces risk of choking. Sitting out of bed promotes independence of individual and increases enjoyment of meal.

 PERFORM THE SKILL

(Please refer to the Standard Steps on p. xii for related rationales.)
Perform hand hygiene.
Apply PPE: gloves, eyewear, mask and gown as appropriate.
Ensure the individual's safety and comfort throughout skill.
Promote independence and involvement of the individual if possible and/or appropriate.
Assess the individual's tolerance to the skill throughout.
Dispose of used supplies, equipment, waste and sharps appropriately.
Remove PPE and discard or store appropriately.
Perform hand hygiene.

Continued

CLINICAL SKILL 30.1 Assisting with eating and drinking—cont'd

Skill activity	Rationale
Ensure that appropriate food and fluid textures are given to individual.	Food texture checked and appropriate texture given to individual to prevent choking or aspiration. Fluid viscosity checked and appropriate viscosity given to individual to avoid aspiration.
Position a chair opposite if assistance with feeding required, so you are sitting face-to-face.	Improves communication and interaction.
Present meal in a safe manner to individual. Ensure meal tray/drink is not placed within individual's reach if it has been identified that the individual requires assistance and/or supervision for eating. Provide assistance to open packaging if required. Ensure individual is alert before commencing feeding. Ask individual for preference for food. Understand the risks associated with assisting an individual to eat and drink (e.g. suspected dysphagia, eating disorders). Assist only as necessary. Allow hot food to cool. Check food is not stuck in buccal region.	Prevents aspiration and/or injury from hot food/fluid. Assists with meal set-up. Promotes independence and involvement if possible. Prepares for potential risks and an emergency situation.
Ensure each mouthful of food is presented in a safe manner to individual. Introduce each mouthful of food verbally and visually to individual, ensuring an appropriate size. Ensure appropriate pacing is employed.	Assesses tolerance to the procedure. Alerts individual to next mouthful of food. Ensures prior mouthful is swallowed prior to next being presented.
Ensure observation is maintained throughout meal. Cease meal if there are any signs of choking, aspiration, reduced level of consciousness, food stuck in cheek, excessive spillage from mouth/drooling, food coming out of nose, not swallowing food after several attempts or regurgitation, vomiting.	Maintains individual's safety.

 AFTER THE SKILL

(Please refer to the Standard Steps on p. xii for related rationales.)
Communicate outcome to the individual, any ongoing care and to report any complications.
Restore the environment.
Report, record and document assessment findings, details of the skill performed and the individual's response.
Report, record and document any abnormalities and/or inability to perform the skill.
Reassess the individual to ensure there are no adverse effects/events from the skill.

Skill activity	Rationale
On completion of meal leave individual sitting upright, clean individual's mouth/face, remove clothes protector.	Ensures individual is treated with respect and courtesy during interactions.
Document in nutrition care plan/fluid balance chart if appropriate. Document and report dietary intake, level of assistance and any swallowing difficulties.	Ensures transfer of nutrition care and appropriate care can be planned and implemented.

(Berman et al 2020; Hall et al 2022; NSW Department of Health 2017)

OBSERVATION CHECKLIST: ASSISTING WITH EATING AND DRINKING

STUDENT NAME: _____

CLINICAL SKILL 30.1: Assisting with eating and drinking

DEMONSTRATION OF: The ability to assist an individual with eating and drinking

If the observation checklist is being used as an assessment tool, the student will need to obtain a scale of independence for each of the performance criteria/evidence.

Independent (I)
Supervised (S)
Assisted (A)
Marginal (M)
Dependent (D)

COMPETENCY ELEMENTS	PERFORMANCE CRITERIA/EVIDENCE	I	S	A	M	D
Preparation for the activity	Identifies indications and rationale for performing the activity Identifies the individual using three individual identifiers Ensures therapeutic interaction Gains the individual's consent Checks facility/organisation policy Validates the order in the individual's record (if applicable) Locates and gathers equipment					
Performs activity informed by evidence	Assists the individual into high Fowler's position out of bed, or elevates head of bed >30 degrees Ensures individual is centred in midline position, head flexed forwards and down Ensures meal is presented in a safe manner to individual Ensures meal tray/drink is not placed within individual's reach if the individual requires assistance and/or supervision when eating Provides assistance opening packaging if required Ensures individual is alert before commencing feeding Asks individual for food preference Understands the risks associated with assisting an individual to eat and drink (e.g. suspected dysphagia, eating disorders) Assists only as necessary Allows hot food to cool Checks food is not stuck in buccal region Ensures each mouthful of food is presented in a safe manner to individual Introduces each mouthful of food verbally and visually, ensuring an appropriate size Ensures appropriate pacing is employed Ensures observation is maintained throughout meal Ceases meal if there are any signs of choking, aspiration, reduced level of consciousness, food stuck in buccal region, excessive spillage from mouth/drooling, food coming out of individual's nose, not swallowing food after several attempts, regurgitation or vomiting Ensures on completion of meal the individual is sitting upright, mouth/face/hands are clean, clothes protector is removed, call bell is within reach					

Continued

COMPETENCY ELEMENTS	PERFORMANCE CRITERIA/EVIDENCE	I	S	A	M	D
Applies critical thinking and reflective practice	Is able to link theory to practice Demonstrates current best practice in the care provided Demonstrates critical thinking (e.g. level of consciousness, position of individual, dysphagia, chronic diseases that require dietary management, food allergies, appetite, assistance needed [personnel and equipment], social and psychological issues that may affect eating, appetite or food and drink choices, food texture, fluid viscosity, whether individual is wearing dentures) Assesses own performance					
Practises within safety and quality assurance guidelines	Reviews against facility/organisation policy Performs hand hygiene, dons appropriate PPE as per infection control protocols Ensures that appropriate food and fluid textures are given to individual Raises the individual's bed to appropriate working position based on nurse's height and lowers at completion of activity Cleans and disposes of equipment and waste appropriately					
Documentation and communication	Explains and communicates the activity clearly to the individual Engages with individual and their carers about their food and nutrition care Reports any concerns/abnormalities regarding safety, food and nutrition care immediately to the RN/medical officer Reports to RN dietary intake, level of assistance and any swallowing difficulties Completes nutrition care plan/fluid balance chart if appropriate, documents in individual's healthcare record Ensures nutrition care information is included in clinical handover					

Educator/Facilitator Feedback:

Educator/Facilitator Score: Competent   Needs further development

How would you rate your overall performance while undertaking this clinical activity? (use a ✓ & initial)

Unsatisfactory   Satisfactory   Good   Excellent

Student Reflection: (discuss how you would approach your practice differently or more effectively)

EDUCATOR/FACILITATOR NAME/SIGNATURE:

STUDENT NAME/SIGNATURE: DATE:

CLINICAL SKILL 30.2 Inserting a nasogastric tube

Please adhere to the policy and procedures of the facility/organisation prior to undertaking the skill. Ensure this skill is in your scope of practice.

NMBA Decision-making Framework considerations (refer to NMBA Decision-making framework for nursing and midwifery 2020):	Equipment:
1. Am I educated? 2. Am I authorised? 3. Am I competent? If you answer 'no' to any of these, do not perform that activity. Seek guidance and support from your teacher/a nurse team leader/clinical facilitator/educator.	Appropriate-sized nasogastric tube (large or fine bore tube) Nasofix or hypoallergenic tape (approx. 7 cm × 2.5 cm split in half for 5 cm of its length to look 'Y-shaped' Lubricant (KY gel) if tube not self-lubricating 10 mL and 20 mL syringes Water or moist cotton buds (if permitted) Kidney dish Disposable gloves Protective eyewear Yankauer sucker and suction Emesis bag/bowl Tissues Protective sheet Plastic bag Equipment for observations (O_2 saturation) Safety pin Spigot or drainage bag if required pH indicator paper/strip

 PREPARE FOR THE SKILL

(Please refer to the Standard Steps on p. xii for related rationales.)
Mentally review the steps of the skill.
Discuss the skill with your instructor/supervisor/team leader, if required.
Confirm correct facility/organisation policy/safe operating procedures.
Validate the order in the individual's record.
Identify indication and rationale for performing the activity.
Assess for any contraindications.
Locate and gather equipment.
Perform hand hygiene.
Ensure therapeutic interaction.
Identify the individual using three individual identifiers.
Gain the individual's consent.
Assess for pain relief.
Prepare the environment.
Provide and maintain privacy.
Assist the individual to assume an appropriate position of comfort.

Skill activity	Rationale
Critically think through the assessment data and problem-solving—special precautions for nasogastric tube insertion.	Evaluate each aspect and its relationship to other data to help identify specific problems and modifications of the procedure that may be needed for the individual.
Assist the individual into the high Fowler's position with neck flexed unless contraindicated. Spinal and neurological individuals must be positioned as per medical orders.	Facilitates tube insertion and reduces risk of gastro-oesophageal reflux and aspiration. Avoids neck extension as it closes oesophagus, opens trachea and promotes aspiration.

 PERFORM THE SKILL

(Please refer to the Standard Steps on p. xii for related rationales.)
Perform hand hygiene.
Apply PPE: gloves, eyewear, mask and gown as appropriate.
Ensure the individual's safety and comfort throughout skill.
Promote independence and involvement of the individual if possible and/or appropriate.
Assess the individual's tolerance to the skill throughout.
Dispose of used supplies, equipment, waste and sharps appropriately.
Remove PPE and discard or store appropriately.
Perform hand hygiene.

CLINICAL SKILL 30.2 Inserting a nasogastric tube—cont'd

Skill activity	Rationale
Clean nares if necessary and examine nostrils for deformity/obstruction and nasal surgery to determine best side for insertion. If nasogastric tube is being reinserted the other nostril should be used.	Asking the individual to breathe through one nostril while occluding the other will help ascertain if one nostril has an occlusion. Minimises risk of irritation and pressure necrosis around the nose.
Measure the portion of tube to be inserted by extending it from the tip of the individual's nose to the earlobe and from the earlobe to the xiphoid process. Note length and mark this measurement on the tube.	Determines the insertion length of the tube to ensure the tube is inserted an adequate distance so that the distal tip rests in the stomach.
Flush fine bore nasogastric tube with 10 mL of water to activate the Hydromer coating.	Ensures easy removal of stylet after insertion and confirms correct positioning.
Lubricate the first 5–10 cm of the tube with water-soluble lubricant. **Note:** Some small-bore tubes self-lubricate when dipped in water.	The use of lubricant will ease insertion by decreasing friction.
Grasp the tube with your hand and gently insert it into the nostril guiding it posteriorly and inferiorly straight back along the floor of the nose. Ask the individual to sniff to ease the passage of the tube from nose to oropharynx. Have an emesis basin and tissues in the individual's lap. Pause a moment if the individual is coughing or gagging.	Insertion of the nasogastric tube can stimulate the gag reflex.
Instruct the individual to tilt the head slightly forwards.	Flexing the head forwards allows the tube to follow the posterior wall of the nasopharynx and enter the oesophagus rather than the trachea.
Instruct the individual to swallow while you gently but steadily advance the tube. Coincide advancement of the tube with the individual swallowing. Sips of water may be given to assist swallowing if safe and not contraindicated.	The muscular movement of swallowing helps advance the tube. Minimises risk of aspiration.
If resistance is met, withdraw the tube 1–2 cm and rotate the tube slowly with downward advancement towards the closest ear. Do not force the nasogastric tube. Abort procedure and attempt other nostril. Withdraw the tube immediately if the individual exhibits signs of distress or a change in respiratory status, if individual begins to cough or change colour or if the tube coils in the individual's mouth. Should two failed attempts occur, cease the procedure and escalate to a more experienced staff member.	Prevents adverse individual outcome such as pneumothorax, aspiration, trauma to surrounding tissues, incorrect tube placement into lungs or cranium.
Advance tube until the pre-measured mark is reached. When the pre-measured mark has been reached secure the tube to the individual's nose using Nasofix or hypoallergenic tape ensuring the tube does not cause pressure on the naris. If inserting a fine-bore nasogastric tube, do not remove stylet until correct placement has been confirmed by X-ray and documented in individual's health record. To prevent tension on the tube, place a piece of tape onto the nasogastric tube (distal end) and attach it to individual's clothing.	Ensures the tube does not move out of the stomach.
Perform and document observations and compare to pre-procedure observations.	Ensures individual has not been compromised by insertion of nasogastric tube.

Continued

CLINICAL SKILL 30.2 Inserting a nasogastric tube—cont'd

Ensure correct position of the nasogastric tube. Aspirate 5 to 10 mL of gastrointestinal fluid. Observe amount and colour and test pH using pH indicator paper/strip. Obtain post-insertion chest/upper abdominal X-ray. The medical officer must document correct placement in the individual's file prior to the administration of any medications, fluids or formula.	Ensures the tube is in the correct location and not in the trachea. Gastric fluid pH is usually 1.0–4.0, indicating the tube is in correct position. pH of pleural fluid is usually >6, indicating incorrect position. Radiological confirmation should be obtained if pH is greater than 5.
Once correct placement has been confirmed and documented, reactivate the Hydromer coating with another 10 mL of water before removing the stylet. The stylet must not be reinserted. If using a large-bore tube for aspiration, attach a spigot or drainage bag to the main lumen of the nasogastric tube.	

AFTER THE SKILL

(Please refer to the Standard Steps on p. xii for related rationales.)
Communicate outcome to the individual, any ongoing care and to report any complications.
Restore the environment.
Report, record and document assessment findings, details of the skill performed and the individual's response.
Report, record and document any abnormalities and/or inability to perform the skill.
Reassess the individual to ensure there are no adverse effects/events from the skill.

Skill activity	Rationale
Document reason for nasogastric tube insertion, nostril used, type and size of tube, insertion distance and the external length of the tube (from nostril to tip).	Ensures transfer of information.

(Berman et al 2020; Crisp et al 2021; Hall et al 2022; LeMone et al 2020; NSW Department of Health 2023; Rebeiro et al 2021)

OBSERVATION CHECKLIST: INSERTING A NASOGASTRIC TUBE

STUDENT NAME: _____

CLINICAL SKILL 30.2: Inserting a nasogastric tube

DEMONSTRATION OF: The ability to insert a nasogastric tube

If the observation checklist is being used as an assessment tool, the student will need to obtain a scale of independence for each of the performance criteria/evidence.

	Scale
Independent (I)	
Supervised (S)	
Assisted (A)	
Marginal (M)	
Dependent (D)	

COMPETENCY ELEMENTS	PERFORMANCE CRITERIA/EVIDENCE	I	S	A	M	D
Preparation for the activity	Identifies indications and rationale for performing the activity Identifies the individual using three individual identifiers Ensures therapeutic interaction Gains the individual's consent Checks facility/organisation policy Validates the medical order in the individual's record and ensures there are no contraindications Locates and gathers equipment					
Performs activity informed by evidence	Assists the individual into the high Fowler's position with neck flexed unless contraindicated Cleans nares if necessary and examines nostrils for deformity/obstruction to determine best side for insertion Measures the portion of the tube to be inserted, notes length and marks this measurement on the tube Flushes fine-bore nasogastric tube with 10 mL of water to activate the Hydromer coating Lubricates the first 5–10 cm of the tube with water-soluble lubricant if not self-lubricating Demonstrates insertion of the tube by grasping the tube and gently inserting it into the nostril, guiding it posteriorly and inferiorly straight back along the floor of the nose Instructs the individual to sniff to ease the passage of the tube Instructs the individual to tilt their head slightly forwards and to swallow while the tube is advanced Coincides advancement of the tube with the individual swallowing Ensures nasogastric tube is not forced Withdraws tube immediately if the individual exhibits signs of distress, a change in respiratory status, begins to cough or changes colour or if the tube coils in the individual's mouth Ensures the tube is advanced until the pre-measured mark is reached Secures the tube to the individual's nose using Nasofix or hypoallergenic tape, ensuring the tube does not cause pressure on the naris Ensures stylet is not removed on fine-bore tube until correct placement has been confirmed by X-ray and documented in individual's healthcare record Attaches a piece of tape onto the nasogastric tube to prevent tension on the tube and attaches to individual's clothing Performs and documents observations and compares to pre-procedure observations Ensures correct position of the nasogastric tube using pH indicator paper Ensures post-insertion chest/upper abdominal X-ray is attended					

Continued

COMPETENCY ELEMENTS	PERFORMANCE CRITERIA/EVIDENCE	I	S	A	M	D
Performs activity informed by evidence *cont'd*	Ensures medical officer has documented correct placement prior to the administration of any medications, fluids or formula and the stylet being removed Ensures the main lumen of the nasogastric tube has a spigot or drainage bag attached if using the large-bore tube for aspiration					
Applies critical thinking and reflective practice	Is able to link theory to practice Demonstrates current best practice in the care provided Demonstrates critical thinking and problem-solving (e.g. individual's health status, contraindications and special precautions for nasogastric tube insertion, privacy, comfort measures) Assesses own performance					
Practises within safety and quality assurance guidelines	Reviews against facility/organisation policy Performs hand hygiene, dons appropriate PPE as per infection control protocols Raises the bed to the appropriate working position based on nurse's height and lowers at completion of activity while maintaining the individual in an upright position Cleans and disposes of equipment and waste appropriately					
Documentation and communication	Explains and communicates the activity clearly to the individual Communicates outcome and ongoing care to the individual and significant others Communicates abnormal findings to appropriate personnel Reports and documents all relevant information and any complications correctly in the healthcare record Reports any complications and/or inability to perform the procedure to the RN and/or medical officer Asks the individual to report any complications during and post procedure					

Educator/Facilitator Feedback:

Educator/Facilitator Score: Competent   Needs further development

How would you rate your overall performance while undertaking this clinical activity? (use a ✓ & initial)

Unsatisfactory   Satisfactory   Good   Excellent

Student Reflection: (discuss how you would approach your practice differently or more effectively)

EDUCATOR/FACILITATOR NAME/SIGNATURE:

STUDENT NAME/SIGNATURE: **DATE:**

CLINICAL SKILL 30.3 Enteral feed

Please adhere to the policy and procedures of the facility/organisation prior to undertaking the skill. Ensure this skill is in your scope of practice.

NMBA Decision-making Framework considerations (refer to NMBA Decision-making framework for nursing and midwifery 2020):	**Equipment:**
1. Am I educated? 2. Am I authorised? 3. Am I competent? If you answer 'no' to any of these, do not perform that activity. Seek guidance and support from your teacher/a nurse team leader/clinical facilitator/educator.	Enteral feeding pump Enteral feeding set Prescribed enteral feed or ready-to-hang formula IV pole Disposable gloves 20 mL oral/enteral syringe pH indicator paper/strip Stethoscope Glucometer to obtain blood glucose by finger-stick

 PREPARE FOR THE SKILL

(Please refer to the Standard Steps on p. xii for related rationales.)
Mentally review the steps of the skill.
Discuss the skill with your instructor/supervisor/team leader, if required.
Confirm correct facility/organisation policy/safe operating procedures.
Validate the order in the individual's record.
Identify indication and rationale for performing the activity.
Assess for any contraindications.
Locate and gather equipment.
Perform hand hygiene.
Ensure therapeutic interaction.
Identify the individual using three individual identifiers.
Gain the individual's consent.
Assess for pain relief.
Prepare the environment.
Provide and maintain privacy.
Assist the individual to assume an appropriate position of comfort.

Skill activity	Rationale
Critically think through assessment data and problem-solving—correct position of nasogastric tube, documentation of order, individual's baseline weight and laboratory values, electrolyte and metabolic abnormalities such as hyperglycaemia and fluid volume excess or deficit and auscultate for bowel sounds.	Evaluates each aspect and its relationship to other data to help identify specific problems and modifications of the procedure that may be needed for the individual. Baseline objective data is used to measure the effectiveness of the feeds. Absent bowel sounds may indicate decreased ability of GI tract to digest or absorb nutrients.
Confirm documentation of enteral feeding regimen (type, route, volume and flow rate) by medical officer and dietitian. Ensure correct position of nasogastric tube has been confirmed by a post-insertion chest/upper abdominal X-ray and documented by medical officer in individual's health records prior to administration of medications or fluids.	Ensures correct feeding regimen. Ensures correct position of nasogastric tube prior to administration of medication or fluids.

 PERFORM THE SKILL

(Please refer to the Standard Steps on p. xii for related rationales.)
Perform hand hygiene.
Apply PPE: gloves, eyewear, mask and gown as appropriate.
Ensure the individual's safety and comfort throughout skill.
Promote independence and involvement of the individual if possible and/or appropriate.
Assess the individual's tolerance to the skill throughout.
Dispose of used supplies, equipment, waste and sharps appropriately.
Remove PPE and discard or store appropriately.
Perform hand hygiene.

CLINICAL SKILL 30.3 Enteral feed—cont'd

Skill activity	Rationale
Check the tube length measurement at the nostril is unchanged compared to the documented correct tube length confirmed by the medical officer by post-insertion X-ray.	Checks correct tube placement prior to commencement of the formula.
Placement on chest/upper abdominal X-ray must be confirmed and documented by a medical officer where there is suspicion of tube displacement or if the individual has been retching, vomiting or violent coughing. With a torch, examine the back of the individual's mouth to ensure tube has not curled up in the back of the throat. Aspirate gastric contents to check for gastric residual. Return aspirated contents to stomach unless the volume exceeds 150 mL. Measure pH of aspirated gastrointestinal contents. Test pH by using pH indicator paper/strips. Gastric aspirate has a pH <5. Observe the aspirate appearance.	Presence of gastric secretions indicates that the distal end of the tube is in the stomach. Residual volume of greater than 150 mL may indicate gastric emptying is delayed. The pH of fluid aspirated from tube of fasting individuals is helpful in differentiating between gastric and respiratory placement and gastric and small bowel placement. Gastric fluid is usually cloudy and grassy green or tan to off-white in colour.
Individual should be positioned in high Fowler's position or elevate head of bed >30 degrees. Where this is contraindicated, the individual should be positioned laterally (left side) to protect the airway during and for at least 60 minutes post cessation of enteral feeding.	Reduces risk of gastro-oesophageal reflux and aspiration by ensuring individual is safely positioned prior to commencement of feeding.
A closed enteral feeding system ready to hang is generally used; it has a maximum 24-hour hang time post connection with a giving set. Giving set must be changed at time of a closed enteral feeding system being hung. Decanted formula should not be hung for more than 8 hours. Ensure non-touch technique when preparing and handling formula and nasogastric tube. Enteral feeding delivery set must be replaced at least every 24 hours. Time and date should be specified on giving set label.	Ensures correct enteral feed and hang time. Prevents contamination of formula and nasogastric tube. Tubing and formula must be free of contamination to prevent bacterial growth.
Ensure formula is at room temperature. Shake formula container well. Close roller clamp at lower end of spike giving set to prevent air entering the tube. Connect tubing to container or prepare ready-to-hang container and fill container and tubing with formula. Connect distal end of tubing to the proximal end of the feeding tube. Hang pack on IV pole and adjust height. Connect tubing through enteral feed pump, prime line as per manufacturer's instruction. Set flow rate as ordered.	Ensures correct administration of formula. Cold formula may cause gastric cramping and discomfort.

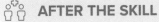 **AFTER THE SKILL**

(Please refer to the Standard Steps on p. xii for related rationales.)
Communicate outcome to the individual, any ongoing care and to report any complications.
Restore the environment.
Report, record and document assessment findings, details of the skill performed and the individual's response.
Report, record and document any abnormalities and/or inability to perform the skill.
Reassess the individual to ensure there are no adverse effects/events from the skill.

Continued

CLINICAL SKILL 30.3 Enteral feed—cont'd

Skill activity	Rationale
Assess individual while feeding is in progress for signs of intolerance to enteral feeding (e.g. vomiting, reflux, nausea, diarrhoea, distension, large residual aspirate volumes).	Ensures formula is tolerated by individual.
During continual enteral feeding, the nasogastric tube should be flushed with 30 mL of tap water three times a day unless clinical indication prevents this volume of fluid. Chart the amount of water used to flush on fluid balance chart. Consult with RN if the feeding tube is blocked. Measure amount of residual aspirate every 4 hours. When tube feedings are not being administered, cap or clamp the proximal end of the feeding tube after flushing the tube with 30 mL water.	Continuous feeding delivers a prescribed hourly rate of feeding which reduces risk of abdominal discomfort. Flushing the tube with water reduces the risk of sediment forming and blocking the tubing. Individuals receiving continuous feeding should have tube placement confirmed and residual aspirate checked every 4 hours. Prevents air entering the stomach between feeds.
Monitor the cleanliness and effectiveness of the tape securing the nasogastric tube to the nose. Tape should be replaced daily. During tape change observe for signs of pressure necrosis around the nose.	Ensures the correct tube placement and absence of pressure areas.
Monitor blood glucose level (BGL) as per facility/ organisation policy. Document intake on fluid balance chart. Monitor intake and output every 24 hours. Weigh individual daily until administration rate is reached for 24 hours then three times per week. Observe return of normal laboratory values. Record and report amount and type of feed, individual's tolerance of feed, adverse effects and patency and placement of tube.	Monitors individual's tolerance of glucose. Ensures accurate intake is recorded. Intake and output are indications of fluid balance or fluid volume excess or deficit. Weight gain is an indicator of improved nutritional status. Sudden gain of more than 900 g in 24 hours may indicate fluid retention. Improving laboratory values indicate improved nutritional status.

(Berman et al 2020; Crisp et al 2021; Hall et al 2022; LeMone et al 2020; NSW Department of Health 2023; Rebeiro et al 2021)

OBSERVATION CHECKLIST: ENTERAL FEED

STUDENT NAME: _____

CLINICAL SKILL 30.3: Enteral feed

DEMONSTRATION OF: The ability to administer enteral feed

If the observation checklist is being used as an assessment tool, the student will need to obtain a scale of independence for each of the performance criteria/evidence.

Independent (I)

Supervised (S)

Assisted (A)

Marginal (M)

Dependent (D)

COMPETENCY ELEMENTS	PERFORMANCE CRITERIA/EVIDENCE	I	S	A	M	D
Preparation for the activity	Identifies indications and rationale for performing the activity Identifies the individual using three individual identifiers Ensures therapeutic interaction Gains the individual's consent Checks facility/organisation policy Validates the order in the individual's record Locates and gathers equipment					
Performs activity informed by evidence	Confirms documentation of enteral feeding regimen (type, route, volume and flow rate) Ensures correct position of nasogastric tube has been confirmed by X-ray and documented by medical officer in individual's healthcare record Ensures tube length measurement at the nostril is unchanged compared to the documented correct tube length Ensures tube has not curled up in the back of the throat Aspirates gastric contents to check for gastric residual and measures amount of residual aspirate every 4 hours (if required) Observes and measures pH of aspirated gastrointestinal contents Positions individual in high Fowler's position or elevates head of bed >30 degrees Connects enteral feeding system with a giving set Ensures giving set is changed at time of a closed enteral feeding system being hung Ensures decanted formula is not hung for more than 8 hours Ensures non-touch technique when preparing and handling formula and nasogastric tube Ensures enteral feeding delivery set is replaced at least every 24 hours, ensuring time and date are specified on giving set label Ensures formula is at room temperature and shaken prior to use Connects tubing to container or prepares ready-to-hang container and fills container and tubing with formula Connects distal end of tubing to the proximal end of the feeding tube Connects tubing through enteral feed pump, primes line as per manufacturer's instruction Sets flow rate as ordered Ensures tube is flushed with 30 mL of tap water three times a day, documents on fluid balance chart Ensures tube is clamped at the proximal end of the feeding tube after flushing the tube with 30 mL water when tube feeds are not being administered Ensures individual is left clean and comfortable Weighs individual as per orders Replaces nose tape daily Observes nose for signs of pressure necrosis					

Continued

COMPETENCY ELEMENTS	PERFORMANCE CRITERIA/EVIDENCE	I	S	A	M	D
Applies critical thinking and reflective practice	Is able to link theory to practice Demonstrates current best practice in the care provided Demonstrates critical thinking and problem-solving (e.g. privacy, correct position of nasogastric tube, documentation of order, individual's baseline weight and laboratory values, electrolyte and metabolic abnormalities, such as hyperglycaemia and fluid volume excess or deficit, and auscultates for bowel sounds) Assesses individual while feeding is in progress for signs of intolerance to enteral feeding (e.g. vomiting, reflux, nausea, diarrhoea, distension, large residual aspirate volumes) Assesses own performance					
Practises within safety and quality assurance guidelines	Reviews against facility/organisation policy Performs hand hygiene, dons appropriate PPE as per infection control protocols Raises the bed to the appropriate working position based on nurse's height and lowers at completion of activity while maintaining the individual in an upright position Cleans and disposes of equipment and waste appropriately					
Documentation and communication	Explains and communicates the activity clearly to the individual and significant others Communicates outcome and ongoing care to individual and significant others Communicates abnormal findings to appropriate personnel Reports and documents all relevant information and any complications correctly in the healthcare record Reports any complications and/or inability to perform the procedure to the RN and/or medical officer Asks the individual to report any complications during and post procedure					

Educator/Facilitator Feedback:

Educator/Facilitator Score: Competent   Needs further development

How would you rate your overall performance while undertaking this clinical activity? (use a ✓ & initial)

Unsatisfactory   Satisfactory   Good   Excellent

Student Reflection: (discuss how you would approach your practice differently or more effectively)

EDUCATOR/FACILITATOR NAME/SIGNATURE:

STUDENT NAME/SIGNATURE: **DATE:**

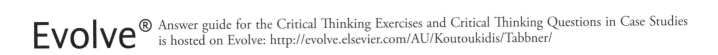

Evolve® Answer guide for the Critical Thinking Exercises and Critical Thinking Questions in Case Studies is hosted on Evolve: http://evolve.elsevier.com/AU/Koutoukidis/Tabbner/

References

Berman, A., Snyder, S., Levett-Jones, T., et al., 2020. *Kozier and Erb's fundamentals of nursing*, 4th ed. Pearson Australia, Frenchs Forest.

Crisp, J., Douglas, S., Rebeiro, G., et al., (eds.), 2021. *Potter and Perry's fundamentals of nursing*, 6th ed. Elsevier, Sydney.

Hall, H., Glew, P., Rhodes, J., 2022. *Fundamentals of nursing and midwifery: A person-centered approach to care*, 4th ed. Australian and New Zealand ed. Lippincott, Williams and Wilkins Australia, Sydney.

LeMone, P., Burke, K., Bauldoff, G., et al., 2020. *Medical–surgical nursing: Critical thinking for person-centred care*, 4th ed. Pearson, Melbourne.

NSW Health, 2023. Guideline: Insertion and management of nasogastric and orogastric tubes in adults. Policy directive: Fine bore nasogastric feeding tubes for adult patients. PD2009_019. Available at: <https://www1.health.nsw.gov.au/pds/Pages/doc.aspx?dn=GL2023_001>.

NSW Department of Health, 2017. Policy directive: Nutrition care. Pd2017_041. NSW Health, Sydney. Available at: <https://www1.health.nsw.gov.au/pds/ActivePDSDocuments/PD2017_041.pdf>.

Nursing and Midwifery Board of Australia (NMBA), 2020. Decision-making framework summary for nursing and midwifery. Available at: <https://www.nursingmidwiferyboard.gov.au/Codes-Guidelines-Statements/Frameworks.aspx>.

Rebeiro, G., Wilson, D., Fuller, S., et al., 2021. *Fundamentals of nursing: Clinical skills workbook*, 4th ed. Elsevier, Chatswood.

URINARY HEALTH

Marie V Long

Overview

The urinary system is responsible for maintaining homeostasis and eliminating waste products of body metabolism through the excretion of urine. Many factors can affect the formation of urine and the subsequent excretion of urine, including normal ageing. Urinary elimination problems can have a significant impact on the person's quality of life and wellbeing. Recognising the impacts on the person and maintaining the person's dignity is a major focus of care planning.

A nursing assessment should be undertaken prior to any procedure, and many procedures related to urinary tract dysfunction require a formal request from a medical practitioner, Nurse Practitioner or Registered Nurse. Urinary catheterisation is an invasive procedure that can cause significant complications. Prevention of hospital-acquired infection, such as catheter-associated urinary tract infections (CAUTIs), is one of the priority areas identified in the National Safety and Quality Health Service (NSQHS) Standards (Australian Commission on Safety and Quality in Health Care 2021). This chapter explores the clinical skills required to meet the specific needs and requirements of a person's care relating to the urinary system, including assisting with toileting, routine urinalysis, mid-stream urine collection, applying a sheath/condom drainage device, urinary catheterisation, emptying of a urinary drainage bag and removal of an indwelling urinary catheter.

CASE STUDY 31.2

Mrs Jane Smith is an 85-year-old woman who resides in an aged-care home. She is in good health and has always been very friendly and talkative with the staff. During handover, you are informed that Mrs Smith has been experiencing urge frequency and incontinence. You have commenced your shift and, upon entering the room, you notice that Mrs Smith is unusually quiet and will not make eye contact with you. She has been incontinent of urine and you notice that her urine smells malodourous. Her observations are BP 145/90 mmHg, RR 22 breaths/min, temp 38.5°, HR 115 beats/min. Mrs Smith is diaphoretic, and she starts to become agitated.

1. What clinical assessments could indicate that Mrs Smith has a delirium?
2. What clinical assessment intervention/skill should be undertaken to determine if Mrs Smith has a UTI?
3. What are your responsibilities as an EN in this situation?

CRITICAL THINKING EXERCISE 31.1

You have accepted care from the morning shift of a person with an IDC in situ post an abdominal hysterectomy. You note at 1400 hrs that there is no urine in the catheter bag. IV fluids are running at 100 mL/hr. The last documented urine output was at 0600 hrs and the bag was emptied of 40 mL at that time. The person you are caring for is confused, febrile, hypertensive, has shortness of breath, is nauseous and is complaining of left flank and chest pain.

1. What is your first response?
2. What is the medical terminology for this volume of urine output?
3. What could the observations and symptoms indicate?

CRITICAL THINKING EXERCISE 31.2

Consider your own values and beliefs about incontinence and how you feel about caring for a person who is incontinent.

1. Write down your thoughts and feelings.
2. Reflect on how these thoughts and feeling may impact on how you care for people who have a continence problem.

CLINICAL SKILL 31.1 Routine urinalysis

Please adhere to the policy and procedures of the facility/organisation prior to undertaking the skill. Ensure this skill is in your scope of practice.

NMBA Decision-making Framework considerations (refer to NMBA Decision-making framework for nursing and midwifery 2020):	Equipment:
1. Am I educated? 2. Am I authorised? 3. Am I competent? If you answer 'no' to any of these, do not perform that activity. Seek guidance and support from your teacher/a nurse team leader/clinical facilitator/educator.	Urinalysis reagent testing strip (dipstick)—check use-by date Paper towel Urine collection container Disposable gloves Watch or timer to measure time required for reaction to occur on the test strip (from immediate to 60 seconds)

 PREPARE FOR THE SKILL

(Please refer to the Standard Steps on p. xii for related rationales.)
Mentally review the steps of the skill.
Discuss the skill with your instructor/supervisor/team leader, if required.
Confirm correct facility/organisation policy/safe operating procedures.
Validate the order in the individual's record.
Identify indication and rationale for performing the activity.
Assess for any contraindications.
Locate and gather equipment.
Perform hand hygiene.
Ensure therapeutic interaction.
Identify the individual using three individual identifiers.
Gain the individual's consent.
Assess for pain relief.
Prepare the environment.
Provide and maintain privacy.
Assist the individual to assume an appropriate position of comfort.

Skill activity	Rationale
Collect a fresh urine specimen from the person in appropriate container (may be a bedpan or urinal) and taken to the pan room for testing.	A fresh specimen is more likely to yield accurate results.

 PERFORM THE SKILL

(Please refer to the Standard Steps on p. xii for related rationales.)
Perform hand hygiene.
Apply PPE: gloves, eyewear, mask and gown as appropriate.
Ensure the individual's safety and comfort throughout use of the skill.
Promote independence and involvement of the individual if possible and/or appropriate.
Assess the individual's tolerance to the skill throughout.
Dispose of used supplies, equipment, waste and sharps appropriately.
Remove PPE and discard or store appropriately.
Perform hand hygiene.

Skill activity	Rationale
Inspect urine for colour, amount, odour and clarity.	Abnormalities in the appearance of the urine may indicate abnormalities.
Prepare testing area by placing absorbent paper towel onto benchtop.	Paper towel will absorb any urine spilt.
Check test strips are within the use-by date.	Out-of-date test strips or inaccurate timing may not give an accurate result.
Uncap bottle and remove reagent strip from bottle. Recap bottle.	Prevents contamination of remaining strips in bottle.

CLINICAL SKILL 31.1 Routine urinalysis—cont'd

Note the time the reagent strip is inserted into the urine.	Not all tests are read at the same time.
Dip reagent strip into the collected urine, making sure to cover all testing areas on the strip.	Ensures the chemical reaction will occur on each test patch area of the strip.
Lift the test strip out of the urine and blot the side of the stick on the paper towel.	Reduces the risk of urine dripping on the test strip container when reading the results.
Holding the reagent strip container on its side, without touching the test strip against the bottle, match the test areas of the reagent strip against the chart on the container. Wait the required time from dipping the strip in the urine to reading the result (from immediate to 60 seconds). Each individual test has a required time for the reaction to complete. Note the results on the chart as the time elapses.	Test results are noted against colour matching on the reagent test strip container chart. Touching the strip against the bottle will lead to cross-contamination. Timing of the reaction for each test ensures accuracy of the results.
Dispose of urine sample, test strip and absorbent towel into correct receptacles.	Correct disposal prevents cross-contamination and spread of infection.

 AFTER THE SKILL

(Please refer to the Standard Steps on p. xii for related rationales.)
Communicate outcome to the individual, any ongoing care and to report any complications
Restore the environment.
Report, record and document assessment findings, details of the skill performed and the individual's response.
Report, record and document any abnormalities and/or inability to perform the skill.
Reassess the individual to ensure there are no adverse effects/events from the skill.

(Patton et al 2024; Watt 2021)

OBSERVATION CHECKLIST: ROUTINE URINALYSIS

STUDENT NAME: _____

CLINICAL SKILL 31.1: Routine urinalysis

DEMONSTRATION OF: The ability to test urine using a reagent strip

If the observation checklist is being used as an assessment tool, the student will need to obtain a scale of independence for each of the performance criteria/evidence.

Independent (I)
Supervised (S)
Assisted (A)
Marginal (M)
Dependent (D)

COMPETENCY ELEMENTS	PERFORMANCE CRITERIA/EVIDENCE	I	S	A	M	D
Preparation for the activity	Identifies indications and rationale for performing the activity Identifies the person using three individual identifiers Ensures therapeutic interaction Gains the person's consent Locates and gathers equipment					
Performs activity informed by evidence	Performs hand hygiene Dons disposable gloves Collects urine specimen in appropriate clean container Inspects urine for colour, volume, odour and clarity Removes reagent strip from container Recaps reagent strip container Notes the time the reagent strip is inserted into the urine Dips reagent strip into the collected urine, covering all testing areas on the strip Correctly matches the test areas of the reagent strip against side of container without contaminating the container or chart Accurately times for each test result					
Applies critical thinking and reflective practice	Is able to link theory to practice Demonstrates current best practice in the skill Seeks assistance if required Checks test strips are in date Checks how to read strip and time required for a result prior to commencing urinalysis Reflects on and assesses own performance					
Practises within safety and quality assurance guidelines	Performs hand hygiene, dons appropriate PPE as per standard infection control guidelines Cleans and disposes of equipment and waste appropriately					
Documentation and communication	Explains and communicates the activity clearly to the person Communicates results of urinalysis appropriately to the person Communicates abnormal findings to appropriate personnel Documents all relevant information and any complications correctly in the healthcare record/charts Reports any complications and/or inability to perform the procedure to the RN					

Educator/Facilitator Feedback:

Educator/Facilitator Score: Competent   Needs further development

How would you rate your overall performance while undertaking this clinical activity? (use a 3 & initial)

Unsatisfactory   Satisfactory   Good   Excellent

Student Reflection: (discuss how you would approach your practice differently or more effectively)

EDUCATOR/FACILITATOR NAME/SIGNATURE:

STUDENT NAME/SIGNATURE: DATE:

CLINICAL SKILL 31.2 Mid-stream urine collection

Please adhere to the policy and procedures of the facility/organisation prior to undertaking the skill. Ensure this skill is in your scope of practice.

NMBA Decision-making Framework considerations (refer to NMBA Decision-making framework for nursing and midwifery 2020):	Equipment:
1. Am I educated? 2. Am I authorised? 3. Am I competent? If you answer 'no' to any of these, do not perform that activity. Seek guidance and support from your teacher/a nurse team leader/clinical facilitator/educator.	Sterile specimen container with wide opening and lid Commercially produced water wipe or mild soap and water to wash genital area Laboratory request form (signed by a medical practitioner or Nurse Practitioner—may be an electronic document) Disposable gloves Biohazard specimen transport bag

 PREPARE FOR THE SKILL

(Please refer to the Standard Steps on p. xii for related rationales.)
Mentally review the steps of the skill.
Discuss the skill with your instructor/supervisor/team leader, if required.
Confirm correct facility/organisation policy/safe operating procedures.
Validate the order in the individual's record.
Identify indication and rationale for performing the activity.
Assess for any contraindications.
Locate and gather equipment.
Perform hand hygiene.
Ensure therapeutic interaction.
Identify the individual using three individual identifiers.
Gain the individual's consent.
Assess for pain relief.
Prepare the environment.
Provide and maintain privacy.
Assist the individual to assume an appropriate position of comfort.

Skill activity	Rationale
Mid-stream urine (MSU) specimen obtains a urine specimen that is not contaminated by microorganisms from the hands or urethra. Accurate urine collection for an MSU can only be achieved if the individual is able to follow instructions. If the person is unable to follow instructions, the nurse will need to assist to obtain the specimen.	
Explain to the person how to obtain a specimen that is free of toilet paper and stool.	To promote collection of an uncontaminated specimen.

 PERFORM THE SKILL

(Please refer to the Standard Steps on p. xii for related rationales.)
Perform hand hygiene.
Apply PPE: gloves, eyewear, mask and gown as appropriate.
Ensure the individual's safety and comfort throughout use of the skill.
Promote independence and involvement of the individual if possible and/or appropriate.
Assess the individual's tolerance to the skill throughout.
Dispose of used supplies, equipment, waste and sharps appropriately.
Remove PPE and discard or store appropriately.
Perform hand hygiene.

CLINICAL SKILL 31.2 Mid-stream urine collection—cont'd

Skill activity	Rationale
Explain to the person how to: • Perform hand hygiene. • Wash genital area. • Female: hold labia open. Male: draw back foreskin if uncircumcised. • Void a small amount of urine into the toilet (keeping the labia held open with one hand). • While not interrupting the flow of urine, with the other hand, place the specimen container in a position to catch the urine, taking care not to touch the inside of the container or touch the container onto the skin of the genital area. Fill approximately half the container. • Remove the container, replace the lid securely without touching the inside surface and place on a secure surface. • Pass the remaining urine into the toilet, wipe as needed, re-dress and wash hands. For a man—make sure the foreskin is replaced to its normal position covering the glans penis. *Note:* If the person is unable to collect the specimen themselves, the nurse will need to assist (with disposable gloves on). Follow the same procedure as above. It may be easier to collect the urine in a larger sterile container and, when collected, pour the specimen into the smaller sterile container for transport to the laboratory. All other steps are the same.	Promotes cooperation and individual's participation. Where appropriate, the individual can collect a clean-voided specimen independently. All actions are an attempt to collect the most uncontaminated specimen possible.
Specimen container may need wiping with an absorbent paper towel. Label the specimen container with the person's name, date of birth, hospital or patient number and the date and time of the specimen collection.	Ensures that the correct specimen is sent for testing and that it is for the correct person.
Specimen container is placed in the zip lock section of the plastic biohazard bag.	Standard infection control precaution.
Pathology request form is checked for the person's details. The pathology request form is placed in the other section of the bag. Indicate on laboratory slip if individual is menstruating.	Ensures correct form and specimen are sent to pathology department and correct test will be undertaken in the pathology department.

AFTER THE SKILL

(Please refer to the Standard Steps on p. xii for related rationales.)
Communicate outcome to the individual, any ongoing care and to report any complications.
Restore the environment.
Report, record and document assessment findings, details of the skill performed and the individual's response.
Report, record and document any abnormalities and/or inability to perform the skill.
Reassess the individual to ensure there are no adverse effects/events from the skill.

Skill activity	Rationale
The specimen should be transported to the laboratory as soon as possible, or stored in a refrigerator until transport can be arranged.	Decomposition and cell growth occur if urine is left standing, and may provide an inaccurate result.

(Patton et al 2024; Rebeiro et al 2021; Watt 2021)

OBSERVATION CHECKLIST: MID-STREAM URINE COLLECTION

STUDENT NAME: _____

CLINICAL SKILL 31.2: Mid-stream urine collection

DEMONSTRATION OF: The ability to collect a mid-stream urine specimen

If the observation checklist is being used as an assessment tool, the student will need to obtain a scale of independence for each of the performance criteria/evidence.

Independent (I)
Supervised (S)
Assisted (A)
Marginal (M)
Dependent (D)

COMPETENCY ELEMENTS	PERFORMANCE CRITERIA/EVIDENCE	I	S	A	M	D
Preparation for the activity	Identifies indications and rationale for performing the activity Performs hand hygiene Identifies the individual using three individual identifiers Ensures therapeutic interaction Gains the individual's consent Checks facility/organisation policy Locates the medical or Nurse Practitioner request for the collection of the specimen Locates and gathers equipment					
Performs activity informed by evidence	Explains the procedural steps to the person, emphasising the need to collect the mid-stream and not to touch the sterile container interior or the lid interior Identifies the need to assist individual if required Provides person with equipment to cleanse perineum Dons disposable gloves Collects urine specimen and ensures that the lid is secured Ensures that the correct individual's details are labelled on the specimen, including the time of specimen collection, and that specimen is placed in biohazard bag Removes gloves and performs hand hygiene Provides hand hygiene for the individual (if needed)					
Applies critical thinking and reflective practice	Is able to link theory to practice Demonstrates current best practice in the skill Seeks assistance if required Identifies if the person is able to undertake procedure independently Recognises the need to store specimen in refrigerator if a delay of more than 24 hours between collection and transport to the laboratory is expected Reflects on and assesses own performance					
Practises within safety and quality assurance guidelines	Reviews against facility/organisation policy concerning specimen collection Performs hand hygiene, dons appropriate PPE as per standard infection control guidelines Labels specimen correctly Cleans and disposes of equipment and waste appropriately					

COMPETENCY ELEMENTS	PERFORMANCE CRITERIA/EVIDENCE	I	S	A	M	D
Documentation and communication	Explains and communicates the activity clearly to the person Communicates the process of microbiological testing of the specimen and when the results are likely to be available Reports and documents that the specimen has been collected correctly in the healthcare record Reports inability to perform the procedure to the RN					

Educator/Facilitator Feedback:

Educator/Facilitator Score: Competent   Needs further development

How would you rate your overall performance while undertaking this clinical activity? (use a ✓ & initial)

Unsatisfactory   Satisfactory   Good   Excellent

Student Reflection: (discuss how you would approach your practice differently or more effectively)

EDUCATOR/FACILITATOR NAME/SIGNATURE:

STUDENT NAME/SIGNATURE: **DATE:**

CLINICAL SKILL 31.3 Assisting with toileting: bedpan, urinal, commode

Please adhere to the policy and procedures of the facility/organisation prior to undertaking the skill. Ensure this skill is in your scope of practice.

NMBA Decision-making Framework considerations (refer to NMBA Decision-making framework for nursing and midwifery 2020):	Equipment:
1. Am I educated? 2. Am I authorised? 3. Am I competent? If you answer 'no' to any of these, do not perform that activity. Seek guidance and support from your teacher/a nurse team leader/clinical facilitator/educator.	Bedpan traditional or slipper type/urinal/commode chair Pan/urinal cover Waterproof sheet/'bluey'/absorbent pad (if using a bedpan) Disposable gloves Toilet paper Hand hygiene available for the person—water, face washer, towel, disposable wipes If the person can assist with moving themselves onto the bedpan, they will need an overhead trapeze bar. If the person is unable to assist in lifting themselves, another person will be needed to assist with rolling them onto the pan or a lifting machine.

 PREPARE FOR THE SKILL

(Please refer to the Standard Steps on p. xii for related rationales.)
Mentally review the steps of the skill.
Discuss the skill with your instructor/supervisor/team leader, if required.
Confirm correct facility/organisation policy/safe operating procedures.
Validate the order in the individual's record.
Identify indication and rationale for performing the activity.
Assess for any contraindications.
Locate and gather equipment.
Perform hand hygiene.
Ensure therapeutic interaction.
Identify the individual using three individual identifiers.
Gain the individual's consent.
Assess for pain relief.
Prepare the environment.
Provide and maintain privacy.
Assist the individual to assume an appropriate position of comfort.

Skill activity	Rationale
Assist with toileting using bedpan/urinal	
A bedpan or urinal is used to assist an individual with toileting when they are unable to move from the bed to the toilet or a commode chair beside the bed.	
Assist the person to a sitting or semi-Fowler's position if the person's health condition allows.	Provides ease of access to insert bedpan. Enables the person to assist by lifting themselves by the overhead trapeze.

 PERFORM THE SKILL

(Please refer to the Standard Steps on p. xii for related rationales)
Perform hand hygiene.
Apply PPE: gloves, eyewear, mask and gown as appropriate.
Ensure the individual's safety and comfort throughout use of the skill.
Promote independence and involvement of the individual if possible and/or appropriate.
Assess the individual's tolerance to the skill throughout.
Dispose of used supplies, equipment, waste and sharps appropriately.
Remove PPE and discard or store appropriately.
Perform hand hygiene.

Continued

CLINICAL SKILL 31.3 Assisting with toileting: bedpan, urinal, commode—cont'd

Skill activity	Rationale
Place waterproof sheet/'bluey'/absorbent pad under the person's buttock area.	Absorbent pad will collect any spilt urine and prevent bed from becoming wet.
Place bedpan under the person's buttocks, on top of the waterproof pad. A urinal is placed between man's thighs (the handle upwards). The penis is placed into the neck of the urinal.	Ensures that urine or faeces will go into the bedpan/urinal and not soil the bedding.
Assist the person with use of toilet paper.	To remove urine and faecal matter from the perineal area.
Remove bedpan/urinal and place the paper cover.	Prevents contents from being viewed during transportation to pan room/flusher.
Provide for hand hygiene (bowl of warm water, hand wash, towel etc.).	Prevents the spread of infection. Provides hygiene requirements for the person.
Volume measurement, urinalysis, use Bristol Stool Chart for documenting faeces.	Measurement required for maintaining fluid balance.
Place the bedpan/urinal in the pan flusher for cleaning/sterilising.	Standard infection control measure.

Assist with toileting using commode

A commode chair is used to assist an individual with toileting when they are unable to move from the bed to the toilet but are able to sit out of bed with assistance. Use of a commode chair provides a more normal position for toileting than use of a bedpan. However, where possible, the person should be assisted to the toilet.

Commode is placed close to the bed or chair with brakes applied.	Provides ease of access. Brakes prevent chair from moving.
Pan placed into commode chair.	Collects urine or faeces.
Individual is assisted onto the commode (may need more than one person to assist).	Prevents individual from falling.
Provide call bell for individual and allow for privacy.	Dignity and privacy are maintained.
Assist individual with use of toilet paper.	To remove urine and faecal matter from the perineal area.
Assist individual into the bed or chair.	To maintain safety.
Provide for hand hygiene (such as a bowl of warm water, hand wash, towel).	Prevents the spread of infection. Provides hygiene requirements for the person.
Remove commode and transport to the pan room.	Remove from vicinity of individual's bedside. Contents are disposed of in the correct manner.
Volume measurement, urinalysis, use Bristol Stool Chart for documenting faeces.	Measurement required for maintaining fluid balance.

AFTER THE SKILL

(Please refer to the Standard Steps on p. xii for related rationales.)
Communicate outcome to the individual, any ongoing care and to report any complications.
Restore the environment.
Report, record and document assessment findings, details of the skill performed and the individual's response.
Report, record and document any abnormalities and/or inability to perform the skill.
Reassess the individual to ensure there are no adverse effects/events from the skill.

(Patton et al 2024; Potter et al 2023; Watt 2021)

OBSERVATION CHECKLIST: ASSISTING WITH TOILETING: BEDPAN, URINAL, COMMODE

| Independent (I) |
| Supervised (S) |
| Assisted (A) |
| Marginal (M) |
| Dependent (D) |

STUDENT NAME: _____

CLINICAL SKILL 31.3: Assisting with toileting: bedpan, urinal, commode

DEMONSTRATION OF: The ability to assist the individual with toileting

If the observation checklist is being used as an assessment tool, the student will need to obtain a scale of independence for each of the performance criteria/evidence.

COMPETENCY ELEMENTS	PERFORMANCE CRITERIA/EVIDENCE	I	S	A	M	D
Preparation for the activity	Identifies indications and rationale for performing the activity Performs hand hygiene Identifies the individual using three individual identifiers Ensures therapeutic interaction Makes an assessment of whether more than one nurse is needed to assist the person Identifies if volume measurement, urinalysis or specimen collection is required Gains the person's consent Locates and gathers required equipment					
Performs activity informed by evidence	Provides privacy—pulls bedside curtains/closes door if appropriate Positions the person in an appropriate position Places bedpan, urinal or commode in correct position Checks the person's comfort Provides call bell and allows for privacy Dons disposable gloves Assists individual with use of toilet paper Takes bedpan, urinal, commode to pan room for inspection, volume measurement, urinalysis etc. if required Disposes of contents in pan flusher and starts the cleaning cycle Removes gloves, performs hand hygiene Provides hand hygiene for the individual Obtains assistance if required to re-dress Documents assessment findings on relevant chart/s. Reports abnormal results if needed					
Applies critical thinking and reflective practice	Is able to link theory to practice Demonstrates current best practice in the care provided Identifies and responds to risks Collects and stores specimens appropriately (if required) Reflects and assesses own performance					
Practises within safety and quality assurance guidelines	Performs hand hygiene, dons appropriate PPE as per standard infection control guidelines Applies brakes to commode chair Adheres to standard infection control precautions Cleans and disposes of equipment and waste appropriately					
Documentation and communication	Explains and communicates the activity clearly to the person Communicates abnormal findings to appropriate personnel Documents all relevant information and any complications correctly in the healthcare record					

Educator/Facilitator Feedback:

Educator/Facilitator Score: Competent   Needs further development

How would you rate your overall performance while undertaking this clinical activity? (use a ✓ & initial)

Unsatisfactory   Satisfactory   Good   Excellent

Student Reflection: (discuss how you would approach your practice differently or more effectively)

EDUCATOR/FACILITATOR NAME/SIGNATURE:

STUDENT NAME/SIGNATURE: **DATE:**

CLINICAL SKILL 31.4 Applying a sheath/condom drainage device

Please adhere to the policy and procedures of the facility/organisation prior to undertaking the skill. Ensure this skill is in your scope of practice.

NMBA Decision-making Framework considerations (refer to NMBA Decision-making framework for nursing and midwifery 2020):	Equipment:
1. Am I educated? 2. Am I authorised? 3. Am I competent? If you answer 'no' to any of these, do not perform that activity. Seek guidance and support from your teacher/a nurse team leader/clinical facilitator/educator.	Silicone sheath/condom catheters in a variety of sizes and sizing guide Disposable razor or personal hair clippers (individual supplied) Urine drainage bag or leg bag and straps Disposable gloves Basin with warm water, soap, washcloth, towel

 PREPARE FOR THE SKILL

(Please refer to the Standard Steps on p. xii for related rationales.)
Mentally review the steps of the skill.
Discuss the skill with your instructor/supervisor/team leader, if required.
Confirm correct facility/organisation policy/safe operating procedures.
Validate the order in the individual's record.
Identify indication and rationale for performing the activity.
Assess for any contraindications.
Locate and gather equipment.
Perform hand hygiene.
Ensure therapeutic interaction.
Identify the individual using three individual identifiers.
Gain the individual's consent.
Assess for pain relief.
Prepare the environment.
Provide and maintain privacy.
Assist the individual to assume an appropriate position of comfort.

Skill activity	Rationale
A sheath/condom catheter is used for a male who is incontinent but can void on his own and who prefers this method rather than continence pads. It should not be used when the person has any skin disease or irritation on the penis or if they have allergies to adhesives, or in men who have a very short retracted penis (the sheath will not stay in place).	
Assess the condition of the skin on the penis. Use a disposable sizing guide to measure the circumference of penis—assess for shaft length. Select an appropriately sized sheath.	Urinary incontinence increases the risk of skin breakdown or irritation. Enables the correct size to be used and reduces the risk of leakage of urine.

 PERFORM THE SKILL

(Please refer to the Standard Steps on p. xii for related rationales.)
Perform hand hygiene.
Apply PPE: gloves, eyewear, mask and gown as appropriate.
Ensure the individual's safety and comfort throughout use of the skill.
Promote independence and involvement of the individual if possible and/or appropriate.
Assess the individual's tolerance to the skill throughout.
Dispose of used supplies, equipment, waste and sharps appropriately.
Remove PPE and discard or store appropriately.
Perform hand hygiene.

Continued

CLINICAL SKILL 31.4 Applying a sheath/condom drainage device—cont'd

Skill activity	Rationale
Ask the man to wash and dry the penis and surrounding skin, including the penile glans (in an uncircumcised man). Hand hygiene provided for individual (such as a bowl of warm water, hand wash, towel). If the man cannot assist, the nurse can do this for him. Make sure that the foreskin is replaced back to its normal position. If needed, clip as much hair as possible from the base of the penis.	Cleanses the skin before application of the condom device. Moisture will reduce the adhesion. Prevents the spread of infection. Provides hygiene requirements for the person. The foreskin must be replaced to its normal position or it can swell and form a constriction ring, which will be painful and can impact on the penile circulation. Assists in the adherence of the sheath.
Prepare the urinary drainage bag for easy attachment to the sheath.	Prepares the system for use.
Grasp the penis along the shaft. The foreskin should be in its natural position (or very slightly extended so that when the condom is fitted, as the foreskin resumes its normal location, the condom is drawn closer to the body). Place the sheath at the tip of the penis and smoothly roll the sheath onto the penis, leaving a small amount of space between the tip of the penis and the drainage tube of the condom sheath. When applied, gently grip the condom around the penile shaft and squeeze for a few seconds to assist adhesion.	Positions the condom catheter on the penis. Inspects the applied condom to ensure it is the right size. It should appear neither too tight nor too loose. Reduces irritation and discomfort. The adhesive is on the inside of the silicone sheath.
Connect the sheath to the urine drainage bag tubing and check for kinks. Apply fixation device to upper thigh. Fit the drainage bag to a hanger for attachment to, for example, a bed rail, or to a stand on the floor.	Allows urine to flow into the collection bag. Secures tubing and limits tension on the condom.

 AFTER THE SKILL

(Please refer to the Standard Steps on p. xii for related rationales.)
Communicate outcome to the individual, any ongoing care and to report any complications.
Restore the environment.
Report, record and document assessment findings, details of the skill performed and the individual's response.
Report, record and document any abnormalities and/or inability to perform the skill.
Reassess the individual to ensure there are no adverse effects/events from the skill.

Skill activity	Rationale
Explain how the sheath works, how the male can manage it himself and what to be aware of (pain, irritation, change in urine etc.). Provide written information on care of sheath drainage.	Health education is empowering and encourages independence.
Document the date, reason for the procedure, condition of the genital area, size and type of sheath applied, type of drainage bag attached to the sheath and if there were any difficulties applying the sheath.	Medicolegal requirement. Allows for the planning and implementation of care.
Check the penis after 30 minutes to ensure that the system is comfortable, not restricting penile blood flow and not leaking.	Assessment reduces risk of complications.

(Patton et al 2024; Rebeiro et al 2021; Watt 2021)

OBSERVATION CHECKLIST: APPLYING A SHEATH/CONDOM DRAINAGE DEVICE

STUDENT NAME: _____

CLINICAL SKILL 31.4: Applying a sheath/condom drainage device

DEMONSTRATION OF: The ability to apply condom drainage

If the observation checklist is being used as an assessment tool, the student will need to obtain a scale of independence for each of the performance criteria/evidence.

Independent (I)
Supervised (S)
Assisted (A)
Marginal (M)
Dependent (D)

COMPETENCY ELEMENTS	PERFORMANCE CRITERIA/EVIDENCE	I	S	A	M	D
Preparation for the activity	Identifies indications and rationale for performing the activity Identifies the individual using three individual identifiers Ensures therapeutic interaction Gains the person's consent Checks facility/organisation policy Confirms the use of sheath/condom drainage in the person's health record Locates and gathers equipment Assists the individual into an appropriate position					
Performs activity informed by evidence	Performs hand hygiene Dons disposable gloves Assesses the condition of the skin on the penis Correctly measures the circumference of penis using a commercial disposable measuring device Selects an appropriately sized sheath/condom Prepares the urinary drainage bag and condom sheath Washes and dries the penis and surrounding skin (or assists the man to do so) Clips hair as needed at the base of the penis Correctly applies the condom sheath on the penis Connects drainage bag and secures this appropriately Removes gloves and performs hand hygiene States the need to assess blood flow to the penis after approx. 30 min and then once per day					
Applies critical thinking and reflective practice	Is able to link theory to practice Demonstrates current best practice in the care provided Assesses the individual's need for/willingness to use a sheath/condom and understanding of the use of a sheath condom Seeks assistance if required Reflects on and assesses own performance					
Practises within safety and quality assurance guidelines	Reviews against facility/organisation policy Performs hand hygiene, dons appropriate PPE as per infection control guidelines Raises the bed to the appropriate working position based on nurse's height and lowers at completion of activity Cleans and disposes of equipment and waste appropriately					

Continued

COMPETENCY ELEMENTS	PERFORMANCE CRITERIA/EVIDENCE	I	S	A	M	D
Documentation and communication	Explains and communicates the activity clearly to the individual Communicates outcome and ongoing care to individual and significant others Communicates abnormal findings to appropriate personnel Reports and documents all relevant information and any complications correctly in the healthcare record Reports any complications and/or inability to perform the procedure to the RN Asks the individual to report any complications during and post procedure					

Educator/Facilitator Feedback:

Educator/Facilitator Score: Competent   Needs further development

How would you rate your overall performance while undertaking this clinical activity? (use a ✓ & initial)

Unsatisfactory   Satisfactory   Good   Excellent

Student Reflection: (discuss how you would approach your practice differently or more effectively)

EDUCATOR/FACILITATOR NAME/SIGNATURE:

STUDENT NAME/SIGNATURE: **DATE:**

CLINICAL SKILL 31.5 Emptying a urine drainage bag

Please adhere to the policy and procedures of the facility/organisation prior to undertaking the skill. Ensure this skill is in your scope of practice.

NMBA Decision-making Framework considerations (refer to NMBA Decision-making framework for nursing and midwifery 2020):	**Equipment:**
1. Am I educated? 2. Am I authorised? 3. Am I competent? If you answer 'no' to any of these, do not perform that activity. Seek guidance and support from your teacher/a nurse team leader/clinical facilitator/educator.	Disposable gloves Alcohol wipe Urine jug Protective eyewear Paper towel × 2 (to prevent spillage of urine on the floor; to cover urine jug while taking it to the pan room or bathroom)

 PREPARE FOR THE SKILL

(Please refer to the Standard Steps on p. xii for related rationales.)
Mentally review the steps of the skill.
Discuss the skill with your instructor/supervisor/team leader, if required.
Confirm correct facility/organisation policy/safe operating procedures.
Validate the order in the individual's record.
Identify indication and rationale for performing the activity.
Assess for any contraindications.
Locate and gather equipment.
Perform hand hygiene.
Ensure therapeutic interaction.
Identify the individual using three individual identifiers.
Gain the individual's consent.
Assess for pain relief.
Prepare the environment.
Provide and maintain privacy.
Assist the individual to assume an appropriate position of comfort.

Skill activity	Rationale
Drainage bags need to be emptied at regular intervals (often once per eight hours) from the drainage port at the base of the drainage bag. The closed system (drainage bag tubing connected to the urethral catheter) should not be broken to reduce the risk of catheter-associated urinary tract infection (CAUTI).	

 PERFORM THE SKILL

(Please refer to the Standard Steps on p. xii for related rationales.)
Perform hand hygiene.
Apply PPE: gloves, eyewear, mask and gown as appropriate.
Ensure the individual's safety and comfort throughout use of the skill.
Promote independence and involvement of the individual if possible and/or appropriate.
Assess the individual's tolerance to the skill throughout.
Dispose of used supplies, equipment, waste and sharps appropriately.
Remove PPE and discard or store appropriately.
Perform hand hygiene.

Skill activity	Rationale
Cleanse the end of the valve at the base of the drainage bag with the alcohol wipe and allow to dry. Place the jug below the valve and open valve, avoid splashing and prevent contact of the drainage valve with the urine jug.	Allows urine to drain from the bag into the jug. Reduces the risk of bacterial contamination of the urine drainage bag.
When the bag is empty, close the valve.	Prevents subsequent drainage of urine out of the bag.
Remove the jug, cover with a piece of paper towel. Remove the paper towel on the floor and dispose of appropriately. Take the urine to the pan room.	Safe transport of a bodily fluid.

CLINICAL SKILL 31.5 Emptying a urine drainage bag—cont'd

Inspect the urine for colour, clarity and odour. Measure the volume.	The person is at risk of CAUTI. Maintain fluid balance chart.
Empty urine from jug into pan flusher or toilet, rinse the jug, place the jug in the pan washer.	Prevents cross-contamination.

 AFTER THE SKILL

(Please refer to the Standard Steps on p. xii for related rationales.)
Communicate outcome to the individual, any ongoing care and to report any complications.
Restore the environment.
Report, record and document assessment findings, details of the skill performed and the individual's response.
Report, record and document any abnormalities and/or inability to perform the skill.
Reassess the individual to ensure there are no adverse effects/events from the skill.

(ACSQHC 2021; Patton et al 2024; Watt 2021)

OBSERVATION CHECKLIST: EMPTYING A URINE DRAINAGE BAG

STUDENT NAME: _____

CLINICAL SKILL 31.5: Emptying a urine drainage bag

DEMONSTRATION OF: The ability to empty a urine drainage bag

If the observation checklist is being used as an assessment tool, the student will need to obtain a scale of independence for each of the performance criteria/evidence.

Independent (I)

Supervised (S)

Assisted (A)

Marginal (M)

Dependent (D)

COMPETENCY ELEMENTS	PERFORMANCE CRITERIA/EVIDENCE	I	S	A	M	D
Preparation for the activity	Identifies indications and rationale for performing the activity Performs hand hygiene Identifies the individual using three individual identifiers Ensures therapeutic interaction Locates and gathers equipment Assesses if drainage bag requires emptying					
Performs activity informed by evidence	Dons disposable gloves and PPE goggles Uses a clean collecting container Places absorbent paper towel on floor under drainage bag valve Cleans end of drainage bag valve with alcohol swab Prevents contact of the drainage valve with the non-sterile collecting container Closes valve Leaves urinary drainage bag in correct position: • Side of bed • Below bladder • Not on floor—on hanger Checks for kinks in tubing, catheter securing device is in correct position Empties urine in pan, flushes and cleans urine collection container Removes gloves and performs hand hygiene Records inspection of urine and volume on fluid balance chart					
Applies critical thinking and reflective practice	Is able to link theory to practice Demonstrates current best practice in the care provided Follows infection control guidelines Uses a jug large enough to avoid spillage Reflects on and assesses own performance					
Practises within safety and quality assurance guidelines	Reviews against facility/organisation policy Performs hand hygiene, dons appropriate PPE as per infection control guidelines Cleans and disposes of equipment and waste appropriately					
Documentation and communication	Explains and communicates the activity clearly to the individual Communicates abnormal findings to appropriate personnel Reports and documents all relevant information and any complications correctly in the healthcare record, including: • Urine, colour and volume drained Reports any complications and/or inability to perform the procedure to the RN					

Educator/Facilitator Feedback:

Educator/Facilitator Score: Competent   Needs further development

How would you rate your overall performance while undertaking this clinical activity? (use a ✓ & initial)

Unsatisfactory   Satisfactory   Good   Excellent

Student Reflection: (discuss how you would approach your practice differently or more effectively)

EDUCATOR/FACILITATOR NAME/SIGNATURE:

STUDENT NAME/SIGNATURE: **DATE:**

CLINICAL SKILL 31.6 Urinary catheterisation (female)

Please adhere to the policy and procedures of the facility/organisation prior to undertaking the skill. Ensure this skill is in your scope of practice.

NMBA Decision-making Framework considerations (refer to NMBA Decision-making framework for nursing and midwifery 2020):	Equipment:
1. Am I educated? 2. Am I authorised? 3. Am I competent? If you answer 'no' to any of these, do not perform that activity. Seek guidance and support from your teacher/a nurse team leader/clinical facilitator/educator.	Procedure trolley/suitable clean surface if in community setting Catheter pack (basic) containing: • Gloves (extra pair optional) • Drapes, one fenestrated • Lubricant (usually water-based or xylocaine gel [2%] in a pre-filled syringe) • Antiseptic cleaning solution (aqueous chlorhexidine), normal saline or sterile water • Gauze swabs • Forceps • Syringe with sterile water to inflate the balloon of indwelling catheter • Receptacle or basin (usually bottom of disposable catheterisation tray) Catheter of correct size and type for procedure (i.e. intermittent or indwelling) Sterile urine drainage bag Catheter strap or other catheter fixation device Urine drainage bag bedside hanger Protective eyewear Blanket/large towel to cover individual Disposable waterproof pad Procedure light/torch

 PREPARE FOR THE SKILL

(Please refer to the Standard Steps on p. xii for related rationales.)
Mentally review the steps of the skill.
Discuss the skill with your instructor/supervisor/team leader, if required.
Confirm correct facility/organisation policy/safe operating procedures.
Validate the order in the individual's record.
Identify indication and rationale for performing the activity.
Assess for any contraindications.
Locate and gather equipment.
Perform hand hygiene.
Ensure therapeutic interaction.
Identify the individual using three individual identifiers.
Gain the individual's consent.
Assess for pain relief.
Prepare the environment.
Provide and maintain privacy.
Assist the individual to assume an appropriate position of comfort.

Skill activity	Rationale
Make an assessment of the need for another nurse to assist (e.g. if the person is confused or uncooperative, or unable to position their legs during the procedure).	Reduces anxiety. Provides assistance.
Assist the person to a semi-Fowler's position. Assist them to remove underwear, place a disposable waterproof pad under the buttocks and drape with a blanket or towel. Position extra lighting if needed.	Promotes comfort and facilitates performance of the procedure. Assists visualisation.

CLINICAL SKILL 31.6 Urinary catheterisation (female)—cont'd

 PERFORM THE SKILL

(Please refer to the Standard Steps on p. xii for related rationales.)
Perform hand hygiene.
Apply PPE: gloves, eyewear, mask and gown as appropriate.
Ensure the individual's safety and comfort throughout use of the skill.
Promote independence and involvement of the individual if possible and/or appropriate.
Assess the individual's tolerance to the skill throughout.
Dispose of used supplies, equipment, waste and sharps appropriately.
Remove PPE and discard or store appropriately.
Perform hand hygiene.

Skill activity	Rationale
Open the outer cover of the catheterisation pack, ensuring aseptic technique is maintained, and slide the pack onto the top shelf of the trolley.	Maintains the sterile field. Reduces risk of transmission of infection.
Using a non-touch technique, open each side of the sterile cover of the catheter pack. Carefully open and place other sterile equipment onto the sterile field, ensuring aseptic technique is maintained (depending on what equipment is in the catheter pack): • Sterile, self-retaining urinary catheter • Urinary drainage bag	Prepares equipment. Maintains the sterile field and therefore reduces the risk of CAUTI.
Organise catheter pack contents and other equipment on sterile field, ensuring aseptic technique is maintained— for example, draw up sterile water into syringe (amount usually 10 mL—check on the catheter balloon port), open lubricant and squeeze out near the edge of one of the plastic trays, open cleansing solution and moisten gauze swabs on the other tray, ready for cleansing the urethral meatus. Remove the top part of the plastic covering the catheter. Place a small amount of lubricating gel on the tip of the catheter and leave on one of the sterile plastic trays.	Maintains an asepsis, which will reduce the risk of CAUTI.
Ask the person (or another nurse) to position the knees so they are flexed and separated, and feet slightly apart on the bed.	Provides a clear view of the urethral meatus.
Carefully pick up the sterile plastic tray with cleansing solution and moistened gauze and place between person's legs.	Makes it easier to perform cleansing procedure.
With the non-dominant hand, separate the labia minora so that the urethral meatus is visualised. Cleanse both the labia and around the urethral orifice with sterile cleansing solution, using single downward strokes. Keep the labia open with non-dominant hand (or leave a sterile piece of gauze in the labia).	Reduces risk of introducing microorganisms from the genital/anal area into the urinary tract. Provides better access to the urethral orifice and helps to prevent labial contamination of the catheter.
Remove used tray and drop into waste bag/bin without contaminating the gloved hand.	Prevents cross-contamination and decreases risk of contaminating the field.
Apply fenestrated drape to genital area.	Creates and extends protective field.
Place sterile paper drape across the person's thighs.	Reduces risk of equipment becoming contaminated during the procedure and extends sterile area.

Continued

CLINICAL SKILL 31.6 Urinary catheterisation (female)—cont'd

Place the second sterile tray with the catheter in it onto the sterile drape between the person's legs. Pick up the lubricated catheter with dominant hand and insert in the urethral meatus. Gently advance the catheter along the urethra until urine flows out into the tray. Insert the catheter approximately 2 cm further.	Gives a good view of the meatus and minimises the risk of contamination of the urethra. Inadvertent inflation of the balloon in the urethra causes pain and urethral trauma. Length of catheter inserted must be in relation to the anatomical structure of the urethra.
Connect the syringe with the correct amount of sterile water (usually 10 mL) to the balloon port of the catheter, ensure syringe is firmly in place and inflate the balloon slowly with a gentle constant force.	The inflated balloon keeps the catheter in the bladder. Inadvertent inflation with the balloon in the urethra causes trauma and pain. Use of less or more than recommended volume can result in an asymmetrically inflated balloon, the catheter falling out or bursting of the balloon.
Connect the sterile drainage bag tubing and ensure it is securely connected.	Ensures the closed system is maintained, reducing the risk of CAUTI.
Make sure the person's genital area is dry. Remove fenestrated drape and equipment from bed. The person's legs may be straightened.	Ensures comfort.
Attach the drainage bag to a bedside hanger and frequently check for kinks in the tubing. Ensure bag is not touching the floor. Ensure the drainage bag is kept lower than the catheter and the person's bladder.	Failure to keep drainage bag below the level of the bladder, or looped or kinked tubing, can slow the flow of urine, causing discomfort and backflow within the system.
Secure the catheter to the individual's inner thigh using a catheter strap device. The securement should be placed where the catheter is stiffest, typically just below the bifurcation. Ensure that the catheter does not become pulled when person is moving.	Stabilising urethral catheters can reduce adverse events such as dislodgement, tissue trauma, inflammation and UTI. Movement-induced trauma (urethral erosion) can lead to UTIs and tissue necrosis.
Depending on the reason for catheterisation, measurement of the amount of urine drained shortly after catheterisation may be required.	In cases of urinary retention.

 AFTER THE SKILL

(Please refer to the Standard Steps on p. xii for related rationales.)
Communicate outcome to the individual, any ongoing care and to report any complications.
Restore the environment.
Report, record and document assessment findings, details of the skill performed and the individual's response.
Report, record and document any abnormalities and/or inability to perform the skill.
Reassess the individual to ensure there are no adverse effects/events from the skill.

Skill activity	Rationale
Document reason for catheterisation or changing catheter, catheter type and size, balloon size and amount of sterile water in the balloon, batch number/lot number (on the outside label of the catheter packaging), expiry date, date and time of insertion. Description of urine, colour and volume drained.	To provide a point of reference or comparison in the event of later queries. It may be helpful to keep the product identification section from the catheter packaging.
If the person is to go home with the catheter, commence a health education program, including troubleshooting and signs and symptoms that indicate they need to seek professional advice. Provide written information about catheter care and management of the urine bag.	The person is likely to have more confidence. Encourages the person to report any problems that may occur while catheter in situ.

(ACSQHC 2021; Cooper & Gosnell 2023; Rebeiro et al 2021; Watt 2021)

OBSERVATION CHECKLIST: URINARY CATHETERISATION (FEMALE)

Independent (I)	
Supervised (S)	
Assisted (A)	
Marginal (M)	
Dependent (D)	

STUDENT NAME: _____

CLINICAL SKILL 31.6: Urinary catheterisation (female)

DEMONSTRATION OF: Ability to undertake catheterisation of females

If the observation checklist is being used as an assessment tool, the student will need to obtain a scale of independence for each of the performance criteria/evidence.

COMPETENCY ELEMENTS	PERFORMANCE CRITERIA/EVIDENCE	I	S	A	M	D
Preparation for the activity	Identifies indications and rationale for performing the activity Identifies the individual using three individual identifiers Ensures therapeutic interaction Explains the procedure and gains the person's consent Checks for sensitivities/allergies Checks facility/organisation policy Confirms the request to insert an indwelling urinary catheter in the individual's health record Identifies the need for another nurse to assist with the procedure (lack of the individual's cooperation or inability to assume an appropriate position) Performs hand hygiene Locates and gathers equipment, including selection of appropriate size and type of catheter Assists the person into an appropriate position and appropriately drapes the person Places waterproof sheet under buttocks					
Performs activity informed by evidence	Performs hand hygiene Opens and assembles equipment aseptically Sets up sterile field and adds any extra equipment aseptically Dons sterile gloves Cleans urethral meatus Drapes the person with fenestrated drape Lubricates catheter tip Inserts catheter into urethra until urine appears Inflates balloon with correct amount of sterile water Collects specimen if necessary Connects to drainage tubing aseptically Removes gloves Secures catheter to inner thigh Positions drainage bag correctly and checks that urine is draining Assists the person to a comfortable position					
Applies critical thinking and reflective practice	Is able to link theory to practice Demonstrates current best practice in the care provided Ensures correct type of catheter and catheter size and bag have been chosen (i.e. short- or long-term use) Obtains assistance if: • Individual is unable to maintain position • Extra light source is required • Individual needs further reassuring Reflects on and assesses own performance					

Continued

COMPETENCY ELEMENTS	PERFORMANCE CRITERIA/EVIDENCE	I	S	A	M	D
Practises within safety and quality assurance guidelines	Reviews against facility/organisation policy Performs hand hygiene, dons appropriate PPE as per standard infection control guidelines Raises the bed to the appropriate working position based on nurse's height and lowers at completion of activity Cleans and disposes of equipment and waste appropriately					
Documentation and communication	Explains and communicates the activity clearly Communicates outcome and ongoing care to person and significant others Communicates abnormal findings to appropriate personnel Reports and documents all relevant information and any complications correctly in the health record, including: • Reason for catheterisation • Size and type of catheter used • Balloon size and amount of sterile water in the balloon • Batch number/lot number (on the outside label of the catheter packaging) • Expiry date • Description of urine, colour and volume drained • Any difficulty with insertion • Plan for how long the catheter is to remain in situ • If a specimen was collected and where it was sent (name pathology) Reports any complications and/or inability to perform the procedure to the RN Establishes a fluid balance chart if required Asks the individual to report any complications during and post procedure					

Educator/Facilitator Feedback:

Educator/Facilitator Score: Competent   Needs further development

How would you rate your overall performance while undertaking this clinical activity? (use a ✓ & initial)

Unsatisfactory   Satisfactory   Good   Excellent

Student Reflection: (discuss how you would approach your practice differently or more effectively)

EDUCATOR/FACILITATOR NAME/SIGNATURE:

STUDENT NAME/SIGNATURE: **DATE:**

CLINICAL SKILL 31.7 Urinary catheterisation (male)

Please adhere to the policy and procedures of the facility/organisation prior to undertaking the skill. Ensure this skill is in your scope of practice.

NMBA Decision-making Framework considerations (refer to NMBA Decision-making framework for nursing and midwifery 2020):	Equipment:
1. Am I educated? 2. Am I authorised? 3. Am I competent? If you answer 'no' to any of these, do not perform that activity. Seek guidance and support from your teacher/a nurse team leader/clinical facilitator/educator.	Procedure trolley/suitable clean surface if in community setting Catheter pack (basic) containing: • Gloves (extra pair optional) • Drapes, one fenestrated • Lubricant (usually water-based or xylocaine gel [2%] in a pre-filled syringe) • Antiseptic cleaning solution (aqueous chlorhexidine), normal saline or sterile water • Gauze swabs • Forceps • Syringe with sterile water to inflate the balloon of indwelling catheter • Receptacle or basin (usually bottom of disposable catheterisation tray) Catheter of correct size and type for procedure (i.e. intermittent or indwelling) Sterile urine drainage bag Catheter strap or other catheter fixation device Urine drainage bag bedside hanger Protective eyewear Blanket/large towel to cover individual Disposable waterproof pad Procedure light/torch

 PREPARE FOR THE SKILL

(Please refer to the Standard Steps on p. xii for related rationales.)
Mentally review the steps of the skill.
Discuss the skill with your instructor/supervisor/team leader, if required.
Confirm correct facility/organisation policy/safe operating procedures.
Validate the order in the individual's record.
Identify indication and rationale for performing the activity.
Assess for any contraindications.
Locate and gather equipment.
Perform hand hygiene.
Ensure therapeutic interaction.
Identify the individual using three individual identifiers.
Gain the individual's consent.
Assess for pain relief.
Prepare the environment.
Provide and maintain privacy.
Assist the individual to assume an appropriate position of comfort.

Skill activity	Rationale
Make an assessment of the need for another nurse to assist (e.g. if the person is confused or uncooperative, or unable to position their legs during the procedure).	Reduces anxiety. Provides assistance.
Assist the person to a supine position with legs extended and flat on bed. Assist them to remove underwear, place a disposable waterproof pad under the buttocks and drape with a blanket or towel. Position extra lighting if needed.	Promotes comfort and facilitates performance of the procedure. Assists visualisation.

CLINICAL SKILL 31.7 Urinary catheterisation (male)—cont'd

 PERFORM THE SKILL

(Please refer to the Standard Steps on p. xii for related rationales.)
Perform hand hygiene.
Apply PPE: gloves, eyewear, mask and gown as appropriate.
Ensure the individual's safety and comfort throughout use of the skill.
Promote independence and involvement of the individual if possible and/or appropriate.
Assess the individual's tolerance to the skill throughout.
Dispose of used supplies, equipment, waste and sharps appropriately.
Remove PPE and discard or store appropriately.
Perform hand hygiene.

Skill activity	Rationale
Open the outer cover of the catheterisation pack, ensuring aseptic technique is maintained, and slide the pack onto the top shelf of the trolley.	Maintains the sterile field. Reduces risk of transmission of infection.
Using a non-touch technique, open each side of the sterile cover of the catheter pack. Carefully open and place other sterile equipment onto the sterile field, ensuring aseptic technique is maintained (depending on what equipment is in the catheter pack): • Sterile, self-retaining urinary catheter • Urinary drainage bag	Prepares equipment. Maintains the sterile field and therefore reduces the risk of CAUTI.
Organise catheter pack contents and other equipment on sterile field, ensuring aseptic technique is maintained; for example, draw up sterile water into syringe (amount usually 10 mL—check on the catheter balloon port), open lubricant and squeeze out near the edge of one of the plastic trays, open cleansing solution and moisten gauze swabs on the other tray, ready for cleansing the urethral meatus. Remove the top part of the plastic covering the catheter. Place a small amount of lubricating gel on the tip of the catheter and leave on one of the sterile plastic trays.	Maintains an asepsis, which will reduce the risk of CAUTI.
Carefully pick up the sterile plastic tray keeping cleansing solution and moistened gauze close to the individual, either on/near the thigh.	Makes it easier to perform cleansing procedure.
With the non-dominant hand, grasp the penis just below the glans and hold upright. If the individual is uncircumcised, retract the foreskin. With the dominant hand, clean the glans around the urethral orifice with sterile cleansing solution in a circular motion. Keep the penis in non-dominant hand.	Reduces risk of introducing microorganisms into the urinary tract. The urethra has two curves in it as it passes through the penis and can be straightened out by lifting the penis in an upright position. Provides better access to the urethral orifice and helps to prevent contamination of the catheter.
Remove used tray and drop into waste bag/bin without contaminating the gloved hand.	Prevents cross-contamination and decreases risk of contaminating the field.
Apply fenestrated drape to genital area.	Creates and extends protective field.
Place sterile paper drape across the person's thighs.	Reduces risk of equipment becoming contaminated during the procedure and extends sterile area.

Continued

CLINICAL SKILL 31.7 Urinary catheterisation (male)—cont'd

Place the second sterile tray with the catheter in it onto the sterile drape between the person's legs. With the non-dominant hand gently straighten and stretch the penis to an angle of 60 to 90 degrees. A pre-filled syringe of lidocaine (uro-jet) can be used to anaesthetise the urinary canal. Pick up the lubricated catheter with dominant hand and insert in the urethral meatus. Gently advance the catheter along the urethra until urine flows out into the tray (to the Y section of the catheter). Replace foreskin if uncircumcised.	Gives a good view of the meatus and minimises the risk of contamination of the urethra. Local anaesthetic to minimise discomfort. Inadvertent inflation of the balloon in the urethra causes pain and urethral trauma. Length of catheter inserted must be in relation to the anatomical structure of the urethra.
Connect the syringe with the correct amount of sterile water (usually 10 mL) to the balloon port of the catheter, ensure syringe is firmly in place, inflate the balloon slowly with a gentle constant force.	The inflated balloon keeps the catheter in the bladder. Inadvertent inflation with the balloon in the urethra causes trauma and pain. Use of less or more than recommended volume can result in an asymmetrically inflated balloon, the catheter falling out or bursting of the balloon.
Connect the sterile drainage bag tubing and ensure it is securely connected.	Ensures the closed system is maintained, reducing the risk of CAUTI.
Make sure the person's genital area is dry. Remove fenestrated drape and equipment from bed.	Ensures comfort.
Attach the drainage bag to a bedside hanger and frequently check for kinks in the tubing. Ensure bag is not touching the floor. Ensure the drainage bag is kept lower than the catheter and the person's bladder.	Failure to keep drainage bag below the level of the bladder, or looped or kinked tubing, can slow the flow of urine, causing discomfort and backflow within the system.
Secure the catheter to the individual's inner thigh using a catheter strap device. The securement should be placed where the catheter is stiffest, typically just below the bifurcation. Ensure that the catheter does not become pulled when person is moving.	Stabilising urethral catheters can reduce adverse events such as dislodgement, tissue trauma, inflammation and UTI. Movement-induced trauma (urethral erosion) can lead to UTIs and tissue necrosis.

 AFTER THE SKILL

(Please refer to the Standard Steps on p. xii for related rationales.)
Communicate outcome to the individual, any ongoing care and to report any complications.
Restore the environment.
Report, record and document assessment findings, details of the skill performed and the individual's response.
Report, record and document any abnormalities and/or inability to perform the skill.
Reassess the individual to ensure there are no adverse effects/events from the skill.

Skill activity	Rationale
Document reason for catheterisation or changing catheter, catheter type and size, balloon size and amount of sterile water in the balloon, batch number/lot number (on the outside label of the catheter packaging), expiry date, date and time of insertion. Description of urine, colour and volume drained.	To provide a point of reference or comparison in the event of later queries. It may be helpful to keep the product identification section from the catheter packaging.
If the person is to go home with the catheter, commence a health education program, including troubleshooting and signs and symptoms that indicate they need to seek professional advice. Provide written information about catheter care and management of the urine bag.	The person is likely to have more confidence. Encourages the person to report any problems that may occur while catheter in situ.

(ACSQHC 2021; Cooper & Gosnell 2023; Rebeiro et al 2021; Watt 2021)

OBSERVATION CHECKLIST: URINARY CATHETERISATION (MALE)

STUDENT NAME: _____

CLINICAL SKILL 31.7: Urinary catheterisation (male)

DEMONSTRATION OF: Ability to undertake catheterisation of males

If the observation checklist is being used as an assessment tool, the student will need to obtain a scale of independence for each of the performance criteria/evidence.

Independent (I)
Supervised (S)
Assisted (A)
Marginal (M)
Dependent (D)

COMPETENCY ELEMENTS	PERFORMANCE CRITERIA/EVIDENCE	I	S	A	M	D
Preparation for the activity	Identifies indications and rationale for performing the activity Identifies the individual using three individual identifiers Ensures therapeutic interaction Explains the procedure and gains the person's consent Checks for sensitivities/allergies Checks facility/organisation policy Confirms the request to insert an indwelling urinary catheter in the individual's health record Identifies the need for another nurse to assist with the procedure (lack of the individual's cooperation or inability to assume an appropriate position) Performs hand hygiene Locates and gathers equipment including selection of appropriate size and type of catheter Assists the person into an appropriate position and appropriately drapes the person Places waterproof sheet under buttocks					
Performs activity informed by evidence	Performs hand hygiene Opens and assembles equipment aseptically Sets up sterile field and adds any extra equipment aseptically Dons sterile gloves Cleans urethral meatus Drapes the person with fenestrated drape Lubricates catheter tip Inserts catheter into urethra until urine appears Inflates balloon with correct amount of sterile water Collects specimen if necessary Connects to drainage tubing aseptically Removes gloves Secures catheter to inner thigh Positions drainage bag correctly and checks that urine is draining Assists the person to a comfortable position					
Applies critical thinking and reflective practice	Is able to link theory to practice Demonstrates current best practice in the care provided Ensures correct type of catheter and catheter size and bag have been chosen (i.e. short- or long-term use) Obtains assistance if: • Individual is unable to maintain position • Extra light source is required • Individual needs further reassuring Reflects on and assesses own performance					

Continued

COMPETENCY ELEMENTS	PERFORMANCE CRITERIA/EVIDENCE	I	S	A	M	D
Practises within safety and quality assurance guidelines	Reviews against facility/organisation policy Performs hand hygiene, dons appropriate PPE as per standard infection control guidelines Raises the bed to the appropriate working position based on nurse's height and lowers at completion of activity Cleans and disposes of equipment and waste appropriately					
Documentation and communication	Explains and communicates the activity clearly Communicates outcome and ongoing care to person and significant others Communicates abnormal findings to appropriate personnel Reports and documents all relevant information and any complications correctly in the health record including: • Reason for catheterisation • Size and type of catheter used • Balloon size and amount of sterile water in the balloon • Batch number/lot number (on the outside label of the catheter packaging) • Expiry date • Description of urine, colour and volume drained • Any difficulty with insertion • Plan for how long the catheter is to remain in situ • If a specimen was collected and where it was sent (name pathology) Reports any complications and/or inability to perform the procedure to the RN Establishes a fluid balance chart if required Asks the individual to report any complications during and post procedure					

Educator/Facilitator Feedback:

Educator/Facilitator Score: Competent   Needs further development

How would you rate your overall performance while undertaking this clinical activity? (use a ✓ & initial)

Unsatisfactory   Satisfactory   Good   Excellent

Student Reflection: (discuss how you would approach your practice differently or more effectively)

EDUCATOR/FACILITATOR NAME/SIGNATURE:

STUDENT NAME/SIGNATURE: **DATE:**

CLINICAL SKILL 31.8 Removal of indwelling urinary catheter

Please adhere to the policy and procedures of the facility/organisation prior to undertaking the skill. Ensure this skill is in your scope of practice.

NMBA Decision-making Framework considerations (refer to NMBA Decision-making framework for nursing and midwifery 2020):	Equipment:
1. Am I educated? 2. Am I authorised? 3. Am I competent? If you answer 'no' to any of these, do not perform that activity. Seek guidance and support from your teacher/a nurse team leader/clinical facilitator/educator.	Disposable gloves Protective eyewear Sterile syringe for deflating balloon Disposable bed protector pad Waste bin or bag

 PREPARE FOR THE SKILL

(Please refer to the Standard Steps on p. xii for related rationales.)
Mentally review the steps of the skill.
Discuss the skill with your instructor/supervisor/team leader, if required.
Confirm correct facility/organisation policy/safe operating procedures.
Validate the order in the individual's record.
Identify indication and rationale for performing the activity.
Assess for any contraindications.
Locate and gather equipment.
Perform hand hygiene.
Ensure therapeutic interaction.
Identify the individual using three individual identifiers.
Gain the individual's consent.
Assess for pain relief.
Prepare the environment.
Provide and maintain privacy.
Assist the individual to assume an appropriate position of comfort.

Skill activity	Rationale
Self-retaining urinary catheters need to have the balloon deflated before removal. It is important to make sure that the full amount of water is removed so that the removal does not cause trauma to the urethra or pain. Make sure that the drainage bag is emptied before you start the procedure.	
Check volume of water that was inflated into the balloon (this will be written in nursing progress note from insertion and is also located on the port for balloon inflation/deflation).	To confirm how much water is in the balloon. To ensure balloon is completely deflated before removing catheter.

 PERFORM THE SKILL

(Please refer to the Standard Steps on p. xii for related rationales.)
Perform hand hygiene.
Apply PPE: gloves, eyewear, mask and gown as appropriate.
Ensure the individual's safety and comfort throughout use of the skill.
Promote independence and involvement of the individual if possible and/or appropriate.
Assess the individual's tolerance to the skill throughout.
Dispose of used supplies, equipment, waste and sharps appropriately.
Remove PPE and discard or store appropriately.
Perform hand hygiene.

Skill activity	Rationale
Place bed protector pad under the person's buttocks. Remove the catheter securing device from the person's thigh.	Comfort of the person.

CLINICAL SKILL 31.8 Removal of indwelling urinary catheter—cont'd

Open syringe and insert the tip into the balloon port. Allow the pressure within the port to force the plunger back and fill the syringe with water. Do not use suction on the syringe but allow the sterile water to come back spontaneously (or if needed only use minimal suction to get the flow started).	Reduces the likelihood of damaging the balloon port or tubing.
Check amount of fluid in syringe corresponds to the amount used at insertion. Remove syringe.	Ensures balloon is completely deflated before removing catheter.
Ask individual to breathe in and then out: as individual exhales, gently remove the catheter. Inspect the catheter to make sure that it is intact and place it on the waterproof sheet for wrapping and disposal. *Note:* If catheter does not easily come out, stop the procedure, reassure the individual and inform the RN. **Do not** place a needle in the tubing or cut the tubing.	Distracts the person while the tubing is being removed. Failure of balloon to deflate. Ruins the integrity of the catheter.

 AFTER THE SKILL

(Please refer to the Standard Steps on p. xii for related rationales.)
Communicate outcome to the individual, any ongoing care and to report any complications.
Restore the environment.
Report, record and document assessment findings, details of the skill performed and the individual's response.
Report, record and document any abnormalities and/or inability to perform the skill.
Reassess the individual to ensure there are no adverse effects/events from the skill.

Skill activity	Rationale
Ask the person to notify a nurse when they feel the desire to void and that they must void into a container for measurement. Encourage them to increase their fluid intake (approx. 250 mL per hour until normal voiding pattern is established unless contraindicated). If the person is voiding small amounts of urine, has symptoms of UTI or voiding frequently, report to the RN.	Assesses whether the person has returned to a normal voiding frequency and volume.
Document time of removal, description of urine, colour and volume drained, time of first void post removal and frequency of voiding.	Accurate recording of individual's progress. Assists with the planning and implementation of care.

(Patton et al 2024; Watt 2021)

OBSERVATION CHECKLIST: REMOVAL OF INDWELLING URINARY CATHETER

STUDENT NAME: _____

CLINICAL SKILL 31.8: Removal of indwelling urinary catheter

DEMONSTRATION OF: The ability to remove an indwelling urinary catheter

If the observation checklist is being used as an assessment tool, the student will need to obtain a scale of independence for each of the performance criteria/evidence.

Independent (I)
Supervised (S)
Assisted (A)
Marginal (M)
Dependent (D)

COMPETENCY ELEMENTS	PERFORMANCE CRITERIA/EVIDENCE	I	S	A	M	D
Preparation for the activity	Identifies indications and rationale for performing the activity Performs hand hygiene Identifies the individual using three individual identifiers Ensures therapeutic interaction Gains the individual's consent Checks facility/organisation policy Confirms the request to remove the indwelling catheter in the person's health record Locates and gathers equipment Assists the person to an appropriate position Checks amount of water instilled into balloon					
Performs activity informed by evidence	Dons disposable gloves Empties drainage bag Places waterproof pad between thighs Removes catheter securing device Inserts syringe into balloon inflation port and allows the fluid to drain into the syringe (small amount of withdrawal pressure only if needed) Withdraws the entire amount of sterile water used to inflate the balloon Asks the individual to breathe deeply and slowly and gently removes the catheter Checks the catheter tip to ensure it is complete and places it on and wraps in the waterproof pad Assists the person to cleanse and dry themself Removes gloves and performs hand hygiene					
Applies critical thinking and reflective practice	Is able to link theory to practice Demonstrates current best practice in the care provided Reflects on and assesses own performance					
Practises within safety and quality assurance guidelines	Reviews against facility/organisation policy Performs hand hygiene, dons appropriate PPE as per infection control guidelines Raises the bed to the appropriate working position based on nurse's height and lowers at completion of activity Cleans and disposes of equipment and waste appropriately					

COMPETENCY ELEMENTS	PERFORMANCE CRITERIA/EVIDENCE	I	S	A	M	D
Documentation and communication	Explains and communicates the activity clearly Communicates outcome and ongoing care to individual and significant others Communicates abnormal findings to appropriate personnel Reports and documents all relevant information and any complications correctly in the healthcare record, including date and time of catheter removal, and is able to identify the need to assess the person's voiding pattern post catheter removal Reports any complications and/or inability to perform the procedure to the RN Asks the individual to report any complications during and post procedure					

Educator/Facilitator Feedback:

Educator/Facilitator Score: Competent   Needs further development

How would you rate your overall performance while undertaking this clinical activity? (use a ✓ & initial)

Unsatisfactory   Satisfactory   Good   Excellent

Student Reflection: (discuss how you would approach your practice differently or more effectively)

EDUCATOR/FACILITATOR NAME/SIGNATURE:

STUDENT NAME/SIGNATURE: **DATE:**

Evolve® Answer guide for the Critical Thinking Exercises and Critical Thinking Questions in Case Studies is hosted on Evolve: http://evolve.elsevier.com/AU/Koutoukidis/Tabbner/

References

Australian Commission on Safety and Quality in Health Care, 2021. *National Safety and Quality Health Service Standards*, 2nd ed. ACSQHC, Sydney.

Cooper, K., Gosnell, K., 2023. *Adult health nursing*, 9th ed. Elsevier, Missouri.

Nursing and Midwifery Board of Australia (NMBA), 2020. Decision-making framework for nursing and midwifery. Available at: <https://www.nursingmidwiferyboard.gov.au/Codes-Guidelines-Statements/Frameworks.aspx>.

Patton, K.T., Bell, F., Thompson, T., Williamson, P., 2024. *The human body in health and disease*, 8th ed. Elsevier, Missouri pp. 571–598.

Potter, P., Perry, A.G., Stockert, P.A., et al., 2023. *Fundamentals of nursing*, 11th ed. Elsevier, Missouri.

Rebeiro, G., Wilson, D., Fuller, S., 2021. *Potter & Perry's fundamentals of nursing workbook*, 4th ed. Elsevier, Chatswood.

Watt, E., 2021. Maintaining continence. In: Crisp, J., Douglas, C., Rebeiro, G., et al. (eds.), 2021. *Potter and Perry's fundamentals of nursing*, 6th ed. Elsevier, Sydney pp. 1043–1089.

Online Resources and Recommended Reading

Continence Foundation of Australia, 2021. Continence in Australia: a snapshot. Continence Foundation of Australia, Melbourne. Available at: <https://continence.org.au/data/files/Reports/Continence_in_Australia_Snapshot.pdf>.

Crisp, J., Douglas, C., Rebeiro, G., et al., (eds.), 2021. *Potter and Perry's fundamentals of nursing*, 6th ed. Elsevier, Sydney.

Gersch, C., 2021. Concepts of care for patients with urinary problems. In: Ignatavicius, D., Workman, L., Rebar, C., et al. *Medical-surgical nursing: concepts for interprofessional collaborative care*. Elsevier, Missouri pp. 1325—1354.

Marieb, E., & Keller, S., 2021. *Essentials of human anatomy & physiology*, 13th ed. Pearson Global, New York.

UroToday, 2019. Urinary catheters. Available at: <https://www.urotoday.com/urinary-catheters.html>.

BOWEL HEALTH

Heather Wakefield

Overview

Any condition that causes a change in an individual's bowel elimination pattern can have a detrimental impact on the person's health and quality of life. Healthy bowel function is maintained by routine elimination habits, a nutritional diet with the recommended amount of fibre and fluid intake, and daily mild exercise to stimulate colonic motility.

Observation of the individual's ability to eliminate faeces, together with observation of the faeces, provides the nurse with an objective assessment of the individual's bowel elimination status. The frequency of bowel actions depends on the individual. A normal range can be from 2–3 times a day to 2–3 times a week (Sorrentino & Remmert 2020). Faecal matter varies significantly in colour, volume and consistency, depending on diet and health. The individual's elimination status is assessed by obtaining information about elimination practices, bowel actions and their medical and surgical history. A list of any medications the individual is taking should also be perused as some medications can affect bowel elimination (Crisp et al 2021).

The nurse should inquire about the individual's usual pattern of defecation and whether they have experienced any recent changes to this pattern. Information should also be obtained about the individual's usual exercise levels and fluid and dietary intake so that, whenever possible, it can be maintained or improved to facilitate better elimination. The nurse should identify early signs and symptoms of any problems associated with elimination so that appropriate care can be implemented to assist the individual to meet their elimination needs.

A program to promote bowel elimination is an important part of the nursing care plan for an individual. The goal of a bowel management program is to assist the individual to evacuate the bowel comfortably, completely and in a timely manner without laxative support by promoting privacy, regular mild exercise, high-fibre foods and an adequate fluid intake. It is important for nurses to support the individual with their bowel elimination while hospitalised as failure to do so may result in a delayed discharge (Williams 2022). As a result of certain disorders such as obstruction or tumours in the bowel, the passage of faeces through the rectum and anus may not be possible (Gulanick & Myers 2022). In these instances, the surgical creation of an artificial opening, called a stoma, takes place.

Care of the individual with a stoma includes the selection and management of appliances, care of the stoma and surrounding skin, meeting nutritional needs and providing psychological support and education (Lataillade & Chabal 2021).

When planning care, considerations concerning the individual's altered body image and/or the impact on intimate relationships need to be responded to in a sensitive, private and dignified manner.

CASE STUDY 32.2

Michael Kramer, a 71-year-old gentleman, has been admitted to your ward for revision of his Parkinson's medication. Michael has a colostomy that was formed two years ago. Michael is quite self-caring of the colostomy; however, when you observe him change the appliance, you notice that the surrounding skin in very excoriated and in fact the appliance was not sticking to the skin in places. When questioned, Michael admits that it has been like that for a while.

1. What factors may contribute to excoriated peristomal skin?
2. Outline nursing interventions that may promote skin healing.
3. Discuss any education you will give Michael regarding his stoma and care.

CRITICAL THINKING EXERCISE 32.1

Jason, aged 22, is admitted to your unit with dehydration and diarrhoea after returning from a backpacking holiday around Indonesia. Jason says the diarrhoea started two weeks prior. What are the nursing implications of this? Describe appropriate nursing interventions for Jason.

CLINICAL SKILL 32.1 Changing an ostomy appliance

Please adhere to the policy and procedures of the facility/organisation prior to undertaking the skill. Ensure this skill is in your scope of practice.

NMBA Decision-making Framework considerations (refer to NMBA Decision-making framework for nursing and midwifery 2020):	Equipment:
1. Am I educated? 2. Am I authorised? 3. Am I competent? If you answer 'no' to any of these, do not perform that activity. Seek guidance and support from your teacher/a nurse team leader/clinical facilitator/educator.	One piece, adhesive, clear drainable colostomy/ileostomy appliance in correct size Pouch closure device Adhesive remover Disposable gloves Deodorant if indicated Gauze pads or washcloth Towel or disposable waterproof pad Basin with warm water Scissors Skin barrier paste Skin barrier wipes

 PREPARE FOR THE SKILL

(Please refer to the Standard Steps on p. xii for related rationales.)
Mentally review the steps of the skill.
Discuss the skill with your instructor/supervisor/team leader, if required.
Confirm correct facility/organisation policy/safe operating procedures.
Validate the order in the individual's record.
Identify indication and rationale for performing the activity.
Assess for any contraindications.
Locate and gather equipment.
Perform hand hygiene.
Ensure therapeutic interaction.
Identify the individual using three individual identifiers.
Gain the individual's consent.
Assess for pain relief.
Prepare the environment.
Provide and maintain privacy.
Assist the individual to assume an appropriate position of comfort.

Skill activity	Rationale
Review care plan and current treatment orders to determine type, size of device and length of time in place.	Provides information about individual's treatment, equipment/supplies needed. To minimise skin irritation, avoid unnecessary changing of entire system.

 PERFORM THE SKILL

(Please refer to the Standard Steps on p. xii for related rationales.)
Perform hand hygiene.
Apply PPE: gloves, eyewear, mask and gown as appropriate.
Ensure the individual's safety and comfort throughout skill.
Promote independence and involvement of the individual if possible and/or appropriate.
Assess the individual's tolerance to the skill throughout.
Dispose of used supplies, equipment, waste and sharps appropriately.
Remove PPE and discard or store appropriately.
Perform hand hygiene.

Skill activity	Rationale
Place towel or disposable waterproof pad under the person. Remove the old appliance gently and place it in a plastic bag.	Promotes comfort. Avoids damage to surrounding skin surface.

Continued

CLINICAL SKILL 32.1 Changing an ostomy appliance—cont'd

Wipe the stoma and surrounding skin, using gauze pads or washcloth and warm water. Pat dry.	Cleanses the skin of mucus and faecal drainage.
Inspect the stoma and surrounding skin. The stoma should be pink or red, and free from excoriation.	Deviations from normal must be reported immediately so that appropriate action can be planned.
Apply the skin barrier wipe to the surrounding skin.	Protects the skin from excoriation when applying and removing appliance.
Remove the adhesive backing and place the new appliance over the stoma. Ensure that it is secured firmly in position with no gaps exposing the skin around the base of the stoma, and that the stoma is not being 'choked'.	Prevents leakage of faeces.
Ensure opening of the appliance is distal to the stoma.	To facilitate drainage.

 AFTER THE SKILL

(Please refer to the Standard Steps on p. xii for related rationales.)
Communicate outcome to the individual, any ongoing care and to report any complications.
Restore the environment.
Report, record and document assessment findings, details of the skill performed and the individual's response.
Report, record and document any abnormalities and/or inability to perform the skill.
Reassess the individual to ensure there are no adverse effects/events from the skill.

(Australian Council of Stoma Associations Inc. 2021; Rebeiro et al 2021; Tollefson et al 2022)

OBSERVATION CHECKLIST: CHANGING AN OSTOMY APPLIANCE

STUDENT NAME: _____

CLINICAL SKILL 32.1: Changing an ostomy appliance

DEMONSTRATION OF: The ability to change an ostomy appliance

If the observation checklist is being used as an assessment tool, the student will need to obtain a scale of independence for each of the performance criteria/evidence.

Independent (I)
Supervised (S)
Assisted (A)
Marginal (M)
Dependent (D)

COMPETENCY ELEMENTS	PERFORMANCE CRITERIA/EVIDENCE	I	S	A	M	D
Preparation for the activity	Identifies indications and rationale for performing the activity Identifies the individual using three individual identifiers Ensures therapeutic interaction Gains the individual's consent Checks facility/organisation policy Validates the order in the individual's record Locates and gathers equipment Assists the individual into an appropriate position					
Performs activity informed by evidence	Places absorbent sheet/towel under individual Removes used appliance and skin barrier Cleans and dries surrounding skin Applies skin barrier and new appliance Ensures appliance fits correctly					
Applies critical thinking and reflective practice	Is able to link theory to practice Demonstrates current best practice in the care provided Identifies changes in the stoma appearance Assesses own performance					
Practises within safety and quality assurance guidelines	Reviews against facility/organisation policy Performs hand hygiene, dons appropriate PPE as per infection control protocols Raises the bed to the appropriate working position based on nurse's height and lowers at completion of activity Adheres to infection control/ANTT principles Cleans and disposes of equipment and waste appropriately					
Documentation and communication	Explains and communicates the activity clearly to the individual Communicates outcome and ongoing care to individual and significant others Communicates abnormal findings to appropriate personnel Reports and documents all relevant information and any complications correctly in the healthcare record Reports any complications and/or inability to perform the procedure to the RN and/or medical officer Asks the individual to report any complications during and post procedure					

Educator/Facilitator Feedback:

Educator/Facilitator Score:　　　　　Competent　　　Needs further development

How would you rate your overall performance while undertaking this clinical activity? (use a ✓ & initial)

Unsatisfactory　　　　　　　　　　Satisfactory　　　Good　　　　Excellent

Student Reflection: (discuss how you would approach your practice differently or more effectively)

EDUCATOR/FACILITATOR NAME/SIGNATURE:

STUDENT NAME/SIGNATURE:　　　　　　　　　　　　　　　　　**DATE:**

CLINICAL SKILL 32.2 Stool assessment/collection

Please adhere to the policy and procedures of the facility/organisation prior to undertaking the skill. Ensure this skill is in your scope of practice.

NMBA Decision-making Framework considerations (refer to NMBA Decision-making framework for nursing and midwifery 2020):	Equipment:
1. Am I educated? 2. Am I authorised? 3. Am I competent? If you answer 'no' to any of these, do not perform that activity. Seek guidance and support from your teacher/a nurse team leader/clinical facilitator/educator.	Faecal specimen container Laboratory request form (signed by a medical practitioner or Nurse Practitioner—may be an electronic document) Biohazard specimen transport bag Bedpan/collection pan Disposable gloves

 PREPARE FOR THE SKILL

(Please refer to the Standard Steps on p. xii for related rationales.)
Mentally review the steps of the skill.
Discuss the skill with your instructor/supervisor/team leader, if required.
Confirm correct facility/organisation policy/safe operating procedures.
Validate the order in the individual's record.
Identify indication and rationale for performing the activity.
Assess for any contraindications.
Locate and gather equipment.
Perform hand hygiene.
Ensure therapeutic interaction.
Identify the individual using three individual identifiers.
Gain the individual's consent.
Assess for pain relief.
Prepare the environment.
Provide and maintain privacy.
Assist the individual to assume an appropriate position of comfort.

Skill activity	Rationale
Provide the individual with a bedpan/collection pan. Explain to the person how to obtain a specimen that is free of toilet paper and urine: encourage the individual to void prior to providing the stool sample.	Ideally, the stool sample should be uncontaminated by urine, although this might not always be possible.

 PERFORM THE SKILL

(Please refer to the Standard Steps on p. xii for related rationales.)
Perform hand hygiene.
Apply PPE: gloves, eyewear, mask and gown as appropriate.
Ensure the individual's safety and comfort throughout skill.
Promote independence and involvement of the individual if possible and/or appropriate.
Assess the individual's tolerance to the skill throughout.
Dispose of used supplies, equipment, waste and sharps appropriately.
Remove PPE and discard or store appropriately.
Perform hand hygiene.

Skill activity	Rationale
Visually assess the stool sample. The size, shape, colour and consistency of the stool should be observed.	Changes in the size, shape, colour and consistency of the stool can be a sign of an underlying medical condition.
Specimen container may need wiping with an absorbent paper towel. Label the specimen container with the person's name, date of birth, hospital or patient number and the date and time of the specimen collection.	Ensures that the correct specimen is sent for testing and that it is for the correct person.

Continued

CLINICAL SKILL 32.2 Stool assessment/collection—cont'd

Using the scooped lid of the faecal specimen container, place a portion of the stool into the container. Place the lid on the container.	All stool samples must be placed into the faecal specimen container.
Specimen container is placed in the ziplock section of the plastic biohazard bag.	Standard infection control precaution.
Pathology request form is checked for the person's details. The pathology request form is placed in the other section of the bag.	Ensures correct form and specimen are sent to pathology department and correct test will be undertaken in the pathology department.

AFTER THE SKILL

(Please refer to the Standard Steps on p. xii for related rationales.)
Communicate outcome to the individual, any ongoing care and report any complications.
Restore the environment.
Report, record and document assessment findings, details of the skill performed and the individual's response.
Report, record and document any abnormalities and/or inability to perform the skill.
Reassess the individual to ensure there are no adverse effects/events from the skill.

Skill activity	Rationale
The specimen should be transported to the laboratory as soon as possible, or stored in a refrigerator until transport can be arranged.	Decomposition and cell growth occur if faeces is left standing, and may provide an inaccurate result.

(Linton & Matteson 2023)

OBSERVATION CHECKLIST: STOOL ASSESSMENT/ COLLECTION

STUDENT NAME: _____

CLINICAL SKILL 32.2: Stool assessment/collection

DEMONSTRATION OF: The ability to undertake a stool assessment/collection

If the observation checklist is being used as an assessment tool, the student will need to obtain a scale of independence for each of the performance criteria/evidence.

Independent (I)
Supervised (S)
Assisted (A)
Marginal (M)
Dependent (D)

COMPETENCY ELEMENTS	PERFORMANCE CRITERIA/EVIDENCE	I	S	A	M	D
Preparation for the activity	Identifies indications and rationale for performing the activity Identifies the individual using three individual identifiers Ensures therapeutic interaction Gains the individual's consent Checks facility/organisation policy Validates the order in the individual's record Locates and gathers equipment Assists the individual into an appropriate position					
Performs activity informed by evidence	Provides pan for stool collection Labels specimen container with individual's identifying details and date and time of collection Scoops stool into container Assesses stool for colour, consistency, amount, odour					
Applies critical thinking and reflective practice	Is able to link theory to practice Demonstrates current best practice in the care provided Identifies abnormal appearance of the stool (if applicable) Assesses own performance					
Practises within safety and quality assurance guidelines	Reviews against facility/organisation policy Performs hand hygiene, dons appropriate PPE as per infection control protocols Cleans and disposes of equipment and waste appropriately					
Documentation and communication	Explains and communicates the activity clearly to the individual Communicates outcome and ongoing care to individual and significant others Communicates abnormal findings to appropriate personnel Reports and documents all relevant information and any complications correctly in the healthcare record Reports any complications and/or inability to perform the procedure to the RN and/or medical officer Asks the individual to report any complications during and post procedure					

Educator/Facilitator Feedback:

Educator/Facilitator Score: Competent   Needs further development

How would you rate your overall performance while undertaking this clinical activity? (use a ✓ & initial)

Unsatisfactory   Satisfactory   Good   Excellent

Student Reflection: (discuss how you would approach your practice differently or more effectively)

EDUCATOR/FACILITATOR NAME/SIGNATURE:

STUDENT NAME/SIGNATURE: **DATE:**

Evolve®

Answer guide for the Critical Thinking Exercises and Critical Thinking Questions in Case Studies is hosted on Evolve: http://evolve.elsevier.com/AU/Koutoukidis/Tabbner/

References

Australian Council of Stoma Associations Inc., 2021. Colostomy hints and tips. Available at: <http://australianstoma.com.au/wp-content/uploads/HInts-and-Tips-for-Colostomy.pdf>.

Crisp, J., Douglas, C., Rebeiro, G., et al., 2021. *Potter & Perry's fundamentals of nursing*, 6th ed. Elsevier, Sydney.

Gulanick, M., Myers, J.L., 2022. *Nursing care plans: Diagnoses, interventions, and outcomes*, 10th ed. Elsevier Mosby, St Louis.

Lataillade, L., Chabal, L. 2021. Therapeutic patient education: A multifaceted approach to ostomy care. *Advances in Skin & Wound Care* 34(1), 36–42.

Linton, A.D., Matteson, M.A., 2023. *Medical-surgical nursing*, 8th ed. Elsevier Saunders, St Louis.

Nursing and Midwifery Board of Australia (NMBA), 2020. Decision-making framework for nursing and midwifery. Available at: <https://www.nursingmidwiferyboard.gov.au/codes-guidelines-statements/frameworks.aspx>.

Rebeiro, G., Wilson, D., Fuller, S., 2021. *Potter and Perry's fundamentals of nursing workbook*, 4th ed. Elsevier, Chatswood.

Sorrentino, S.A., Remmert, L.N., 2020. *Mosby's textbook for nursing assistants*, 10th ed. Elsevier, St Louis.

Tollefson, J., Watson, G., Jelly, E., Tambree, K., 2022. *Essential clinical skills: Enrolled nurses*, 5th ed. Cengage, South Melbourne.

Williams, P., 2022. *Basic geriatric nursing*, 8th ed. Elsevier, St Louis.

PAIN

Andrea Zivin and Jasmin Rigby-Day

Overview

According to the International Association for the Study of Pain (IASP) (2021), pain is defined as 'an unpleasant sensory and emotional experience associated with, or resembling that associated with, actual or potential tissue damage'. It is imperative to remember pain is always subjective and an understanding that 'pain' is whatever the person reports.

There are many pain assessment tools that nurses can use to measure the level and severity of pain that a patient is experiencing. The numerical rating scale (Brown et al 2020) and the Abbey Pain Scale (Crisp et al 2021) are examples of tools that quantify the severity of the person's pain. These tools can be used to inform an appropriate approach to pain management (Knight et al 2023).

The key to effective pain management is a focused pain assessment. Pain assessment is considered to be the fifth vital sign. It is imperative that pain is routinely and regularly assessed. Therefore, it is considered a core assessment skill along with the classic vital signs of blood pressure, heart rate, respiration rate, and temperature (Crisp et al 2021). A head-to-toe assessment is required to provide a full understanding of the individual's pain being experienced. The recommended mnemonic to use for focused pain assessment is PQRSTU. This includes provoking/palliative factors, quality, region and radiation, severity, times (onset, duration and pattern) and understanding to the person (Crisp et al 2021). With further in-depth subjective and objective data being obtained, appropriate pain management and administration of medications can be achieved.

According to Knights et al (2023), a 'stepwise' flowchart approach is utilised for pain management and medication administration. This includes step 1, mild pain (1–3): the use of non-opioid analgesia such as paracetamol or a non-steroidal anti-inflammatory such as ibuprofen; step 2, moderate pain (4–6): the use of an oral opioid such as codeine or tramadol with or without non-opioid medications; and step 3, strong pain (7–10): the use of 'strong' opioids, such as morphine or fentanyl with or without non-opioid medications. The use of pain management guidelines provides consistency and effective pain management for individuals who are experiencing pain.

When measuring pain in an individual, the nurse should observe the following points (Brown et al 2020):

- Ensure the equipment is gathered, appropriate and functioning.
- Have knowledge of the individual's usual or previous range of pain.
- Know and understand the individual's medical history, therapies and medications prescribed.
- Perform measurements in an appropriate environment that will have minimal effect on pain.
- Have an organised, systematic approach.

- Have the knowledge to interpret the significance of a pain score and consequently make decisions about individual care.
- Determine the frequency of pain measurement based on the individual's condition.
- Have the knowledge to analyse results.
- Be aware of other physical signs and symptoms of pain.
- Verify and communicate findings and changes of an individual's condition to the relevant Registered Nurse (RN) or medical officer.

The skill presented in this chapter addresses a focused pain assessment using the PQRSTU mnemonic.

 CASE STUDY 33.1

Mrs Corowa, 86 years old, is an Aboriginal and Torres Strait Islander woman. Two months ago, her family decided to move her into a residential aged-care home since they could no longer care for her in the home. The facility is called ACES and is dedicated to Aboriginal and Torres Strait Islander cultured individuals. Mrs Corowa has a medical history of dementia, uncontrolled type 2 diabetes mellitus, osteoarthritis and rheumatic heart disease. Chronic pain is a major ongoing issue for her, and she is not inclined to take medication. Describe the assessment and management of Mrs Corowa's pain.

CRITICAL THINKING EXERCISE 33.2

Discuss the rationale for ensuring that pain assessment is undertaken in a non-judgmental manner.

CLINICAL SKILL 33.1 Focused pain assessment

Please adhere to the policy and procedures of the facility/organisation prior to undertaking the skill. Ensure this skill is in your scope of practice.

NMBA Decision-making Framework considerations (refer to NMBA Decision-making framework for nursing and midwifery 2020):	Equipment:
1. Am I educated? 2. Am I authorised? 3. Am I competent? If you answer 'no' to any of these, do not perform that activity. Seek guidance and support from your teacher/a nurse team leader/clinical facilitator/educator.	Appropriate pain assessment scale such as: • Pain intensity scale • Pain distress scale • Visual analogue scale (VAS) • Facial pain scale • FLACC • Abbey Pain Scale Vital sign equipment: • Sphygmomanometer • Pulse oximeter • Thermometer probe

 PREPARE FOR THE SKILL

(Please refer to the Standard Steps on p. xii for related rationales.)
Mentally review the steps of the skill.
Discuss the skill with your instructor/supervisor/team leader, if required.
Confirm correct facility/organisation policy/safe operating procedures.
Validate the order in the individual's record.
Identify indication and rationale for performing the activity.
Assess for any contraindications.
Locate and gather equipment.
Perform hand hygiene.
Ensure therapeutic interaction.
Identify the individual using three individual identifiers.
Gain the individual's consent.
Assess for pain relief.
Prepare the environment.
Provide and maintain privacy.
Assist the individual to assume an appropriate position of comfort.

Skill activity	Rationale
Collate known history from healthcare record (including paper-based and/or electronic records) including: • Pain history & correlated BP, HR, RR, SaO_2 and temperature • Recent invasive procedures (e.g. blood tests, surgery) • Current medical conditions and comorbidities (including cognitive capabilities) • Person's previous response to analgesia (both pharmaceutical and non-pharmaceutical).	Subjective and objective data identify key information to focus your pain assessment and enable safe guidance with effective dosing of pain medication and implementation of non-pharmacological pain-management interventions. It can provide baseline information and the bigger picture of the person's health status.
Verify the indication for the pain assessment including selecting the most appropriate pain tool. This may take into consideration person's age, culture and language/cognition.	It is important that the nurse understands why the individual is receiving this assessment and uses the most appropriate tool to achieve the most accurate data.

Continued

CLINICAL SKILL 33.1 Focused pain assessment—cont'd

 PERFORM THE SKILL

(Please refer to the Standard Steps on p. xii for related rationales.)
Perform hand hygiene.
Apply PPE: gloves, eyewear, mask and gown as appropriate.
Ensure the individual's safety and comfort throughout skill.
Promote independence and involvement of the individual if possible and/or appropriate.
Assess the individual's tolerance to the skill throughout.
Dispose of used supplies, equipment, waste and sharps appropriately.
Remove PPE and discard or store appropriately.
Perform hand hygiene.

Skill activity	Rationale
Assess person, family and caregiver knowledge of health including: • Prior experience with pain • Prior experience with pain management • Understanding and feelings about completing this assessment.	Ensures that the person, family and/or caregiver have the capacity to gather, communicate, process and understand health information. Reveals any clarification, instructions and/or supports required.
Conduct a pain history, assessing each of the following characteristics of the pain using the PQRSTU mnemonic: **P—Provoking/Palliative** *What were you doing when the pain started?* *What makes the pain worse?* *Is there something that helps relieve the pain?* *What caused it?*	This is a simple mnemonic to remember when obtaining a pain history. PQRSTU identifies the nature, source and aggravating factors of pain and what is beneficial to the person in reducing this discomfort. It is important to understand the person's perspective on their pain.
Q—Quality *What does the pain feel like? Try to describe in own words.*	This information is helpful in understanding the underlying pain mechanism (e.g. neuropathic or nociceptive) and may assist in the type of pain treatment chosen. Some words that may be used by the individual include gripping, knife-like, burning, prickling, tingling, dull, ache, cramping, throbbing, stabbing, shooting etc.
R—Region/Radiation *Where is the pain located?* *Does the pain travel anywhere else?* *Do you feel it is related to any other pain? If so, tell me more.*	The location(s) and distribution of the pain are helpful in determining the pain mechanism. It may be demonstrated through words or pointing to oneself.
S—Severity *How severe is the pain?* *Can you rate the pain from 0–10?* (Use a numerical scale or faces scale or any other tool that is appropriate for the individual.) Use the assessment scales here (e.g. NRS, VAS, Abbey Pain Scale etc.).	Understanding the level of pain directly from the person enables the nurse to plan management and implement appropriate interventions. Body language and facial expressions can also be a good indicator.
T—Time (onset, duration and pattern) *When did the pain start?* *How long has the pain been present?* *Is the pain consistent or intermittent?*	May provide further detail about whether the pain is acute or chronic and the pathophysiological background of the pain.
U—Understanding *How does the pain affect you?* *What treatments have been tried?* *What is the goal of treatment?*	Assesses what the individual understands about their own attitudes and beliefs towards: pain, treatment options and overarching goals of management of pain. Determines the success of other pain interventions. Provides important information to enable relevant, realistic and appropriate education.

CLINICAL SKILL 33.1 Focused pain assessment—cont'd

When pain is self-reported, assess physical, behavioural and emotional signs and symptoms, including non-verbal indicators of pain: • Moaning, crying, whimpering, groaning, vocalisations • Decreased activity • Facial expressions (e.g. grimace, clenched teeth) • Change in usual behaviour (e.g. less active, irritable) • Abnormal gait (e.g. shuffling) and posture (e.g. bent, leaning) • Guarding a body part; functional impairment such as decreased range of motion (ROM) • Diaphoresis • Depression, hopelessness, anger, fear, social withdrawal • Assess for decreased gastrointestinal (GI) motility, constipation, nausea and vomiting • Assess for insomnia, anorexia and fatigue.	Signs and symptoms may reveal source and nature of pain. Non-verbal responses to pain are useful in assessing pain in individuals who are cognitively impaired or unable to self-report. Experiencing pain may decrease opportunities to engage in activities, experiences or relationships, causing a negative affect that contributes to feelings of depression, hopelessness, anger, fear and social withdrawal. Constipation can occur with most pain medications; however, it is most common with opioid therapy. Co-occurrence of pain and insomnia or fatigue is common and is strongly associated with reduced functional ability.
Examine site of pain or discomfort when possible: inspect for discoloration, swelling or drainage; palpate for change in temperature, area of altered sensation, painful area or areas that trigger pain; assess range of motion of involved joints.	Reveals nature of pain and directs towards appropriate interventions.
Assess vital signs (objective data): • Blood pressure • Heart rate • Respiratory rate • Oxygen saturation • Temperature.	Can indicate (while not always sensitive) the presence of pain and provide further insight to any other potential concerns underlying in the person. Also provides continuity to observe for trends over time.
Analyse and interpret the findings from the above assessment. Is intervention required? If so, discuss with the individual. Make an appropriate decision in conjunction with the person on what would be most beneficial for them: • Pharmacological intervention • Non-pharmacological intervention.	Based on the PQRSTU findings, and in conjunction with the person, decide the best course of management. Take into consideration allergens, previous responses to interventions and the severity/location of the pain.

 AFTER THE SKILL

(Please refer to the Standard Steps on p. xii for related rationales.)
Communicate outcome to the individual, any ongoing care and to report any complications.
Restore the environment.
Report, record and document assessment findings, details of the skill performed and the individual's response.
Report, record and document any abnormalities and/or inability to perform the skill.
Reassess the individual to ensure there are no adverse effects/events from the skill.

Skill activity	Rationale
Plan for next assessment of effectiveness of intervention, and pain assessment. For example, reassess pain level 30–60 minutes post intervention. Provide education as needed.	It is important to continually reassess pain, to keep the person as comfortable as possible and determine if the chosen intervention is effective. Keeps individual informed and creates an opportunity to initiate education.

(Brown et al 2020; Crisp et al 2021; Rebeiro et al 2021)

OBSERVATION CHECKLIST: FOCUSED PAIN ASSESSMENT

STUDENT NAME: _____

CLINICAL SKILL 33.1: Comprehensive pain assessment

DEMONSTRATION OF: The ability to perform a focused pain assessment safely and correctly.

If the observation checklist is being used as an assessment tool, the student will need to obtain a scale of independence for each of the performance criteria/evidence.

Independent (I)

Supervised (S)

Assisted (A)

Marginal (M)

Dependent (D)

COMPETENCY ELEMENTS	PERFORMANCE CRITERIA/EVIDENCE	I	S	A	M	D
Preparation for the activity	Identifies indication and rationale for undertaking the activity Identifies the individual using three individual identifiers Ensures therapeutic interaction Gains the individual's consent Checks facility/organisation policy Validates the order in the individual's record Locates and gathers equipment Assists the individual into an appropriate position Assesses person, family and caregiver knowledge					
Performs activity informed by evidence	Performs pain assessment: using PQRSTU to gather information appropriately, communicating with open-ended questions P: Provoking/Palliative Q: Quality R: Region/Radiation S: Severity T: Time (onset, duration, pattern) U: Understanding Performs assessment of physical, emotional and behavioural signs and symptoms Performs vital observations: BP, HR, RR, SaO_2 and temperature Interprets findings of the assessment, and plans response such as: pharmacological and non-pharmacological interventions Concludes encounter: provides education as needed and follow-up plan with the individual					
Applies critical thinking and reflective practice	Is able to link theory to practice Demonstrates current best practice in the care provided Plans for analgesia and/or non-pharmacological interventions (as required) Establishes a plan for ongoing pain assessment Considers involvement of other healthcare professions (if appropriate) Assesses own performance and interaction with the individual					
Practises within safety and quality assurance guidelines	Reviews against facility/organisation policy Performs hand hygiene Cleans and disposes of equipment appropriately					

COMPETENCY ELEMENTS	PERFORMANCE CRITERIA/EVIDENCE	I	S	A	M	D
Documentation and communication	Explains and communicates the assessment clearly to the individual Communicates outcome of assessment and ongoing care to individual and significant others Reports any concerns of findings to the RN and/or medical officer Documents all relevant information correctly in the healthcare record Educates the individual to report any changes or concerns to the nurse					

Educator/Facilitator Feedback:

Educator/Facilitator Score: Competent   Needs further development

How would you rate your overall performance while undertaking this clinical activity? (use a ✓ & initial)

Unsatisfactory   Satisfactory   Good   Excellent

Student Reflection: (discuss how you would approach your practice differently or more effectively)

EDUCATOR/FACILITATOR NAME/SIGNATURE:

STUDENT NAME/SIGNATURE:

DATE:

Evolve®
Answer guide for the Critical Thinking Exercises and Critical Thinking Questions in Case Studies is hosted on Evolve: http://evolve.elsevier.com/AU/Koutoukidis/Tabbner/

References

Brown, D., Edwards, H., Buckley, T., et al., 2020. *Lewis's medical-surgical nursing*, 5th ed. Elsevier, Sydney.

Crisp, J., Douglas, C., Rebeiro, G., et al., 2021. *Potter and Perry's fundamentals of nursing*, 6th ed. Elsevier, Sydney.

International Association for the Study of Pain (IASP), 2021. IASP terminology—pain terms. Available at: <https://www.iasp-pain.org/Education/Content.aspx?ItemNumber=1698>.

Knights, K., Darroch, S., Rowland, A., et al., 2023. *Pharmacology for health professionals*, 6th ed. Elsevier, Sydney.

Nursing and Midwifery Board of Australia (NMBA), 2020. Decision-making framework summary for nursing and midwifery. Available at: <https://www.nursingmidwiferyboard.gov.au/Codes-Guidelines-Statements/Frameworks.aspx>.

Rebeiro, G., Wilson, D., Fuller, S., 2021. *Fundamentals of nursing: Clinical skills workbook*, 4th ed. Elsevier, Chatswood.

SENSORY HEALTH

Megan Christophers

Overview

The sensory abilities of taste, smell, touch, sight and hearing enable the person to 'sense' changes in their external and internal environments. This is an essential requirement for maintaining homeostasis, so we can interact with the world around us (Waugh 2023).

Perception of stimuli has its origin within the five special sense organs, which are adapted to receive specific stimuli: tongue (taste), nose (smell), skin (touch), eyes (sight) and ears (hearing and maintenance of balance). The eye is the means by which light is reflected from objects and travels to the retina so that an image is formed. Nerve endings in the retina transmit electrical impulses along the optic nerve to the brain for interpretation. As the eyes are one of the major structures by which an individual receives information about the external environment, this chapter focuses on the care of the eyes.

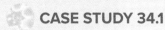 **CASE STUDY 34.1**

Henry Goldfield is a 48-year-old man working as a car salesman. Over the past two months Henry progressively had trouble hearing clients talking on the telephone. Henry also complained to his boss that he is feeling dizzy and suggested he should not take clients for a test drive until the dizziness stops. This week Henry was admitted to the hospital with left-sided facial pain, discharge from the left ear and a reduced sense of taste.

1. What do you think is happening to Henry?
2. What are some of the nursing care considerations you need to take into account when caring for Henry?

CRITICAL THINKING EXERCISE 34.1

Maria Russo is a 73-year-old woman who presented to the GP and Nurse Practitioner with progressive central blurred vision. She has a medical history of obesity and is a current smoker.

1. What health education would you provide to her within the clinic appointment?
2. Provide an explanation of the cause of her symptoms.

CLINICAL SKILL 34.1 Application of eye pad

Please adhere to the policy and procedures of the facility/organisation prior to undertaking the skill. Ensure this skill is in your scope of practice.

NMBA Decision-making Framework considerations (refer to NMBA Decision-making framework for nursing and midwifery 2020):	Equipment:
1. Am I educated? 2. Am I authorised? 3. Am I competent? If you answer 'no' to any of these, do not perform that activity. Seek guidance and support from your teacher/a nurse team leader/clinical facilitator/educator.	Sterile eye pad Disposable gloves Tape

 PREPARE FOR THE SKILL

(Please refer to the Standard Steps on p. xii for related rationales.)
Mentally review the steps of the skill.
Discuss the skill with your instructor/supervisor/team leader, if required.
Confirm correct facility/organisation policy/safe operating procedures.
Validate the order in the individual's record.
Identify indication and rationale for performing the activity.
Assess for any contraindications.
Locate and gather equipment.
Perform hand hygiene.
Ensure therapeutic interaction.
Identify the individual using three individual identifiers.
Gain the individual's consent.
Assess for pain relief.
Prepare the environment.
Provide and maintain privacy.
Assist the individual to assume an appropriate position of comfort.

Skill activity	Rationale
Ensure that the person is sitting or lying with their head well supported and there is adequate lighting.	Ensures the person is relaxed and comfortable and therefore less likely to move during procedure and cause corneal damage.

 PERFORM THE SKILL

(Please refer to the Standard Steps on p. xii for related rationales.)
Perform hand hygiene.
Apply PPE: gloves, eyewear, mask and gown as appropriate.
Ensure the individual's safety and comfort throughout skill.
Promote independence and involvement of the individual if possible and/or appropriate.
Assess the individual's tolerance to the skill throughout.
Dispose of used supplies, equipment, waste and sharps appropriately.
Remove PPE and discard or store appropriately.
Perform hand hygiene.

Skill activity	Rationale
Before the eye pad is applied, the person is asked to close their eyelid firmly.	Ensures the eye is not directly in contact with the eye pad and prevents corneal damage.
Use gentle unhurried movements and avoid all sudden movements.	Prevents person from moving or flinching to prevent corneal damage.

Continued

CLINICAL SKILL 34.1 Application of eye pad—cont'd

The pad should be applied so that the eyelid cannot be opened. Check medical orders since sometimes double padding is required.	Ensures the eye is not directly in contact with the eye pad and prevents corneal damage.
Pressure should not be applied, unless prescribed by a medical officer.	Pressure can damage the eye.
The eye pad is secured into position using hypoallergenic tape. Place the tape diagonally from forehead to cheek.	Prevents exposure of the eye. Placing tape at an angle reduces the risk of pressure on the eye.
Ask the individual to report any complications during and post procedure if able. Explain that their range of vision and depth perception may be altered.	Provides anticipatory guidance so that the individual takes more care when ambulating or feeding themselves.

AFTER THE SKILL

(Please refer to the Standard Steps on p. xii for related rationales.)
Communicate outcome to the individual, any ongoing care and to report any complications.
Restore the environment.
Report, record and document assessment findings, details of the skill performed and the individual's response.
Report, record and document any abnormalities and/or inability to perform the skill.
Reassess the individual to ensure there are no adverse effects/events from the skill.

(Australian Commission on Safety and Quality in Health Care [ACSQHC] 2021; Berman et al 2021; Tollefson et al 2022)

OBSERVATION CHECKLIST: APPLICATION OF EYE PAD

STUDENT NAME: _____

CLINICAL SKILL 34.1: Application of eye pad

DEMONSTRATION OF: The ability to correctly apply an eye pad to an individual

If the observation checklist is being used as an assessment tool, the student will need to obtain a scale of independence for each of the performance criteria/evidence.

Independent (I)
Supervised (S)
Assisted (A)
Marginal (M)
Dependent (D)

COMPETENCY ELEMENTS	PERFORMANCE CRITERIA/EVIDENCE	I	S	A	M	D
Preparation for the activity	Identifies indications and rationale for performing the activity Identifies the individual using three individual identifiers Ensures therapeutic interaction Gains the individual's consent Checks facility/organisation policy Validates the order in the individual's record Locates and gathers equipment					
Performs activity informed by evidence	Ensures that the person is sitting or lying with their head well supported Asks person to close their eyelid firmly Uses gentle unhurried movements Applies eye pad so that the eyelid cannot be opened Applies pressure only if medically directed Secures eye pad in position using hypoallergenic tape Applies tape diagonally from forehead to cheek					
Applies critical thinking and reflective practice	Is able to link theory to practice Demonstrates current best practice in the care provided Assesses own performance					
Practises within safety and quality assurance guidelines	Reviews against facility/organisation policy Performs hand hygiene, dons appropriate PPE as per infection control protocols Raises the bed to the appropriate working position based on nurse's height and lowers at completion of activity Cleans and disposes of equipment and waste appropriately Performs hand hygiene					
Documentation and communication	Explains and communicates the activity clearly to the individual Communicates outcome and ongoing care to individual and significant others Communicates abnormal findings to appropriate personnel Reports and documents all relevant information and any complications correctly in the healthcare record Reports any complications and/or inability to perform the procedure to the RN and/or medical officer Asks the individual to report any complications during and post procedure					

Educator/Facilitator Feedback:

Educator/Facilitator Score: Competent   Needs further development

How would you rate your overall performance while undertaking this clinical activity? (use a ✓ & initial)

Unsatisfactory   Satisfactory   Good   Excellent

Student Reflection: (discuss how you would approach your practice differently or more effectively)

EDUCATOR/FACILITATOR NAME/SIGNATURE:

STUDENT NAME/SIGNATURE: **DATE:**

CLINICAL SKILL 34.2 Eye irrigation

Please adhere to the policy and procedures of the facility/organisation prior to undertaking the skill. Ensure this skill is in your scope of practice.

NMBA Decision-making Framework considerations (refer to NMBA Decision-making framework for nursing and midwifery 2020):	Equipment:
1. Am I educated? 2. Am I authorised? 3. Am I competent? If you answer 'no' to any of these, do not perform that activity. Seek guidance and support from your teacher/a nurse team leader/clinical facilitator/educator.	Dressing pack or sterile gauze and kidney dish or another receptacle Sterile eye irrigating solution Gloves Towel or absorbent mat

 PREPARE FOR THE SKILL

(Please refer to the Standard Steps on p. xii for related rationales.)
Mentally review the steps of the skill.
Discuss the skill with your instructor/supervisor/team leader, if required.
Confirm correct facility/organisation policy/safe operating procedures.
Validate the order in the individual's record.
Identify indication and rationale for performing the activity.
Assess for any contraindications.
Locate and gather equipment.
Perform hand hygiene.
Ensure therapeutic interaction.
Identify the individual using three individual identifiers.
Gain the individual's consent.
Assess for pain relief.
Prepare the environment.
Provide and maintain privacy.
Assist the individual to assume an appropriate position of comfort.

Skill activity	Rationale
Assist the person into a recumbent position, with the head tilted towards the affected side.	Prevents the solution running either over the cheek into the other eye or out of the affected eye and down the side of the nose.

 PERFORM THE SKILL

(Please refer to the Standard Steps on p. xii for related rationales.)
Perform hand hygiene.
Apply PPE: gloves, eyewear, mask and gown as appropriate.
Ensure the individual's safety and comfort throughout skill.
Promote independence and involvement of the individual if possible and/or appropriate.
Assess the individual's tolerance to the skill throughout.
Dispose of used supplies, equipment, waste and sharps appropriately.
Remove PPE and discard or store appropriately.
Perform hand hygiene.

Skill activity	Rationale
Place a towel under the head on the affected side and across the neck. Place a kidney dish against the person's cheek and ask the individual to hold it in position.	Prevents solution from flowing down the neck.
Pour irrigating solution into the sterile receptacle or open the container of eye wash. Gently hold the eyelid open with one hand.	A person will instinctively try to close the eye.

Continued

CLINICAL SKILL 34.2 Eye irrigation—cont'd

Hold the fluid container 2.5 cm away from the eye.	If the fluid container is held too high, fluid will flow at increased pressure, causing discomfort and possible damage to the eye.
Pour a little solution over the cheek first.	Accustoms the person to the feel of the solution and prevents person moving during procedure.
Direct the flow of solution from the nasal corner outwards.	Because the head is tilted, the stream of irrigating solution will flow over the eyeball and prevent contamination of the other eye.
Avoid directing the stream forcefully onto the eyeball, and avoid touching the eye's structures.	Prevents discomfort and damage to the eye.
Ask the person to look up and down and to either side while irrigating.	Ensures that the whole area is washed.
When the eye has been thoroughly irrigated, ask the person to close the eyes, and use a new gauze swab to dry the lids.	Promotes comfort.
Ask the individual to report any complications during and post procedure, if able.	Provides anticipatory guidance so that the individual takes more care when ambulating or feeding themselves.

AFTER THE SKILL

(Please refer to the Standard Steps on p. xii for related rationales.)
Communicate outcome to the individual, any ongoing care and to report any complications.
Restore the environment.
Report, record and document assessment findings, details of the skill performed and the individual's response.
Report, record and document any abnormalities and/or inability to perform the skill.
Reassess the individual to ensure there are no adverse effects/events from the skill.

(ACSQHC 2021; Berman et al 2021; Stromberg 2023; Tollefson et al 2022)

OBSERVATION CHECKLIST: EYE IRRIGATION

STUDENT NAME: _____

CLINICAL SKILL 34.2: Eye irrigation

DEMONSTRATION OF: The ability to irrigate the eye

If the observation checklist is being used as an assessment tool, the student will need to obtain a scale of independence for each of the performance criteria/evidence.

Independent (I)
Supervised (S)
Assisted (A)
Marginal (M)
Dependent (D)

COMPETENCY ELEMENTS	PERFORMANCE CRITERIA/EVIDENCE	I	S	A	M	D
Preparation for the activity	Identifies indications and rationale for performing the activity Identifies the individual using three individual identifiers Ensures therapeutic interaction Gains the individual's consent Checks facility/organisation policy Validates the order in the individual's record Locates and gathers equipment					
Performs activity informed by evidence	Positions person correctly into a recumbent position, with the head tilted towards the affected side, sitting or lying with their head well supported Places a towel under the head on the affected side and across the neck Places a kidney dish against the person's cheek and asks the person to hold it in position Performs hand hygiene and puts on gloves Prepares irrigation fluid and gently holds the eyelid open with one hand Holds the fluid container 2.5 cm away from the eye Accustoms the person to the feel of the solution by pouring a little solution over the cheek first Directs the flow of solution from the nasal corner outwards, avoiding a direct stream forcefully onto the eyeball, and avoids touching the eye's structures Asks the person to look up and down and to either side while irrigating to ensure that the whole area is washed Asks the person to close the eyes and uses a new gauze swab to dry the lids					
Applies critical thinking and reflective practice	Is able to link theory to practice Demonstrates current best practice in the care provided Assesses own performance					
Practises within safety and quality assurance guidelines	Reviews against facility/organisation policy Performs hand hygiene, dons appropriate PPE as per infection control protocols Raises the bed to the appropriate working position based on nurse's height and lowers at completion of activity Cleans and disposes of equipment and waste appropriately					
Documentation and communication	Explains and communicates the activity clearly to the individual Communicates outcome and ongoing care to individual and significant others Communicates abnormal findings to appropriate personnel Reports and documents all relevant information and any complications correctly in the healthcare record Reports any complications and/or inability to perform the procedure to the RN and/or medical officer Asks the individual to report any complications during and post procedure					

Educator/Facilitator Feedback:

Educator/Facilitator Score: Competent   Needs further development

How would you rate your overall performance while undertaking this clinical activity? (use a ✓ & initial)

Unsatisfactory   Satisfactory   Good   Excellent

Student Reflection: (discuss how you would approach your practice differently or more effectively)

EDUCATOR/FACILITATOR NAME/SIGNATURE:

STUDENT NAME/SIGNATURE: **DATE:**

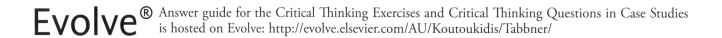 Evolve® Answer guide for the Critical Thinking Exercises and Critical Thinking Questions in Case Studies is hosted on Evolve: http://evolve.elsevier.com/AU/Koutoukidis/Tabbner/

References

Australian Commission on Safety and Quality in Health Care (ACSQHC), 2021. *National safety and quality health service standards*, 2nd ed updated. ACSQHC, Sydney.

Berman, A., Frandsen, G., Snyder, S., et al. 2021. *Kozier and Erb's fundamentals of nursing*, 5th ed. Pearson Education Australia, Melbourne.

Nursing and Midwifery Board of Australia (NMBA), 2020. Decision-making framework for nursing and midwifery. Available at: <https://www.nursingmidwiferyboard.gov.au/Codes-Guidelines-Statements/Frameworks.aspx>.

Stromberg, H., 2023. *Medical-surgical nursing: Concepts and practice*, 5th ed. Elsevier, St Louis.

Tollefson, J., Watson, G., Jelly, E., et al., 2022. *Essential clinical skills of enrolled nurses*, 5th ed. South Melbourne, Melbourne.

Waugh, A., Grant, A., 2023. *Ross and Wilson anatomy and physiology in health and illness: The special senses*, 14th ed. Elsevier, Edinburgh.

NEUROLOGICAL HEALTH

Anne MacLeod

Overview

The nervous system is responsible for the coordination of all other systems. It provides a network for communication within the body, and between the body and its environment. The brain is informed of events occurring both within and outside the body by nerve impulses that originate at a large number of sensory receptors. The receptors, which may be nerve endings, single specialised cells or a group of cells forming a sense organ, convert the energy of a stimulus into impulses that pass to specific areas of the brain. An understanding of this complex and dynamic system underpins many aspects of care, as almost all medical conditions can affect the human nervous system in some way, and it enables healthcare professionals to make accurate neurological assessments of individuals.

This chapter focuses on the assessment of the neurological system including neurological and neurovascular assessment. Neurological assessment includes checking the level of consciousness, the pupils, motor function, sensory function and the vital signs. The frequency with which assessment is performed and documented depends on the individual's condition and on the healthcare facility's policy.

Neurovascular assessment includes skin assessment (colour, temperature, oedema), palpation and assessment of pulses, sensation, motor function and pain. Assessment findings are used to support a diagnosis and determine or modify care interventions.

CASE STUDY 35.2

Mr Ng is a 65-year-old male who has been admitted to the neurology unit following a haemorrhagic stroke. He initially presented by ambulance after a sudden onset of severe headache and right-sided weakness. He has a history of hypertension and was on antihypertensive medication. Mr Ng was confused on arrival and had a blood pressure of 220/100. On initial presentation to the emergency department the following assessment data was obtained:

- GCS 13/15 (E4 V3 M 5)
- PEARL 4
- Respiratory rate 18 breaths/minute
- Blood pressure 220/100 mmHg
- Heart rate 56 beats/minute, regular
- T 37.5°C
- Right hemiplegia
  1. Detail how you would perform your physical assessment of the individual.
  2. What risk factors does Mr Ng have in relation to his stroke and how do the risk factors contribute to stroke?
  3. What are some indications of dysphagia?
  4. What is your management plan for Mr Ng? What medical interventions will be required?

CRITICAL THINKING EXERCISE 35.3

Alex, 21 years old, presented to emergency complaining of a severe headache and stiff neck. On examination, you notice he is febrile, has a rash on his torso and a dislike of bright lights. He is diagnosed with meningitis. What are common symptoms of meningitis in older children and adults?

CLINICAL SKILL 35.1 Performing a neurological assessment

Please adhere to the policy and procedures of the facility/organisation prior to undertaking the skill. Ensure this skill is in your scope of practice.

NMBA Decision-making Framework considerations (refer to NMBA Decision-making framework for nursing and midwifery 2020):	Equipment:
1. Am I educated? 2. Am I authorised? 3. Am I competent? If you answer 'no' to any of these, do not perform that activity. Seek guidance and support from your teacher/a nurse team leader/clinical facilitator/educator.	Sphygmomanometer BP cuff Stethoscope Thermometer Watch (with a second hand) Penlight and pupil gauge Neurological observations chart (must include Glasgow Coma Scale [GCS])

 PREPARE FOR THE SKILL

(Please refer to the Standard Steps on p. xii for related rationales.)
Mentally review the steps of the skill.
Discuss the skill with your instructor/supervisor/team leader, if required.
Confirm correct facility/organisation policy/safe operating procedures.
Validate the order in the individual's record.
Identify indication and rationale for performing the activity.
Assess for any contraindications.
Locate and gather equipment.
Perform hand hygiene.
Ensure therapeutic interaction.
Identify the individual using three individual identifiers.
Gain the individual's consent.
Assess for pain relief.
Prepare the environment.
Provide and maintain privacy.
Assist the individual to assume an appropriate position of comfort.

Skill activity	Rationale
Determine the need for neurological assessment and validate the medical orders in the individual's record.	Ensures correct procedure is about to take place. Physical signs and symptoms such as confusion, decreased level of consciousness and limb weakness may indicate alterations in neurological function.

 PERFORM THE SKILL

(Please refer to the Standard Steps on p. xii for related rationales.)
Perform hand hygiene.
Apply PPE: gloves, eyewear, mask and gown as appropriate.
Ensure the individual's safety and comfort throughout skill.
Promote independence and involvement of the individual if possible and/or appropriate.
Assess the individual's tolerance to the skill throughout.
Dispose of used supplies, equipment, waste and sharps appropriately.
Remove PPE and discard or store appropriately.
Perform hand hygiene.

Continued

CLINICAL SKILL 35.1 Performing a neurological assessment—cont'd

Skill activity	Rationale
Eyes opening (E)	
Assess arousal or wakefulness: • Assess for eye opening by observing the individual as you approach him/her—if he/she opens eyes spontaneously (spontaneous, score 4). • If the individual's eyes remain closed, speak in a clear strong voice by calling the individual by name to elicit a response. If eyes open (to speech, score 3). • If there is no response to speech, exert a painful stimulus (e.g. trapezium squeeze/supra-orbital pressure or sternal rub—used as a last measure). • If eyes open (to pain, score 2).	Altered level of consciousness is a key indicator to brain function. The GCS assesses the individual's level of consciousness. A fully conscious individual responds to questions spontaneously. As level of consciousness decreases individual may show irritability, a shortened attention span or an unwillingness to cooperate. Watch the individual for any response. If no response is gained, the individual is spoken to at first quietly then more loudly. Response is opening the eyes.
• If there is no eye opening following the application of painful stimulus (none, score 1). • Record (C) if the eye is closed due to trauma or swelling. **Note:** Record the best response only in this chart section.	If there is no auditory response, gentle touch is used, then use a central painful stimulus. If the individual has periorbital oedema due to trauma or surgery, a 'c' for closed can be documented next to 'None' (1) column.
Assess best motor response (M)	
Assess overall awareness and ability to respond to external stimuli by recording best arm response: • Ask the individual to perform a simple motor task (e.g. 'raise your arm' or 'squeeze and let go of my hands'). If the individual follows the command even weakly (obeys commands, score 6). • If the individual does not respond to verbal commands, apply a central painful stimulus (e.g. trapezium squeeze/supra-orbital pressure or sternal rub—used as a last measure) to determine the best arm response. • If the individual demonstrates purposeful movement to locate and remove the source of painful stimulus by bringing the hand up to at least nipple line, it is recorded as localising (localise to pain, score 5). • If the individual's hand or body moves away from the source of pain, it is recorded as withdraws (withdraws, score 4). • The individual may respond by flexing an arm demonstrating abnormal posturing (decorticate) (flexion to pain, score 3). • The individual may respond by extending an elbow and internally rotating wrist (decerebrate posturing). This response is recorded as abnormal extension (extension to pain, score 2). • If there is no response to the painful stimulus (none, score 1). **Note:** Record the best response only in this chart section.	When spoken to, a fully conscious individual should reply with an appropriate verbal response. A person with a decreased level of consciousness may respond in a puzzled way or may not respond at all, showing no response even when someone speaks directly into their ear. The individual who is able to respond is asked a series of simple questions (e.g. identify themself, what month, season or year it is). Impaired hearing may affect response. If the individual is not oriented to person, place or time, ascertain their best verbal response. Scores on the GCS are confused, inappropriate words, incomprehensible sounds and no response.
GCS is out of 15 and recorded on neurological observation chart. Overall score or change in score determines need to report to Registered Nurse (RN) and medical officer. Refer to facility/organisation policy regarding clinical review/rapid response criteria.	The GCS allows the evaluation of an individual's neurological status. The higher the score, the more normal the level of neurological functioning.

CLINICAL SKILL 35.1 Performing a neurological assessment—cont'd

Assess pupillary activity:
- Note the size (mm), shape and equality of both the pupils in normal lighting.
- Shine a penlight torch, moving from the outer aspect of the eye to the pupil. Observe the reaction of the pupil.
- Test each eye separately and record reaction:
  - > Yes '+'
  - > No '−'
  - > Closed 'C'
  - > Sluggish 'SL'.
- Pupillary response should be brisk constriction to light.
- Pupils are assessed for equality (are both pupils the same size?).
- Report to RN and medical officer if pupils become unequal or if one becomes more sluggish than the other.

Evaluating the pupils provides vital information about the brain and raised intracranial pressure.

Pupil size (1–8 mm) is determined using the pupil gauge before the light reflex is used.

Pupil shape is determined as round, oval or drawn to indicate abnormality.

Pupil reactivity to light is assessed by bringing the penlight from the lateral side of the individual's head towards the nose. Observe for pupil constriction (direct response) and repeat with the other eye.

Document a lack of consensual reaction (opposite pupil fails to constrict when light is shone in eye) in healthcare record.

Do not confuse a prosthetic eye with a fixed pupil. There will be no response from a blind eye.

If pupils are not the same size, 'unequal' differences are noted between the right and left sections of the chart.

Assess limb strength

Testing limb strength gives an indication of the part of the brain that is affected as opposed to testing level of consciousness.

Bilateral upper limb muscle strength:
- Instruct individual to move arms, lift limb against gravity, move limb against your resistance.
- Ask the individual to squeeze both the assessor's hands followed by asking the individual to:
  - > Pull your hands towards them against resistance.
  - > Push your hands away against resistance (normal power).
- Active movement of body part against gravity with some resistance (mild weakness).
- Active movement of body part against gravity (severe weakness).
- Active movement of body part when effect of gravity is removed (spastic flexion).
- Only a trace or flicker of movement is seen or felt in the muscle (extension).
- No detectable muscle contraction (no response).

Bilateral lower limb muscle strength:
- Instruct individual to move legs laterally on bed; lift limb against gravity; move limb against your resistance.

Note: Record the response for each limb separately in this section of the chart as per upper limb muscle assessment:
- (normal power)
- (mild weakness)
- (severe weakness)
- (extension)
- (no response).

Assessment of limb strength usually focuses on the arms and legs, and the identification of significant changes are important for denoting improvement, stabilisation or deterioration in the individual's condition. The techniques used to evaluate limb strength depend on the individual's level of consciousness.

Each extremity is assessed unless contraindicated.

The individual is given clear commands such as 'squeeze my hands' or 'push against my hands'. Compare both sides. Record right (R) and left (L) separately if there is a difference between the two sides.

Response is recorded as normal, mild weakness, severe weakness, flexion, extension or no response.

Continued

CLINICAL SKILL 35.1 Performing a neurological assessment—cont'd

Assess vital signs

Initially, vital signs are monitored every 15 minutes until stable then hourly or as per organisational/facility guidelines.	Vital sign changes are late changes in brain deterioration. A drop in level of consciousness is the earliest sign of neurological deterioration. Change in vital signs can indicate a worsening neurological condition, and therefore vital signs are always recorded at the same time as other neurological observations. Change in vital signs may also provide clues as to other medical problems in an unconscious individual who cannot tell staff what symptoms they are experiencing. Vital sign changes associated with raised intracranial pressure: • Bradycardia • Tachycardia (very late sign) • Hypertension (typically, an elevated systolic blood pressure combined with a widening pulse pressure) • Irregular respirations.

AFTER THE SKILL

(Please refer to the Standard Steps on p. xii for related rationales.)
Communicate outcome to the individual, any ongoing care and to report any complications.
Restore the environment.
Report, record and document assessment findings, details of the skill performed and the individual's response.
Report, record and document any abnormalities and/or inability to perform the skill.
Reassess the individual to ensure there are no adverse effects/events from the skill.

(ACSQHC 2021; Berman et al 2021; Crisp et al 2021; Hall et al 2022; LeMone et al 2020; Rebeiro et al 2021)

OBSERVATION CHECKLIST: PERFORMING A NEUROLOGICAL ASSESSMENT

STUDENT NAME: _____

CLINICAL SKILL 35.1: Performing a neurological assessment

DEMONSTRATION OF: The ability to effectively perform a neurological assessment

If the observation checklist is being used as an assessment tool, the student will need to obtain a scale of independence for each of the performance criteria/evidence.

Independent (I)
Supervised (S)
Assisted (A)
Marginal (M)
Dependent (D)

COMPETENCY ELEMENTS	PERFORMANCE CRITERIA/EVIDENCE	I	S	A	M	D
Preparation for the activity	Identifies indications and rationale for performing the activity Identifies the individual using three individual identifiers Ensures therapeutic interaction Gains the individual's consent Checks facility/organisation policy Validates the order in the individual's record Locates and gathers equipment Assists the individual into an appropriate position					
Performs activity informed by evidence	**Eyes opening (E)** *Score 1–4* Assesses for eye opening—if individual opens eyes spontaneously (score 4) If eyes open to speech (score 3) If eyes open to pain (score 2) If there is no eye opening following the application of painful stimulus (score 1) Record (C) if the eye is closed due to trauma or swelling **Assess verbal response (V)** *Score 1–5* Obtains the individual's attention and allows time for the individual to respond Asks questions to assess orientation to person, place and time (e.g. asks the individual their full name, what the month or year is, and where they are). If correct answers are elicited to all three questions the individual is oriented (score 5) The individual is confused if answers incorrectly to any of the above three questions (score 4) Record 'X' if culturally and linguistically diverse If the individual uses inappropriate words or phrases that make little or no sense (score 3) If the individual makes incomprehensible sounds, moaning or groaning (score 2) If the individual makes no attempt to speak and no sounds are made in response to the painful stimulus (score 1) Record 'T' if unable to speak due to tracheostomy or ETT **Assess best motor response (M)** *Score 1–6* Asks the individual to perform a simple motor task (e.g. 'raise your arm' or 'squeeze and let go of my hands') If the individual obeys commands even weakly (score 6) If the individual does not respond to verbal commands, apply a central painful stimulus to determine the best arm response If the individual demonstrates purposeful movement to locate and remove the source of painful stimulus by bringing the hand up to at least nipple line, it is recorded as localise to pain (score 5)					

Continued

COMPETENCY ELEMENTS	PERFORMANCE CRITERIA/EVIDENCE	I	S	A	M	D
	If the individual's hand or body moves away from the source of pain, it is recorded as withdraws (score 4)					
	If the individual responds to pain by flexing an arm, demonstrating abnormal posturing (decorticate) (score 3)					
	If the individual responds by extending an elbow and internally rotating wrist (decerebrate posturing), record as abnormal extension to pain (score 2)					
	If there is no response to the painful stimulus (score 1)					
	GCS score is out of 15 and recorded on neurological observation chart					
	Assess pupillary activity					
	Notes the size (mm), shape and equality of both the pupils in normal lighting					
	Observes the reaction of the pupil when a torch light is shone					
	Tests each eye separately and records reaction					
	Yes '+'					
	No '−'					
	Closed 'C'					
	Sluggish 'SL'					
	Pupillary response should be brisk constriction to light					
	Pupils are assessed for equality					
	Assess limb strength					
	Bilateral upper limb muscle strength					
	Instructs individual to move arms, to lift limb against gravity and move limb against resistance					
	Asks the individual to squeeze both the assessor's hands then asks the individual to pull nurse's hands towards them against resistance and push nurse's hands away against resistance (normal power)					
	Active movement of body part against gravity with some resistance (mild weakness)					
	Active movement of body part against gravity (severe weakness)					
	Active movement of body part when effect of gravity is removed (spastic flexion)					
	Only a trace or flicker of movement is seen or felt in the muscle (extension)					
	No detectable muscle contraction (no response)					
	Bilateral lower limb muscle strength					
	Instructs individual to move legs laterally on bed; to lift limb against gravity and move limb against nurse's resistance					
	Normal power, mild weakness, severe weakness, extension, no response					
	Assess vital signs					
	Recognises a drop in level of consciousness is the earliest sign of neurological deterioration					
	Records vital signs at the same time as other neurological observations					
	Recognises a change in vital signs may be associated with raised intracranial pressure:					
	• Bradycardia					
	• Tachycardia (very late sign)					
	• Hypertension (typically an elevated systolic blood pressure combined with a widening pulse pressure)					
	• Irregular respirations					

COMPETENCY ELEMENTS	PERFORMANCE CRITERIA/EVIDENCE	I	S	A	M	D
Applies critical thinking and reflective practice	Demonstrates critical thinking and problem-solving (e.g. comfort measures, pain relief) Is able to link theory to practice Demonstrates current best practice in the care provided Identifies any neurological deficits Demonstrates understanding of relationship between neurological deficits and individual's diagnosis Checks current findings to previous observation Describes nursing actions relevant to the individual's current neurological status Explains the rationale for observations and nursing care Assesses own performance					
Practises within safety and quality assurance guidelines	Reviews against facility/organisation policy Performs hand hygiene, dons appropriate PPE as per infection control protocols Raises the bed to the appropriate working position based on nurse's height and lowers at completion of activity Cleans and disposes of equipment and waste appropriately					
Documentation and communication	Explains and communicates the activity clearly to the individual Communicates outcome and ongoing care to individual and significant others Communicates abnormal findings to appropriate personnel Reports and documents all relevant information and any complications correctly in the healthcare record Reports any complications and/or inability to perform the procedure to the RN and/or medical officer Asks the individual to report any complications during and post procedure Reports to RN/medical officer immediately or initiates a clinical review/rapid response if the GCS score drops by 1–2 points					

Educator/Facilitator Feedback:

Educator/Facilitator Score: Competent   Needs further development

How would you rate your overall performance while undertaking this clinical activity? (use a ✓ & initial)

Unsatisfactory   Satisfactory   Good   Excellent

Student Reflection: (discuss how you would approach your practice differently or more effectively)

EDUCATOR/FACILITATOR NAME/SIGNATURE:

STUDENT NAME/SIGNATURE: **DATE:**

CLINICAL SKILL 35.2 Neurovascular assessment

Please adhere to the policy and procedures of the facility/organisation prior to undertaking the skill. Ensure this skill is in your scope of practice.

NMBA Decision-making Framework considerations (refer to NMBA Decision-making framework for nursing and midwifery 2020):	Equipment:
1. Am I educated? 2. Am I authorised? 3. Am I competent? If you answer 'no' to any of these, do not perform that activity. Seek guidance and support from your teacher/a nurse team leader/clinical facilitator/educator.	Neurovascular assessment chart

PREPARE FOR THE SKILL

(Please refer to the Standard Steps on p. xii for related rationales.)
Mentally review the steps of the skill.
Discuss the skill with your instructor/supervisor/team leader, if required.
Confirm correct facility/organisation policy/safe operating procedures.
Validate the order in the individual's record.
Identify indication and rationale for performing the activity.
Assess for any contraindications.
Locate and gather equipment.
Perform hand hygiene.
Ensure therapeutic interaction.
Identify the individual using three individual identifiers.
Gain the individual's consent.
Assess for pain relief.
Prepare the environment.
Provide and maintain privacy.
Assist the individual to assume an appropriate position of comfort.

PERFORM THE SKILL

(Please refer to the Standard Steps on p. xii for related rationales.)
Perform hand hygiene.
Apply PPE: gloves, eyewear, mask and gown as appropriate.
Ensure the individual's safety and comfort throughout skill.
Promote independence and involvement of the individual if possible and/or appropriate.
Assess the individual's tolerance to the skill throughout.
Dispose of used supplies, equipment, waste and sharps appropriately.
Remove PPE and discard or store appropriately.
Perform hand hygiene.

Skill activity	Rationale
Assess the limb distal to the surgery/injury	

Compare affected limb with unaffected limb assessing both limbs for (document affected limb only):
• Colour
   > Visually check colour, document as pink, pale/white or cyanotic, dusky, cyanotic, mottled or purple/black.
• Temperature
   > Check temperature with superficial touch, document as warm, cool or hot.
• Pulses
   > Palpate for presence of peripheral pulses distal to injury.
   > Document pulses as strong, weak, absent.
	Obtains a baseline prior to surgery.
	Assesses the vasculature and nerve supply to a traumatised limb.
	Monitors limb status so that permanent damage or complications are avoided by identifying indicators of problems early and intervening.
	Limb assessed as normal if limb pink in colour, warm to touch, capillary refill of 1–2 seconds, swelling full, strong pulse, normal sensation.
	Limb assessed as inadequate arterial supply if pale/white or cyanotic in colour, cool to touch, capillary refill >2 seconds, swelling hollow or prune-like.

Continued

CLINICAL SKILL 35.2 Neurovascular assessment—cont'd

- Sensation
  - > Touch and assess visual limb surfaces for presence and type of sensation. Document as normal, decreased sensation, loss of sensation, numbness, tingling or pins and needles.
- Motor function
  - > Active movement or passive movement.
- Pain
  - > Assess pain on movement of limb and document pain score: 0 (no pain), 10 (worst pain).
- Swelling and ooze
  - > Visually check for swelling and ooze.
  - > Document swelling as nil, small, moderate.

Limb assessed as inadequate venous return if limb dusky, cyanotic, mottled or purple/black in colour, hot to touch, immediate capillary refill, swelling distended or tense, tissues feel hard.

Capillary refill assessment is evaluated by pressing firmly down on the nail bed of fingers or toes for five seconds. The nail bed will blanch and the colour should return within two seconds once pressure is released.

If pulses are not palpable due to plaster casts, assess closely above parameters.

Individuals may report changes in sensation if neurovascular compromise is present or may be a result of a nerve block or epidural (this should be documented on the neurovascular chart).

Individual assessed as having active movement if able to voluntarily extend and flex an extremity or digit.

Individual assessed as having passive movement if assessor is able to extend and flex an extremity or digit.

If pulse is not present, document and notify medical officer, observe colour, capillary refill and temperature.

Immediately report to medical team if there is any deterioration in neurovascular assessment.

AFTER THE SKILL

(Please refer to the Standard Steps on p. xii for related rationales.)

Communicate outcome to the individual, any ongoing care and to report any complications.

Restore the environment.

Report, record and document assessment findings, details of the skill performed and the individual's response.

Report, record and document any abnormalities and/or inability to perform the skill.

Reassess the individual to ensure there are no adverse effects/events from the skill.

(Berman et al 2021; Crisp et al 2021; Hall et al 2022; LeMone et al 2020)

OBSERVATION CHECKLIST: NEUROVASCULAR ASSESSMENT

| Independent (I) |
| Supervised (S) |
| Assisted (A) |
| Marginal (M) |
| Dependent (D) |

STUDENT NAME: _____

CLINICAL SKILL 35.2: Neurovascular assessment

DEMONSTRATION OF: The ability to perform a neurovascular assessment

If the observation checklist is being used as an assessment tool, the student will need to obtain a scale of independence for each of the performance criteria/evidence.

COMPETENCY ELEMENTS	PERFORMANCE CRITERIA/EVIDENCE	I	S	A	M	D
Preparation for the activity	Identifies indications and rationale for performing the activity Identifies the individual using three individual identifiers Ensures therapeutic interaction Gains the individual's consent Checks facility/organisation policy Validates the order in the individual's record Locates and gathers equipment Assists the individual into an appropriate position					
Performs activity informed by evidence	Assesses the limb distal to the surgery/injury Compares affected limb with unaffected limb, assesses both limbs for: • Colour—visually checks colour, documents as pink, pale/white or cyanotic, dusky, cyanotic, mottled or purple/black • Temperature—checks temperature with superficial touch, documents as warm, cool or hot • Pulses—palpates for presence of peripheral pulses distal to injury. Documents pulses as strong, weak, absent • Sensation—touches and assesses visual limb surface for presence and type of sensation. Documents as normal, decreased sensation, loss of sensation, numbness, tingling or pins and needles • Motor function—active movement or passive movement • Pain—assesses pain on movement of limb, pain score 0–10 • Swelling and ooze—visually checks for swelling and ooze. Documents swelling as nil, small, moderate					
Applies critical thinking and reflective practice	Demonstrates critical thinking and problem-solving (e.g. comfort measures, pain relief) Is able to link theory to practice Demonstrates current best practice in the care provided Identifies any neurovascular deficits Demonstrates understanding of relationship between neurovascular assessment and individual's diagnosis Checks current findings to previous observation Describes nursing actions relevant to the individual's current neurovascular assessment Explains the rationale for observations and nursing care Assesses own performance					

Continued

COMPETENCY ELEMENTS	PERFORMANCE CRITERIA/EVIDENCE	I	S	A	M	D
Practises within safety and quality assurance guidelines	Reviews against facility/organisation policy Performs hand hygiene, dons appropriate PPE as per infection control protocols Raises the bed to the appropriate working position based on nurse's height and lowers at completion of activity Cleans and disposes of equipment and waste appropriately					
Documentation and communication	Explains and communicates the activity clearly to the individual Communicates outcome and ongoing care to individual and significant others Communicates abnormal findings to appropriate personnel Reports and documents all relevant information and any complications correctly in the healthcare record Reports any complications and/or inability to perform the procedure to the RN and/or medical officer Asks the individual to report any complications during and post procedure					

Educator/Facilitator Feedback:

Educator/Facilitator Score: Competent   Needs further development

How would you rate your overall performance while undertaking this clinical activity? (use a ✓ & initial)

Unsatisfactory   Satisfactory   Good   Excellent

Student Reflection: (discuss how you would approach your practice differently or more effectively)

EDUCATOR/FACILITATOR NAME/SIGNATURE:

STUDENT NAME/SIGNATURE: **DATE:**

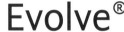 Evolve® Answer guide for the Critical Thinking Exercises and Critical Thinking Questions in Case Studies is hosted on Evolve: http://evolve.elsevier.com/AU/Koutoukidis/Tabbner/

References

Australian Commission on Safety and Quality in Health Care (ACSQHC), 2021. Recognising and responding to acute deterioration. Available at: <https://www.safetyandquality.gov.au/wp-content/uploads/2017/11/Recognising-and-Responding-to-Acute-Deterioration.pdf>.

Berman, A., Frandsen, G., Snyder, S., et al., 2021. *Kozier and Erb's fundamentals of nursing*, 5th ed. Pearson, Melbourne.

Crisp, J., Douglas, C., Rebeiro, D., et al., 2021. *Potter & Perry's fundamentals of nursing*, ANZ ed, 6th ed. Elsevier, Chatswood.

Hall, H., Glew, P., Rhodes, J., 2022. *Fundamentals of nursing & midwifery: A person-centred approach to care*, 4th ed. Lippincott Williams & Wilkins, Sydney.

LeMone, P., Bauldoff, G., Gubrud-Howe, P., et al., 2020. *LeMone and Burke's medical-surgical nursing: Critical thinking for person-centred care*, 4th ed. Pearson, Melbourne.

Nursing and Midwifery Board of Australia (NMBA), 2020. Decision-making framework for nursing and midwifery. Available at: <https://www.nursingmidwiferyboard.gov.au/Codes-Guidelines-Statements/Frameworks.aspx>.

Rebeiro, G., Wilson, D., Fuller, S., 2021. *Potter and Perry's fundamentals of nursing workbook*, 4th ed. Elsevier, Chatswood.

ENDOCRINE HEALTH

Christine Standley

Overview

The endocrine system consists of several small glands that secrete hormones into the blood. Hormones act like chemical messengers that promote different physiological processes such as metabolism, growth, fluid balance and reproduction. Over- or under-production of hormones can have widespread effects on other systems in the body. An understanding of hormone function and the effects of hormone imbalances provides healthcare professionals with the ability to identify and care for individuals with endocrine disorders.

For those individuals with diabetes, who are measuring blood glucose levels, described below is an accurate method of assessing the current blood glucose level, effectiveness of diet, exercise levels and medication therapy. Measuring blood glucose is performed by obtaining a drop of blood which is then applied to a reagent strip and read by one of the many blood glucose meters available. A digital display of the glucose level is provided at the time of measurement.

CASE STUDY 36.2

Anthea, a diabetes nurse educator, introduces 60-year-old Mr Singh to Maddy, the Enrolled Nurse allocated to care for him. Anthea explains that Mr Singh has type 2 diabetes mellitus and that she would like Maddy to assist in educating him about his condition.

Mr Singh feels shy and confused, and says, 'Anthea, is nice, but I don't understand what she is trying to teach me about my diabetes. I am having to test my blood sugar level all the time and take all of these tablets.' He shows Maddy a list of medications that Anthea has indicated he may be required to take.

Maddy begins by asking Mr Singh if he knows what his target blood sugar level should be.

Mr Singh cannot remember, so she reminds him.

1. What is the normal blood glucose range before meals for a person with type 2 diabetes mellitus?
    'What you mean? I can eat, can't I?' Mr Singh asks.

    'Of course you can,' Maddy answers, reassuring him. 'Did Anthea explain to you when you should test your blood?'

    'Yes, in the morning before my breakfast. Why?'

2. Explain why Mr Singh needs to test his blood glucose prior to breakfast each day.
    He sighs and admits, 'This is not easy. She says I have to do many other things, like watch what I eat. It is too complicated.'

3. What dietary advice would Maddy provide Mr Singh to improve self-management of his diabetes?
4. What sort of changes could Mr Singh make to his lifestyle and habits to improve glycaemic control?
    Maddy feels that Mr Singh is overwhelmed, so she comforts him and reassures him that his concerns are normal and that his questions are valid.

5. Other than Anthea, his specific diabetes educator, which other health professionals could Maddy refer Mr Singh to, or at least make him aware of?
    Mr Singh smiles and says, 'Thank you, Maddy. You make it easy for me and now I feel much better.'

CRITICAL THINKING EXERCISE 36.4

A 38-year-old mother of two has been admitted with an adrenal gland tumour. Considering the role of the adrenal gland, what possible endocrine disorders might they have? List the physical manifestations of each potential disorder. How might you explain what she is experiencing?

CLINICAL SKILL 36.1 Measuring blood glucose

Please adhere to the policy and procedures of the facility/organisation prior to undertaking the skill. Ensure this skill is in your scope of practice.

NMBA Decision-making Framework considerations (refer to NMBA Decision-making framework for nursing and midwifery 2020):	Equipment:
1. Am I educated? 2. Am I authorised? 3. Am I competent? If you answer 'no' to any of these, do not perform that activity. Seek guidance and support from your teacher/a nurse team leader/clinical facilitator/educator.	Blood glucose meter Reagent strips Tissues or cotton balls Lancet or peripheral blood access Sharps container Disposable gloves Warm washcloth An appropriate chart for documentation

 PREPARE FOR THE SKILL

(Please refer to the Standard Steps on p. xii for related rationales.)
Mentally review the steps of the skill.
Discuss the skill with your instructor/supervisor/team leader, if required.
Confirm correct facility/organisation policy/safe operating procedures.
Validate the order in the individual's record.
Identify indication and rationale for performing the activity.
Assess for any contraindications.
Locate and gather equipment.
Perform hand hygiene.
Ensure therapeutic interaction.
Identify the individual using three individual identifiers.
Gain the individual's consent.
Assess for pain relief.
Prepare the environment.
Provide and maintain privacy.
Assist the individual to assume an appropriate position of comfort.

Skill activity	Rationale
Assist the individual to wash hands with soap and warm water and dry thoroughly.	Promotes skin cleansing; even the smallest bits of food can alter a reading. Warm water increases the peripheral circulation due to vasodilation, facilitating blood flow at the puncture site. Make sure the site is entirely dry because even water can affect results.

 PERFORM THE SKILL

(Please refer to the Standard Steps on p. xii for related rationales.)
Perform hand hygiene.
Apply PPE: gloves, eyewear, mask and gown as appropriate.
Ensure the individual's safety and comfort throughout skill.
Promote independence and involvement of the individual if possible and/or appropriate.
Assess the individual's tolerance to the skill throughout.
Dispose of used supplies, equipment, waste and sharps appropriately.
Remove PPE and discard or store appropriately.
Perform hand hygiene.

Skill activity	Rationale
Prepare the blood glucose meter as per the manufacturer's instructions. Check the machine has been calibrated with the test strip. Check the date on the reagent strip and ensure the lid is closed securely.	Blood glucose meters may require recalibration to ensure accuracy of result. Reagent strips may have an expiry date and are affected by moisture in the air.

CLINICAL SKILL 36.1 Measuring blood glucose—cont'd

Insert the reagent strip into the blood glucose meter. Follow manufacturer's guidelines regarding when to insert the strip.	This is generally before the blood is applied to the strip.
Prepare the lancet and place firmly against the soft flesh at either side of the top of the finger. Quickly pierce the finger. If a drop of blood does not appear, gently 'milk' the finger, if necessary, by massaging finger from base towards fingertip, ensuring hand is below heart level.	Ensures the skin is pierced. Reduces discomfort. The fingertip is the most accurate test site because it registers changes in blood glucose more quickly than the rest of the body. There are fewer nerve endings on the sides of the fingers; they are therefore less painful. Increases vasodilation and adequate blood flow for accuracy of result. Excessive squeezing of tissues during collection may contribute to pain, bruising, scarring, hematoma formation, or dilution of the sample with serous fluid.
Allow the blood to drop onto the test strip.	This may differ depending on the monitor. The blood should cover the test strip. Some reagent strips fill from the side.
Apply pressure to the puncture site with tissue or cotton swab for 30–60 seconds or until bleeding has stopped.	Prevents further bleeding after the sample has been obtained and prevents haematoma formation.
Timing is determined by the manufacturer.	Ensures accurate results. Most blood glucose meters display a digital readout.
Read the BGL result from the blood glucose meter.	Note and record result to allow comparison with the individual's normal blood glucose level.
Turn off the blood glucose meter, remove the test strip and dispose of supplies appropriately.	Reduces risk of transmission of infection.

 AFTER THE SKILL

(Please refer to the Standard Steps on p. xii for related rationales.)
Communicate outcome to the individual, any ongoing care and to report any complications.
Restore the environment.
Report, record and document assessment findings, details of the skill performed and the individual's response.
Report, record and document any abnormalities and/or inability to perform the skill.
Reassess the individual to ensure there are no adverse effects/events from the skill.

(Australian Commission on Safety and Quality in Health Care 2021; Crawford 2023; Dickson 2023; Miller 2022)

OBSERVATION CHECKLIST: MEASURING BLOOD GLUCOSE

STUDENT NAME: _____

CLINICAL SKILL 36.1: Measuring blood glucose

DEMONSTRATION OF: The ability to safely and correctly measure blood glucose levels

If the observation checklist is being used as an assessment tool, the student will need to obtain a scale of independence for each of the performance criteria/evidence.

Independent (I)
Supervised (S)
Assisted (A)
Marginal (M)
Dependent (D)

COMPETENCY ELEMENTS	PERFORMANCE CRITERIA/EVIDENCE	I	S	A	M	D
Preparation for the activity	Identifies indications and rationale for performing the activity Identifies the individual using three individual identifiers Ensures therapeutic interaction Gains the individual's consent Checks facility/organisation policy Validates the order in the individual's record Locates and gathers equipment Assists the individual into an appropriate position					
Performs activity informed by evidence	Selects appropriate puncture site Stimulates circulation Holds area to be punctured in a dependent position while gently massaging finger towards puncture site Correctly positions lancet and pierces the skin sharply and quickly Correctly applies the blood to the reagent strip Applies pressure to puncture site Places strip in blood glucose meter according to manufacturer's instructions Reads the result					
Applies critical thinking and reflective practice	Demonstrates critical thinking and problem-solving (e.g. individual's health status, skin assessment, contraindications and special precautions for measuring blood glucose, risk factors—bleeding disorders, normal/abnormal results in reading) Is able to link theory to practice Demonstrates current best practice in the care provided Assesses own performance					
Practises within safety and quality assurance guidelines	Reviews against facility/organisation policy Performs hand hygiene, dons appropriate PPE as per infection control and WHS protocols Raises the bed to the appropriate working position based on nurse's height and lowers at completion of activity Cleans and disposes of equipment and waste appropriately					
Documentation and communication	Explains and communicates the activity clearly to the individual Communicates outcome and ongoing care to individual and significant others Communicates abnormal findings to appropriate personnel Reports and documents all relevant information and any complications correctly in the healthcare record Reports any complications and/or inability to perform the procedure to the RN and/or medical officer Asks the individual to report any complications during and post procedure					

Educator/Facilitator Feedback:

Educator/Facilitator Score: Competent   Needs further development

How would you rate your overall performance while undertaking this clinical activity? (use a ✓ & initial)

Unsatisfactory   Satisfactory   Good   Excellent

Student Reflection: (discuss how you would approach your practice differently or more effectively)

EDUCATOR/FACILITATOR NAME/SIGNATURE:

STUDENT NAME/SIGNATURE: **DATE:**

Evolve®

Answer guide for the Critical Thinking Exercises and Critical Thinking Questions in Case Studies is hosted on Evolve: http://evolve.elsevier.com/AU/Koutoukidis/Tabbner/

References

Australian Commission on Safety and Quality in Health Care, 2021. National safety and quality health service standards, 2nd ed. ACSQHC, Sydney. Available at: <https://www.safetyandquality.gov.au/publications-and-resources/resource-library/national-safety-and-quality-health-service-standards-second-edition>.

Crawford, A.H., 2023. Endocrine problems. In: Harding, M.M., Kwong, J., Hagler, D., et al., *Lewis's medical-surgical nursing*, 12th ed. Elsevier, St Louis.

Dickinson, J.K., 2023. Diabetes. In: Harding, M.M., Kwong, J., Hagler, D., et al., *Lewis's medical-surgical nursing*, 12th ed. Elsevier, St Louis.

Miller, B., 2022. Diabetes mellitus – Pathophysiology. In: Banasik, J., *Pathophysiology*, 7th ed. Elsevier, St Louis.

Nursing and Midwifery Board of Australia (NMBA), 2020. Decision-making framework for nursing and midwifery. Available at: <https://www.nursingmidwiferyboard.gov.au/Codes-Guidelines-Statements/Frameworks.aspx>.

Online Sources and Recommended Reading

Diabetes Australia—Vic, 2020. Newly diagnosed type 1: <www.diabetesvic.org.au/newlydiagnosed>.

Diabetes Australia, 2022. Managing diabetes: <https://www.diabetesaustralia.com.au/managing-diabetes/>.

PALLIATIVE CARE

Laura Healey

Overview

Taking care of the person after death, also referred to as 'last offices', is an essential part of the care of individuals and should be performed with respect and dignity. Extremely important to remember is that individuals who are dying and their families/carer have very special needs. The care of a person who is dying is an extremely intimate and private event occurring at a time when a person is at their most vulnerable and deserves to be treated with the utmost respect (Marie Curie 2022c).

The processes that take place after an individual dies are determined by place of death and nature of death (expected or unexpected). Each organisation will have their own policy and procedures for care after death. Remember to check your organisational policy or ask your manager for information on this; it is important to follow local and national guidelines.

Personal care should be provided after the death has been verified and ideally where possible within four hours of the individual dying, to maintain their appearance and condition. Two staff members should be allocated to perform this duty and at least one should be a registered nurse or another healthcare worker with the relevant education.

If the individual has an advance care plan this should be reviewed to ensure the individual's wishes and requests are met. If the individual does not have an advance care plan, check for details of any personal wishes relating to care after death from their family/carer. This ensures awareness of their individual wishes and respect for any spiritual, religious or cultural practices to be performed. This may also be the most appropriate time to check if the person had registered to be an organ donor; where and if applicable.

If appropriate and the death is expected, try to establish with the family/carer if they would like to be present at the time of death and if they wish to be involved in subsequent care. This is highly personal and may be influenced by cultural or religious practices. If they do wish to be involved, it is important to sensitively prepare them for changes to the body after death such as rigor mortis (stiffening of the body) and cooling temperature of the skin. Also discuss any other moving, handling and infection control procedures required if participating in care.

If the family/carer are present at the time of death, they should be supported as required. Every death is unique, and people react differently. It is important to be respectful of the needs of anyone close to the deceased. They might wish for you to take the lead, or they may prefer that you remain in the background. If they were not present at the time of death, they need to be informed sensitively and allowed the time they need with their loved one, and this again is very personal. Check for any care requirements required for children or dependent family members or if arrangements have been made. If not, then advice/support from a social worker may be required.

Be available for the family/carer and listen to them rather than speak. When they are ready, they may require guidance on what happens next; for example, how to register the death or contact a funeral director. They may also require direction to bereavement services. Reassure them that everything has been done to care for the individual and to maintain their dignity. This is especially important during times, such as the pandemic, when people important to the individual may not have been able to spend time with them in the way they would have liked.

It is very important to know the cultural background of any individual you are caring for to meet these needs, as only some religions will nominate a spokesperson for the family at such critical times. Early identification of specific cultural, religious or faith traditions can help engage Aboriginal liaison officers, multicultural health services, accredited hospital chaplains, etc. It is also important to inform individuals and their families/carer about interpreters, chaplains and prayer rooms available within a facility.

If not already occurring, consideration should be given when and where possible to prioritise a single room for ongoing care. Environmental noise should be kept to a minimum; this includes from carers and visitors for the comfort of others. Disruptive visitors, family members or other staff should be managed and asked to be respectful or leave the area. Within the healthcare setting support staff such as domestic staff and food service staff should be aware and know whether to enter the room. All staff should be mindful of 'corridor conversations' and avoid as much as is possible, including personal conversations and those with family/carer members.

Most in-hospital deaths do not require referral to the coroner. Coroners have a legal duty to investigate sudden, unexpected and unnatural deaths to determine the identity, circumstances and any medical cause of death. In some instances, after an investigation the coroner may make recommendations to improve public safety and prevent further deaths. The medical officer certifying the individual's death will advise if a coroner referral is required or not (Coroners Court 2022).

Caring for an individual who has died and their family/carer can be emotionally challenging and distressing to the staff due to the very personal nature of the process. Whilst death is a natural process, caring for a person after death may leave you feeling uncomfortable or you may experience grief. Sometimes, these emotions can be triggered a long time after the person has died. Their death can also bring up memories of people you know who have died. If this happens then speak with your direct line manager about how you are feeling. A debrief session may be beneficial with your line manager and/ or other colleagues. If required, a referral for counselling can be made and your manager may suggest contact with the Employees Assistance Program (EAP). If this is not available or appropriate, or does not make you feel comfortable, then seek assistance from your general practitioner for a referral to see a counsellor or psychologist.

In summary, aspects to consider before caring for the person after death:
- Coroners' referral: being attended or not
- Cultural, religious or faith traditions to be observed
- Family/carer
- Infectious disease status
- Family/friends wish to be involved in care
- Organ donation.

 CASE STUDY 38.3

Joe, 34, has died from metastatic bowel cancer, two days before his 35th birthday. His family want to thank you for all your care and support during his last days. They comment that you are 'the best' and cared for him better than anyone. Reflect upon this comment and your thoughts in response to this. How will this influence your nursing in the future?

CRITICAL THINKING EXERCISE 38.1

In what ways do you think COVID-19 impacted the experience of individuals who were dying and admitted to hospital? How do you think COVID-19 impacted care provided? How might nurses reflect on these challenges and prepare for any future crisis?

CLINICAL SKILL 38.1 Care of the person after death

Please adhere to the policy and procedures of the facility/organisation prior to undertaking the skill. Ensure this skill is in your scope of practice.

NMBA Decision-making Framework considerations (refer to NMBA Decision-making framework for nursing and midwifery 2020):	Equipment:
1. Am I educated? 2. Am I authorised? 3. Am I competent? If you answer 'no' to any of these, do not perform that activity. Seek guidance and support from your teacher/a nurse team leader/clinical facilitator/educator.	PPE—disposable gloves, disposable apron, protective eyewear Identification labels/tags/name bands Forms—Authority for Removal, Death Certificate, Cremation Certificate (and other forms/checklists as applicable to organisational policy) Washbasin, washcloth, warm water, and bath towel Toiletries—mouth care, brush/comb, soap Continence pads Dressings (as applicable) Disposable gown/shroud or clothing according to organisational policy/family/carer(s) wishes Body bag (according to organisational policy) For infectious bodies: Biohazard bags Face mask/shield

 PREPARE FOR THE SKILL

(Please refer to the Standard Steps on p. xii for related rationales.)
Mentally review the steps of the skill.
Discuss the skill with your instructor/supervisor/team leader, if required.
Confirm correct facility/organisation policy/safe operating procedures.
Validate the order in the individual's record.
Identify indications and rationale for performing the activity.
Assess for any contraindications.
Locate and gather equipment.
Perform hand hygiene.
Ensure therapeutic interaction.
Identify the individual using three individual identifiers.
Gain the individual's consent.
Assess for pain relief.
Prepare the environment.
Provide and maintain privacy.
Assist the individual to assume an appropriate position of comfort.

Skill activity	Rationale
Establish infectious risk.	If the deceased is suspected or has a known infectious disease, then they should be cared for with the same precautions as they were in life as this prevents infection and reduces risk of transmission. All staff should be aware of the infectious status of the deceased when organising equipment to prepare the body and when collecting the person for transfer to the mortuary/funeral director. When the deceased has been identified as having/had an infectious disease appropriate care and labelling should be applied (i.e. place an Infectious Disease—Handle with Care label on the outside of the body bag). Remove all disposable PPE and place in biohazard bag and place into a ward clinical waste bin. The mortuary/funeral director is to be notified of infectious status of body at time of collection.

CLINICAL SKILL 38.1 Care of the person after death—cont'd

Review advance care plan/directive for/discuss with family/carer(s) any cultural and/or spiritual/religious rites/ preferences that are in line with the deceased's wishes before handling the body. Determine if family/carer(s) wish to be present or help with care of the person.	Respects individuality of person and family/carer(s) and supports their right to having cultural or religious values and beliefs upheld. Provides closure for those who wish to help with body preparation.

 PERFORM THE SKILL

(Please refer to the Standard Steps on p. xii for related rationales.)
Perform hand hygiene.
Apply PPE: gloves, eyewear, mask and gown as appropriate.
Ensure the individual's safety and comfort throughout use of the skill.
Promote independence and involvement of the individual if possible and/or appropriate.
Assess the individual's tolerance to the skill throughout.
Dispose of used supplies, equipment, waste and sharps appropriately.
Remove PPE and discard or store appropriately.
Perform hand hygiene.

Skill activity	Rationale
Care of the person At time of apparent death: • Lay on back and straighten limbs (if possible). • Place one pillow under the head. • Close the eyes by applying light pressure for 30 seconds. • If the individual had dentures and they were not in the mouth, place them in a labelled denture cup and ensured that they are transported with the person to the mortuary/funeral director. • Cover person with appropriate covers.	To maintain the deceased's dignity, ensure the deceased is lying straight prior to rigor mortis which occurs 2–6 hours after death. Supports alignment and helps the mouth stay closed. Closing the eyes maintains dignity, and for tissue protection in case of corneal donation. Helps to retain the shape of the face. To maintain the deceased's privacy and dignity.
Preparation of the person (if not a coroner's case*): • Wash body, unless requested not to do so for spiritual/religious/cultural reasons. • Family/carer(s) may wish to assist with washing. They must be aware of potential infectious risks and, depending on the place of death, wear PPE as instructed. • Clean mouth and teeth or dentures. • Comb and tidy hair. • Use pads to absorb possible leaks from the urethra, vagina or rectum. • Remove tubes such as cannula and catheters. • Cover drain and wound sites with a clean absorbent dressing and secure with an occlusive dressing. • Dress appropriately before they go to the mortuary or funeral directors. This may be in a shroud or personal clothing depending on the place of death, local policy or wishes of the family/carer(s). • Jewellery/belongings—refer to and follow local organisational requirements.	For hygienic and aesthetic reasons. Prevents infection and reduces risk of transmission. The body can continue to excrete fluids after death. To maintain the deceased's dignity and shows respect for the person. To prevent leakage. Invasive devices including cannulas and catheters are removed (except for persons referred to the coroner). Covering/changing dressings controls odours and creates more acceptable appearance. To ensure the deceased's dignity is always preserved.
Identification—refer to and follow local organisational requirements regarding identification labels/tags/name bands.	To meet legal requirements and key contact's wishes and safekeeping of valuables. To ensure correct identification of the deceased.
Offer the family/carer(s) time to be with the deceased as long as they wish prior to transportation to the mortuary/ funeral director.	Compassionate care provides family members with meaningful experience during early phase of grief. Ensure privacy and a safe environment.

Continued

CLINICAL SKILL 38.1 Care of the person after death—cont'd

Transfer to mortuary/funeral director organised (as per organisational policy) after completion of:
- Care of the person or last offices
- Placement of the person in body bag with label attached to outside of bag
- Local organisational documentation requirements
- Verification of Death form
- Medical Certificate of Cause of Death or Intention to Complete form
- Cremation certificate (if applicable).

After viewing occurs the body is to be transported to the mortuary/funeral director, in a tag sealed body bag (as applicable to setting/local organisational policy).
Note: Individuals who are bariatric are transferred to the mortuary on a bariatric bed.

 AFTER THE SKILL

(Please refer to the Standard Steps on p. xii for related rationales.)
Communicate outcome to the individual, any ongoing care and to report any complications.
Restore the environment.
Report, record and document assessment findings, details of the skill performed and the individual's response.
Report, record and document any abnormalities and/or inability to perform the skill.
Reassess the individual to ensure there are no adverse effects/events from the skill.

* For a Coronial Case, refer to local organisational policy, the MO/RN in Charge for actions to be taken as these will vary to those listed above.
(Crisp et al 2021; Hospice UK 2022; Marie Curie 2022c; Perry et al 2022; Queensland Health 2019)

OBSERVATION CHECKLIST: CARE OF THE PERSON AFTER DEATH

| Independent (I) |
| Supervised (S) |
| Assisted (A) |
| Marginal (M) |
| Dependent (D) |

STUDENT NAME: _____

CLINICAL SKILL 38.1: Care of the person after death

DEMONSTRATION OF: The ability to safely and correctly perform care of the person after death

If the observation checklist is being used as an assessment tool, the student will need to obtain a scale of independence for each of the performance criteria/evidence.

COMPETENCY ELEMENTS	PERFORMANCE CRITERIA/EVIDENCE	I	S	A	M	D
Preparation for the activity	Mentally reviews the steps of the skill Discusses the skill with your instructor/supervisor/team leader, if required Confirms correct facility/organisation policy/safe operating procedures Validates the order in the individual's record Identifies indications and rationale for performing the activity Locates and gathers equipment Performs hand hygiene Ensures therapeutic interaction Identifies the individual using three individual identifiers Gains the family's/carer's consent Prepares the environment Provides and maintains privacy Reviews advance care plan/ directive for/discusses with family/carer(s) any cultural and/or spiritual/religious rites/preferences that are in line with the deceased's wishes before handling the body Determines if family/carer(s) wish to be present or help with care of the person					
Performs activity informed by evidence	Preparation of the body (if not a coroner's case*): • Washes body, unless requested not to do so for spiritual/religious/cultural reasons • Family/carer(s) may wish to assist with washing. They must be aware of potential infectious risks and, depending on the place of death, wear PPE as instructed • Cleans mouth and teeth or dentures • Combs and tidies hair • Uses pads to absorb possible leaks from the urethra, vagina or rectum • Removes tubes such as cannulas and catheters • Covers drain and wound sites with a clean absorbent dressing and secures with an occlusive dressing • Dresses appropriately before they go to the mortuary or funeral directors. This may be in a shroud or personal clothing depending on the place of death, local policy or wishes of the family/carer(s) • Jewellery/belongings—refers to and follows local organisational requirements • Offers the family/carer(s) time to be with the deceased as long as they wish prior to transportation to the mortuary/funeral director					

Continued

COMPETENCY ELEMENTS	PERFORMANCE CRITERIA/EVIDENCE	I	S	A	M	D
	Transfers to mortuary/funeral director organised (as per organisational policy) after completion of: • Care of the person or last offices • Placement of the body in body bag with label attached to outside of bag • Local organisational documentation requirements • Verification of Death form • Medical Certificate of Cause of Death or Intention to Complete form • Cremation certificate (if applicable)					
Applies critical thinking and reflective practice	Demonstrates critical thinking and problem-solving Is able to link theory to practice Demonstrates current best practice in the care provided Assesses own performance					
Practises within safety and quality assurance guidelines	Reviews against facility/organisational policy Performs hand hygiene, dons appropriate PPE as per infection control and WHS protocols Raises the bed to the appropriate working position based on nurse's height and lowers at completion of activity Cleans and disposes of equipment and waste appropriately					
Documentation and communication	Explains and communicates the activity to family/carer Reports, records and documents assessment findings, details of the skill performed Reports any complications and/or inability to perform the procedure to the RN and/or medical officer Restores the environment * For a Coronial Case, refers to local organisational policy, the MO/RN in Charge for actions to be taken as these will vary to those listed above					

Educator/Facilitator Feedback:

Educator/Facilitator Score: Competent   Needs further development

How would you rate your overall performance while undertaking this clinical activity? (use a ✓ & initial)

Unsatisfactory   Satisfactory   Good   Excellent

Student Reflection: (discuss how you would approach your practice differently or more effectively)

EDUCATOR/FACILITATOR NAME/SIGNATURE:

STUDENT NAME/SIGNATURE: **DATE:**

Evolve® Answer guide for the Critical Thinking Exercises and Critical Thinking Questions in Case Studies is hosted on Evolve: http://evolve.elsevier.com/AU/Koutoukidis/Tabbner/

References

Coroners Court NSW, 2022. Understanding the NSW coronial jurisdiction. Available at: <https://coroners.nsw.gov.au/the-coronial-process/what-to-expect-during-the-coronial-process.html>.

Nursing and Midwifery Board of Australia (NMBA), 2020. Decision-making framework for nursing and midwifery. Available at: <https://www.nursingmidwiferyboard.gov.au/Codes-Guidelines-Statements/Frameworks.aspx>.

Online Resources

CareSearch. Care of the body. Considerations regarding care and preparation of the body after someone dies: <https://www.caresearch.com.au/Health-Professionals/Nurses/The-Dying-Patient/After-Death-Care/Care-of-the-Body>.

Victoria Health. Palliative care – grief and loss: <https://www.health.vic.gov.au/patient-care/palliative-care-grief-and-loss>.

NSW Government. Clinical Excellence Commission. Last Days of Life Toolkit: <https://www.cec.health.nsw.gov.au/__data/assets/pdf_file/0009/359271/Information-for-the-multidisciplinary-team.PDF>.

Australian Government Services Australia. What to do when a loved one dies: <https://www.servicesaustralia.gov.au/what-to-do-when-loved-one-dies?context=60101>.

Cancer Council NSW. After the death: <https://www.cancercouncil.com.au/cancer-information/advanced-cancer/end-of-life/for-carers/after-the-death/>.

ACUTE AND PERIOPERATIVE CARE

Lise Martin

Overview

Acute care is defined as any care that is provided for individuals needing care for an acute illness, injury or recovery. This can be achieved within the hospital setting or in the community (Australian Commission on Safety and Quality in Health Care 2021).

Through the evolution of training and the advocacy and standardisation of education by the Australian Nursing and Midwifery Accreditation Council (ANMAC), Enrolled Nurses (ENs) have become an integral part of the assessment, planning, implementation and evaluation processes of acute individuals and are moving into highly acute clinical areas, such as cardiac and respiratory units, emergency departments and neonatal care—areas once reserved only for Registered Nurses (RNs) (McKenna et al 2019).

Today, ENs are able to perform complex and advanced procedures, such as urinary catheterisation, oxygen therapy and tracheostomy care, and perform specialist skills such as venipuncture, oral and pharyngeal suctioning and central venous access device (CVAD) management. This is in addition to needing enhanced critical thinking and problem-solving skills when managing the care of acute patients (McKenna et al 2019).

Teaching of preoperative activities is essential for the prevention of postoperative complications, and involves instructing the individual about how to perform deep breathing and coughing techniques, as well as leg exercises and ways to move and change position to enhance circulation. The person is informed regarding the importance of these activities and is encouraged to practise them regularly so that the techniques will be familiar when they are required postoperatively. If specialised techniques are required to assist with movement in the postoperative period, such as the use of a rolling or turning frame after total hip replacement, an opportunity to practise these techniques should be provided in the preoperative phase.

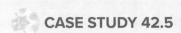

CASE STUDY 42.5

Elective hysterectomy

Ms Hayward, 48 years old, is a non-urgent elective Category 3 individual who is to undergo an abdominal hysterectomy. The surgery has been recommended since she has suffered with increasing blood loss and a lowering of Hb over the past two years, due to fibroids in the uterus.

She will return to the ward with an indwelling catheter (IDC) in situ and a PCA (patient-controlled analgesia) unit.

1. What is the longest time Ms Hayward should have waited for her surgery?
2. What effect could an extended wait have on her health status?
3. Describe some fears or anxiety Ms Hayward may have in regard to her surgery.
4. Identify a psychological issue Ms Hayward could face in regard to body image and self-esteem.
5. What potential problems may Ms Hayward experience immediately on return to the ward?
6. What nursing interventions could be implemented to prevent or reduce these problems?

CRITICAL THINKING EXERCISE 42.1

You are looking after Ian, a 45-year-old man, who has been admitted to the cardiothoracic ward post an acute myocardial infarct (AMI). He is recovering post coronary artery bypass graft surgery. Ian is the main income earner in his family and has two young children under the age of five years and a supportive wife, Lucy, at home.

1. Identify the physical issues Ian may experience.
2. Identify psychosocial issues Ian may experience.
3. List the ongoing care (including allied healthcare) that Ian and his family may require during his recovery.

CLINICAL SKILL 42.1 Venipuncture

Please adhere to the policy and procedures of the facility/organisation prior to undertaking the skill. Ensure this skill is in your scope of practice.

NMBA Decision-making Framework considerations (refer to NMBA Decision-making framework for nursing and midwifery 2022):

1. Am I educated?
2. Am I authorised?
3. Am I competent?

If you answer 'no' to any of these, do not perform that activity. Seek guidance and support from your teacher/a nurse team leader/clinical facilitator/educator.

Equipment:

Disposable gloves
Protective eye wear
Disposable collection tray
Tourniquet
Vacutainer access device/21–23 G needle and syringe/butterfly 21–23 G with vacutainer attachment
Pathology test tubes
Sharps container
Alcohol wipes
Dressing (e.g. pressure dot, cottonwool and tape or bandaid)
Completed pathology request form and pen
Biohazard specimen transport bag

 PREPARE FOR THE SKILL

(Please refer to the Standard Steps on p. xii for related rationales.)
Mentally review the steps of the skill.
Discuss the skill with your instructor/supervisor/team leader, if required.
Confirm correct facility/organisation policy/safe operating procedures.
Validate the order in the individual's record.
Identify indication and rationale for performing the activity.
Assess for any contraindications.
Locate and gather equipment.
Perform hand hygiene.
Ensure therapeutic interaction.
Identify the individual using three individual identifiers.
Gain the individual's consent.
Assess for pain relief.
Prepare the environment.
Provide and maintain privacy.
Assist the individual to assume an appropriate position of comfort during the activity.

 PERFORM THE SKILL

(Please refer to the Standard Steps on p. xii for related rationales.)
Perform hand hygiene.
Apply PPE: gloves, eyewear, mask and gown as appropriate.
Ensure the individual's safety and comfort throughout skill.
Promote independence and involvement of the individual if possible and/or appropriate.
Assess the individual's tolerance to the skill throughout.
Dispose of used supplies, equipment, waste and sharps appropriately.
Remove PPE and discard or store appropriately.
Perform hand hygiene.

Skill activity	Rationale
Place tourniquet about 10 cm above intended puncture site (above the elbow or wrist joint) and clip ends together and tighten firmly, so that two fingers can fit under comfortably. Palpate the distal pulse to ensure the artery is not occluded.	Helps to distend vein. Prevents discomfort due to tourniquet being too tight. Helps prevent complications.
Locate the vein by palpating using the index and middle fingers of your dominant hand. Use distension methods (drop and dangle, heat pack). Once the vein is located, release tourniquet.	Palpating for the vein enables assessment of the vein through touch (bouncy and full of blood). Facilitates filling of the vein and distension. Facilitates refill of the vein.

CLINICAL SKILL 42.1 Venipuncture—cont'd

Cleanse the area with an alcohol wipe using circular motion (inner to outer) from the intended puncture site for 30 seconds and wait 30 seconds for the area to dry. Reapply tourniquet. Stabilise the vein by anchoring (stretching) the skin below the insertion site with your non-dominant hand. Insert needle tip with bevel up into the vein. The needle should be parallel to the vein and above it with the angle of insertion approximately 15–30 degrees. Once the tip of the needle is in the vein, remove your anchor and attach the tubes one by one to the vacutainer and fill each tube with blood. Release the tourniquet once you are getting flow to prevent haemolysis.	Prevents the introduction of microorganisms and ensures proper antiseptic preparation of skin. Enables the smooth entry into the vein and prevents the vein from moving around. Going in too deep can lead to puncturing the vein all the way through and causing a haematoma. Haemolysis can interfere with an accurate result.
Once the required tubes are filled and removed from the vacutainer, the tourniquet is also released; support the insertion site with the cotton ball (do not push down) and withdraw the needle. Apply pressure to the puncture site and ask the individual to continue to put pressure on the site if able. Discard sharp immediately into the sharps container.	Prevents discomfort to the site. Prevents excessive bleeding and a haematoma from forming. Complies with infection control and WHS legislation.
Invert tubes, as per recommendation from manufacturer. Label and sign the tubes of blood and verify the individual's details. Sign the pathology form and place form and tubes in the required pathology biohazard bag.	Mixes blood with additives, avoids incorrect results/re-collections. Abides by organisational guidelines and ensures the correct results for the correct individual. Enables proper transporting of tubes.
Check the puncture site to ensure the bleeding has stopped and change the cotton ball if required and apply tape. Inform individual to notify you of any further bleeding, pain at the site or if a haematoma forms.	Prevents complications from the procedure.
Send blood specimens to pathology in a timely manner.	Ensures blood tests are as fresh as possible for accurate results.

 AFTER THE SKILL

(Please refer to the Standard Steps on p. xii for related rationales.)
Communicate outcome to the individual, any ongoing care and to report any complications.
Restore the environment.
Report, record and document assessment findings, details of the skill performed and the individual's response.
Report, record and document any abnormalities and/or inability to perform the skill.
Reassess the individual to ensure there are no adverse effects/events from the skill.

(Carter & Notter 2024; Crisp et al 2021; Tollefson & Hillman 2021)

OBSERVATION CHECKLIST: VENIPUNCTURE

STUDENT NAME: _____

CLINICAL SKILL 42.1: Venipuncture

DEMONSTRATION OF: The ability to safely and correctly perform venipuncture

If the observation checklist is being used as an assessment tool, the student will need to obtain a scale of independence for each of the performance criteria/evidence.

Independent (I)
Supervised (S)
Assisted (A)
Marginal (M)
Dependent (D)

COMPETENCY ELEMENTS	PERFORMANCE CRITERIA/EVIDENCE	I	S	A	M	D
Preparation for the activity	Identifies indications and rationale for performing the activity Identifies the individual using three individual identifiers Ensures therapeutic interaction Gains the individual's consent Checks facility/organisation policy Validates the order in the individual's record Locates and gathers equipment Assists the individual into an appropriate position Checks the pathology slip for specific tests required					
Performs activity informed by evidence	Ensures correct palpation of vein and application of tourniquet Cleanses the area correctly, ensuring no cross-contamination Inserts the needle as recommended using the correct equipment (i.e. vacutainer device, needle and butterfly/syringe) Applies gauze and pressure to puncture site Labels collection containers with individual's identifying information, date and time of collection as per organisation policy Places filled specimen container/s in specimen bag with request slip Ensures specimens are sent to laboratory in a timely fashion					
Applies critical thinking and reflective practice	Assesses the individual's prior experience of venipuncture Performs any necessary assessments related to the correct performance of venipuncture (i.e. mastectomy site, oedema) Monitors the individual's anxiety related to the procedure Correctly assesses the vein for venipuncture Assesses the individual's ability to cooperate with the procedure and assist when required Assesses the site for any complications Is able to link theory to practice Demonstrates current best practice in the care provided Assesses own performance					

COMPETENCY ELEMENTS	PERFORMANCE CRITERIA/EVIDENCE	I	S	A	M	D
Practises within safety and quality assurance guidelines	Reviews against facility/organisation policy Performs hand hygiene, dons appropriate PPE as per infection control protocols Checks individual's allergies to latex or tape Ensures the appropriate working position based on nurse's height and the person's position (in bed, in chair) and on completion of activity ensures person is safe post procedure (lowers bed) Cleans and disposes of equipment and waste appropriately					
Documentation and communication	Explains and communicates the activity clearly to the individual Communicates outcome and ongoing care to individual and significant others Communicates abnormal findings to appropriate personnel Reports and documents all relevant information and any complications correctly in the healthcare record Reports any complications and/or inability to perform the procedure to the RN and/or medical officer Asks the individual to report any complications during and post procedure					

Educator/Facilitator Feedback:

Educator/Facilitator Score: Competent   Needs further development

How would you rate your overall performance while undertaking this clinical activity? (use a ✓ & initial)

Unsatisfactory   Satisfactory   Good   Excellent

Student Reflection: (discuss how you would approach your practice differently or more effectively)

EDUCATOR/FACILITATOR NAME/SIGNATURE:

STUDENT NAME/SIGNATURE: **DATE:**

CLINICAL SKILL 42.2 Central venous access device (CVAD): Monitoring and management

Please adhere to the policy and procedures of the facility/organisation prior to undertaking the skill. Ensure this skill is in your scope of practice.

NMBA Decision-making Framework considerations (refer to NMBA Decision-making framework for nursing and midwifery 2022):

1. Am I educated?
2. Am I authorised?
3. Am I competent?

If you answer 'no' to any of these, do not perform that activity. Seek guidance and support from your teacher/a nurse team leader/clinical facilitator/educator.

Equipment:

Dressing change:
  Sterile gloves
  Disposable gloves
  Sterile dressing pack
  Occlusive dressing
  Solution (as per healthcare facility policy, usually 2% chlorhexidine and 70% alcohol)
  Sterile bungs/caps
  Stabilisation device
  Extra sterile gauze squares
  Waste bag

Catheter removal:
  Sterile gloves
  Disposable gloves
  Sterile dressing pack
  Occlusive dressing
  Solution (as per healthcare facility policy, usually 2% chlorhexidine and 70% alcohol)
  Extra sterile gauze squares
  Suture remover
  Scissors
  Specimen container
  Completed pathology request form and pen
  Biohazard specimen transport bag
  Waste bag

📋 PREPARE FOR THE SKILL

(Please refer to the Standard Steps on p. xii for related rationales.)
Mentally review the steps of the skill.
Discuss the skill with your instructor/supervisor/team leader, if required.
Confirm correct facility/organisation policy/safe operating procedures.
Validate the order in the individual's record.
Identify indication and rationale for performing the activity.
Assess for any contraindications.
Locate and gather equipment.
Perform hand hygiene.
Ensure therapeutic interaction.
Identify the individual using three individual identifiers.
Gain the individual's consent.
Assess for pain relief.
Prepare the environment.
Provide and maintain privacy.
Assist the individual to assume an appropriate position of comfort during the activity.

PERFORM THE SKILL

(Please refer to the Standard Steps on p. xii for related rationales.)
Perform hand hygiene.
Apply PPE: gloves, eyewear, mask and gown as appropriate.
Ensure the individual's safety and comfort throughout skill.
Promote independence and involvement of the individual if possible and/or appropriate.
Assess the individual's tolerance to the skill throughout.
Dispose of used supplies, equipment, waste and sharps appropriately.
Remove PPE and discard or store appropriately.
Perform hand hygiene.

Continued

CLINICAL SKILL 42.2 Central venous access device (CVAD): Monitoring and management—cont'd

Skill activity	Rationale
Open a sterile dressing pack and place any additional equipment within easy reach.	Prevents cross-infection. Prevents the introduction of microorganisms.

Dressing change

Don disposable gloves and gently peel back old dressing towards the insertion site, anchoring the catheter. Remove stabilisation device (if present). Inspect for signs of infection. Measure length of catheter from the insertion site to the tip.	Prevents cross-infection. Prevents the dislodgement of the catheter. Assesses for complications, which may need further management. Identifies external catheter migration.
Remove gloves, perform hand hygiene (as per policy) and don sterile gloves. Cleanse skin with appropriate cleaning solution as per hospital guidelines. Wait for cleaning solution to dry. Place stabilisation device onto the skin in the correct place (if PICC line). Apply occlusive dressing over the catheter insertion site including the stabilisation device (if used).	Prevents the introduction of microorganisms and ensures asepsis. Prevents cross-contamination. Ensures full antisepsis has been achieved. Secures the catheter to prevent dislodgement. An occlusive dressing allows the area to breathe by preventing moisture under the dressing, preventing infection. Allows monitoring for any signs of infection.

Catheter removal

Confirm medical order for removal of central catheter. Position the individual in a supine position. Don disposable gloves and gently peel back old dressing towards the insertion site, anchoring the catheter. Remove stabilisation device (if used). Inspect for signs of infection.	Abides by legal and organisation guidelines. Reduces the risk for air embolism during catheter removal. Prevents cross-infection. Prevents the dislodgement of the catheter. Used generally on PICC lines. Assesses for complications, which may need further management.
Remove gloves, perform hand hygiene (as per policy) and don sterile gloves. Cleanse skin and visible portion of catheter with cleaning solution in an outward circular motion as per hospital guidelines. Wait for solution to dry. Remove any sutures. Ask the individual to perform the Valsalva manoeuvre. (If unable to comply, remove during expiration.) Place a piece of sterile gauze over the insertion site and gently remove the catheter from the vein in one smooth motion, leaving the gauze in situ once removed. Place the tip of the catheter on the sterile field of the dressing tray. Check the site for any excess bleeding or exudate before covering with an occlusive dressing. **Note:** If the tip is to be sent to pathology, cut the tip with sterile scissors and place tip in a sterile specimen container.	Prevents the introduction of microorganisms and ensures asepsis. Prevents cross-contamination. Ensures full antisepsis has been achieved. Reduces the risk of air embolism during catheter removal. Do not force catheter, as it may break apart. If any resistance, stop the procedure, cover with a sterile dressing and inform the nurse in charge/doctor. Reduces the risk of contamination. Prevents post-removal air embolism and the introduction of microorganisms. The doctor may want to test for any microorganisms.
Label and sign the container and verify the individual's details. Sign the pathology form and place form and specimen container in the required pathology biohazard bag.	Abides by organisational guidelines and ensures the correct results for the correct individual. Enables proper transporting of specimen.
Send specimen container to pathology in a timely manner.	Ensures specimen is as fresh as possible for accurate results.

CLINICAL SKILL 42.2 Central venous access device (CVAD): Monitoring and management—cont'd

 AFTER THE SKILL

(Please refer to the Standard Steps on p. xii for related rationales.)
Communicate outcome to the individual, any ongoing care and to report any complications.
Restore the environment.
Report, record and document assessment findings, details of the skill performed and the individual's response.
Report, record and document any abnormalities and/or inability to perform the skill.
Reassess the individual to ensure there are no adverse effects/events from the skill.

(Crisp et al 2021; The Royal Children's Hospital Melbourne 2020; Tollefson & Hillman 2021)

OBSERVATION CHECKLIST: CENTRAL VENOUS ACCESS DEVICE MANAGEMENT: MONITORING AND MANAGEMENT

| Independent (I) |
| Supervised (S) |
| Assisted (A) |
| Marginal (M) |
| Dependent (D) |

STUDENT NAME: _____

CLINICAL SKILL 42.2: Central venous access device management: monitoring and management

DEMONSTRATION OF: The ability to safely and correctly perform central venous access device management including dressing change, removal and medication administration

If the observation checklist is being used as an assessment tool, the student will need to obtain a scale of independence for each of the performance criteria/evidence.

COMPETENCY ELEMENTS	PERFORMANCE CRITERIA/EVIDENCE	I	S	A	M	D
Preparation for the activity	Identifies indications and rationale for performing the activity Identifies the individual using three individual identifiers Ensures therapeutic interaction Gains the individual's consent Checks facility/organisation policy Validates the order in the individual's record Locates and gathers equipment Assists the individual into an appropriate position					
Performs activity informed by evidence	For dressing change: • Opens and assembles equipment aseptically • Sets up sterile field • Dons disposable gloves • Removes old dressing and stabilisation device (if present) • Inspects for signs of infection • Measures length of catheter from insertion site to tip • Removes gloves and performs hand hygiene • Dons sterile gloves • Cleanses access site with appropriate cleaning solution as per facility guidelines, using a clean swab for each stroke, allows to dry • Applies stabilisation device in correct position (if PICC) • Applies occlusive dressing over the catheter insertion site (including the stabilisation device) • Disposes of waste in appropriate receptacle • Performs hand hygiene For catheter removal: • Confirms medical order for removal of central catheter • Positions the individual in a supine position • Dons disposable gloves and gently peels back old dressing towards the insertion site, anchoring the catheter • Inspects for signs of infection • Removes gloves, performs hand hygiene (as per policy) and dons sterile gloves • Cleanses skin and visible portion of catheter with cleaning solution in an outward circular motion • Waits for solution to dry • Removes sutures and removes stabilisation device (if applicable). Instructs the individual to perform Valsalva manoeuvre (if unable to comply, remove during expiration) • Places a piece of sterile gauze over the insertion site and gently removes the catheter from the vein in one smooth motion, leaving the gauze in situ once removed • Places the tip of the catheter on the sterile field of the dressing tray					

COMPETENCY ELEMENTS	PERFORMANCE CRITERIA/EVIDENCE	I	S	A	M	D
	• Checks the site for any excess bleeding or exudate before covering with an occlusive dressing If tip is to be sent to pathology: • Cuts the tip with sterile scissors and places tip in sterile specimen container • Signs and labels container and completes pathology form correctly Following dressing change or catheter removal: • Places individual into a comfortable position and asks the individual to inform you of any difficulty breathing, pain or oozing from the site • Disposes of equipment in the correct waste receptacle • Performs hand hygiene • Monitors individual for any adverse effects • Communicates any abnormal findings to the RN/medical officer • Reports and documents all relevant information correctly in the healthcare record					
Applies critical thinking and reflective practice	• Assesses the individual's clinical status • Monitors the individual's anxiety related to the procedure • Correctly assesses the site for any complications • Assesses the individual's ability to cooperate with the procedure and assist when required • Is able to link theory to practice • Demonstrates current best practice in the care provided • Assesses own performance					
Practises within safety and quality assurance guidelines	• Reviews against facility/organisation policy • Performs hand hygiene, dons appropriate PPE as per infection control protocols • Adheres to infection control/ANTT principles • Checks individual's allergies to latex, tape or solution • Raises the bed to the appropriate working position based on nurse's height and lowers at completion of activity • Cleans and disposes of equipment and waste appropriately					
Documentation and communication	• Explains and communicates the activity clearly to the individual • Communicates outcome and ongoing care to individual and significant others • Communicates abnormal findings to appropriate personnel • Reports and documents all relevant information and any complications correctly in the healthcare record and CVAD chart (if applicable) • Documents accurately on pathology form and specimen (if tip sent to microbiology) • Reports any complications and/or inability to perform the procedure to the RN and/or medical officer • Asks the individual to report any complications during and post procedure					

Educator/Facilitator Feedback:

Educator/Facilitator Score: Competent   Needs further development

How would you rate your overall performance while undertaking this clinical activity? (use a ✓ & initial)

Unsatisfactory   Satisfactory   Good   Excellent

Student Reflection: (discuss how you would approach your practice differently or more effectively)

EDUCATOR/FACILITATOR NAME/SIGNATURE:

STUDENT NAME/SIGNATURE: **DATE:**

CLINICAL SKILL 42.3 Preoperative and postoperative exercises

Please adhere to the policy and procedures of the facility/organisation prior to undertaking the skill. Ensure this skill is in your scope of practice.

NMBA Decision-making Framework considerations (refer to NMBA Decision-making framework for nursing and midwifery 2022):	Equipment:
1. Am I educated? 2. Am I authorised? 3. Am I competent? If you answer 'no' to any of these, do not perform that activity. Seek guidance and support from your teacher/a nurse team leader/clinical facilitator/educator.	Pillow/rolled towel Tissues Rubbish bin

 PREPARE FOR THE SKILL

(Please refer to the Standard Steps on p. xii for related rationales.)
Mentally review the steps of the skill.
Discuss the skill with your instructor/supervisor/team leader, if required.
Confirm correct facility/organisation policy/safe operating procedures.
Validate the order in the individual's record.
Identify indication and rationale for performing the activity.
Assess for any contraindications.
Locate and gather equipment.
Perform hand hygiene.
Ensure therapeutic interaction.
Identify the individual using three individual identifiers.
Gain the individual's consent.
Assess for pain relief.
Prepare the environment.
Provide and maintain privacy.
Assist the individual to assume an appropriate position of comfort during the activity.

 PERFORM THE SKILL

(Please refer to the Standard Steps on p. xii for related rationales.)
Perform hand hygiene.
Apply PPE: gloves, eyewear, mask and gown as appropriate.
Ensure the individual's safety and comfort throughout skill.
Promote independence and involvement of the individual if possible and/or appropriate.
Assess the individual's tolerance to the skill throughout.
Dispose of used supplies, equipment, waste and sharps appropriately.
Remove PPE and discard or store appropriately.
Perform hand hygiene.

Skill activity	Rationale
Provide health education preoperatively and postoperatively to individuals regarding early mobilisation, repositioning, lung expansion exercises, secretion clearance techniques and limb exercises by effective communication skills and demonstration.	
Deep breathing and coughing	
Deep breathing	Improves pulmonary function. Prevents pneumonia, atelectasis and other postoperative complications. Uses the diaphragm and abdominal muscles to fully ventilate the lungs. Normal breathing pattern can change and become shallower after chest or abdominal surgery, after general anaesthesia or when an individual is inactive.

Continued

CLINICAL SKILL 42.3 Preoperative and postoperative exercises—cont'd

Assess normal breathing pattern	Note depth, rate, volume for baseline data
Assess individual's risk of postoperative complications by reviewing individual's history, past medical history, history of respiratory diseases, vascular disease, previous thrombosis, medications, history of occupation and smoking and any complications previously from anaesthetic.	General anaesthetic (GA) predisposes individuals to respiratory problems due to lungs not being inflated fully; cough reflex is suppressed during surgery, thus secretions collect within airway passage. Post surgery, a decrease in lung volume requires a greater effort to cough. Inadequate lung expansion has potential for common complications such as pneumonia/atelectasis. If individual has known history of respiratory disease, it is more likely that complications may occur. Smoking damages cilia and increases mucus secretions. GA and immobilisation result in decreased contraction in lower extremities, which promotes venous status.
Assess individual's ability to cough/huff/deep-breathe, by having them take a deep breath and observing the movement of their shoulders and chest wall or use of accessory muscles. Measure chest excursion during a deep breath. Ask them to cough after taking a deep breath.	Reveals maximum potential for chest expansion and ability to cough/huff/deep-breathing. Serves as baseline data to perform activity.
Explain the importance to recovery and physiological benefits of postoperative exercises to individual/significant others.	Information allows individual to understand why they are important and allows individual to 'take charge' of information.
Demonstrate to individual/significant others and instruct individual how to attend to exercises.	
Deep breathing (diaphragmatic breathing) Assist/instruct individual into comfortable semi-Fowler's to Fowler's sitting position or to stand.	Upright position facilitates diaphragmatic movement.
Stand or sit facing the individual, close enough so individual can hear and see you.	Allows individual to observe breathing exercises.
Instruct individual to place palms of hands across from each other, down and along lower borders of rib cage, place tips of third fingers lightly together.	Position of hands allows individual to feel chest and abdomen move as the diaphragm descends.
Demonstrate to individual and watch individual do same.	Ascertain individual is giving you their full attention. Allows individual to observe breathing exercises.
Instruct individual to take a slow deep breath inhaling through the nose, instructing individual to feel middle fingers separate during inhalation.	Slow deep breath prevents hyperventilation. Inhaling through nose warms and humidifies air.
Demonstrate and watch individual attend to this step.	Allows individual to observe breathing exercises.
Explain to individual they should feel normal downward motion of diaphragm during inspiration. Explain that abdominal organs descend and chest wall expands.	Explanation and demonstration focus on normal ventilatory movement of chest wall. Individual has understanding of how diaphragmatic breathing occurs and feels.
Watch the individual is not using chest and shoulder muscles.	Using ancillary shoulder muscle and chest muscles increases energy expenditure.
Instruct individual to hold slow deep breath for 2–3 seconds and slowly exhale through the mouth.	Allows for gradual expulsion of air.
Explain middle fingertips will touch as chest wall contracts.	Individual has understanding of expansion of lungs and how it feels.
Repeat whole process together.	Allows individual to observe slow rhythmic breathing patterns.

CLINICAL SKILL 42.3 Preoperative and postoperative exercises—cont'd

Instruct individual to practise so they can be observed.	Repetition of exercises reinforces learning and correct techniques.
Instruct individual these exercises will need to be attended to post surgery 10 times every two hours.	Regular deep breathing prevents postoperative complications.
Controlled coughing Maintain upright position. Nurse to demonstrate skill. Demonstrate/instruct individual on placing pillow/rolled-up towel over wound/invasive devices with the palm of hand with gentle pressure. Take two slow deep breaths in through the nose, hold for 2–3 seconds and exhale through the mouth on the third breath instead of exhaling cough from bottom of lungs. Ensure cough is deep and not clearing the throat. Repeat. Inspect expectoration and record.	Slow expulsion of air frequently initiates the coughing reflex, which facilitates expectoration of mucus and prevents hyperventilation. Clearing throat does not remove mucus from deep in airways. Coughing uses abdominal and accessory respiratory muscles. Splinting supports the incision and surrounding tissues and reduces pain during coughing.
Leg exercises	
Observe individuals closely for respiratory difficulty, chest pain and general discomfort. Decreased muscle mass, degenerative changes in joints and degenerative tissue changes can result in limited range of motion.	Maintains blood circulation. Stimulates blood circulation, thereby preventing thrombophlebitis and thrombus formation. Exercise offers the potential to improve circulation, wound healing outcomes and functional and emotional wellbeing. Physical activity reduces the risk of falls and injuries.
Expose the individual's legs by untucking the sheets at the foot of the bed and folding the sheets to the middle of the bed.	Folding sheets back halfway exposes individual's legs to perform exercises, but maintains privacy.
Calf pumping Dorsiflexion and hyperextension of ankles. Have the individual: 1. Flex ankles and raise toes towards head, stretching posterior calf. 2. Hold for a count of 2. 3. Relax. 4. Repeat five times then proceed to other foot. Perform every hour.	Calf muscle pump improves venous return. The calf muscle pump is the primary mechanism to return blood from the lower limbs to the heart. During exercise, the calf muscles (gastrocnemius and soleus) contract and compress the intramuscular and deep veins, raising venous pressure and propelling blood in the deep venous system to flow towards the heart, while the one-way valve function prevents reflux, thereby preventing blood from pooling. When the gastrocnemius and soleus muscles contract, they expel more than 60% of venous blood into the large popliteal vein.
Foot circles Have the individual: 1. Point the toe and raise the leg slightly off the bed. 2. Use the great toe to trace a circle in the air, first to the right and then to the left. 3. Repeat five times and then proceed to the other foot. Perform every hour.	Moving the ankle joint assists the calf muscles to pump venous blood back up to the heart.
Leg lifts Have the individual: 1. Lie on back or in a semi-sitting position, and raise the leg off the bed. 2. Hold for count of 5. 3. Lower leg to the bed. 4. Repeat five times then proceed to other leg. Perform every hour.	Stimulates blood circulation by contracting the hamstring and quadriceps muscles. Helps prevent circulatory problems, such as thrombophlebitis, by facilitating venous return to the heart. Also decreases postoperative 'gas pains'.

Continued

CLINICAL SKILL 42.3 Preoperative and postoperative exercises—cont'd

Quad exercise Have the individual: 1. Lie in a comfortable position. 2. Press knee into the bed, relax, repeat. 3. Press knee into the bed, lift leg straight, off the bed, hold, gently lower leg, repeat.	Stimulates blood circulation by contracting the hamstring and quadriceps muscles. Helps prevent circulatory problems, such as thrombophlebitis, by facilitating venous return to the heart. Also decreases postoperative 'gas pains'.
While the individual is performing the exercises, assess the person for signs of exertion or discomfort.	Assessment alerts nurse if exercise activity needs to be stopped.
Repositioning/turning in bed	
Instruct an individual who has right-sided incision to turn to the left side of the bed as follows: • Flex the knees. • Splint the wound/invasive devices by holding the left arm and hand or a small pillow or folded towel over the site.	Minimises pressure against the incision and reduces pain. Turning periodically and alternately facilitates better inflation of the uppermost segments of the lungs.
Instruct individual to assume supine position, place left hand over incision/invasive devices. Keep the left leg straight, flex the right knee over the left leg, hold onto the bed rail with right hand and pull while rolling towards left side.	Puts less pressure on the side with the pain/incision.
Special aids such as a trapeze are available on most beds; these should be taught to individual as required.	Specific medical procedures may require the use of aids.

 AFTER THE SKILL

(Please refer to the Standard Steps on p. xii for related rationales.)
Communicate outcome to the individual, any ongoing care and to report any complications.
Restore the environment.
Report, record and document assessment findings, details of the skill performed and the individual's response.
Report, record and document any abnormalities and/or inability to perform the skill.
Reassess the individual to ensure there are no adverse effects/events from the skill.

(Berman et al 2020; Crisp et al 2021; Rebeiro et al 2021)

OBSERVATION CHECKLIST: PRE- AND POSTOPERATIVE EXERCISES

STUDENT NAME: _____

CLINICAL SKILL 42.3: Pre- and postoperative exercises (deep breathing and controlled coughing, leg exercises, passive range of motion exercises)

DEMONSTRATION OF: The ability to instruct/demonstrate preoperatively exercises that must be performed postoperatively

If the observation checklist is being used as an assessment tool, the student will need to obtain a scale of independence for each of the performance criteria/evidence.

Independent (I)

Supervised (S)

Assisted (A)

Marginal (M)

Dependent (D)

COMPETENCY ELEMENTS	PERFORMANCE CRITERIA/EVIDENCE	I	S	A	M	D
Preparation for the activity	Identifies indications and rationale for performing the activity Identifies the individual using three individual identifiers Ensures therapeutic interaction Gains the individual's consent Checks facility/organisation policy Validates the order in the individual's record Locates and gathers equipment Assists the individual into an appropriate position					
Performs activity informed by evidence	**Deep breathing (DB) and coughing** Identifies surgical/invasive sites and informs the individual of the position they will assume in bed after surgery Demonstrates to the individual how to support the surgical site/invasive sites with pillow/folded towel and demonstrates how to press hand firmly into pillow Instructs the individual to turn their head away from the nurse when coughing Instructs individual to cover their mouth with tissue while coughing Identifies on care plan/pathway additional postop orders that may pertain to individual (e.g. bed rest) Identifies how often exercises are to be performed Explains that pain relief will be provided if required using a pain assessment tool **Reposition/turning** Instructs individual to assume right supine position, place left hand over incision, keep left leg straight, flex right knee over the left leg, hold left side rail with right hand, pull and roll towards left side **Leg exercises** Instructs individual to attend to foot circles, dorsiflexion and hyperextension of ankles, leg lifts, quad exercises Places call bell and personal items within reach					

Continued

COMPETENCY ELEMENTS	PERFORMANCE CRITERIA/EVIDENCE	I	S	A	M	D
Applies critical thinking and reflective practice	Assesses individual's ability to cough/huff/DB and perform leg exercises Assesses the individual's pain status Observes individual closely for respiratory difficulty, chest pain, general discomfort, decreased muscle mass, degenerative changes in joints and degenerative tissue changes which can result in limited range of motion Is able to link theory to practice Demonstrates current best practice in the care provided Assesses own performance					
Practises within safety and quality assurance guidelines	Reviews against facility/organisation policy Performs hand hygiene, dons appropriate PPE as per infection control protocols Raises the bed to the appropriate working position based on nurse's height and lowers at completion of activity Cleans and disposes of equipment and waste appropriately					
Documentation and communication	Explains and communicates the activity clearly to the individual Communicates outcome and ongoing care to individual and significant others Communicates abnormal findings to appropriate personnel Reports and documents all relevant information and any complications correctly in the healthcare record, including: • Colour, consistency and amount of sputum if expectorated • Which joint or muscle group was problematic • Normal configuration, range of motion, muscle mass, strength and tone and joints to be exercised Reports any complications and/or inability to perform the procedure to the RN and/or medical officer Asks the individual to report any complications during and post procedure					

Educator/Facilitator Feedback:

Educator/Facilitator Score: Competent   Needs further development

How would you rate your overall performance while undertaking this clinical activity? (use a ✓ & initial)

Unsatisfactory   Satisfactory   Good   Excellent

Student Reflection: (discuss how you would approach your practice differently or more effectively)

EDUCATOR/FACILITATOR NAME/SIGNATURE:

STUDENT NAME/SIGNATURE: **DATE:**

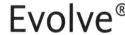 **Evolve®** Answer guide for the Critical Thinking Exercises and Critical Thinking Questions in Case Studies is hosted on Evolve: http://evolve.elsevier.com/AU/Koutoukidis/Tabbner/

References

Australian Commission on Safety and Quality in Health Care (ACSQHC), 2021. National safety and quality health service standards, 2nd ed. ACSQHC, Sydney. Available at: <https://www.safetyandquality.gov.au/publications-and-resources/resource-library/national-safety-and-quality-health-service-standards-second-edition>.

Berman, A., Frandsen, G., Snyder, S., et al., 2020. *Kozier and Erb's fundamentals of nursing*, 5th ed. Pearson, Melbourne.

Burston, A., Corfee, F., 2018. Perioperative nursing. In: Berman, A., Snyder, S., Levett-Jones, T., et al., *Kozier and Erb's fundamentals of nursing: Concepts, process and practice*, 3rd ed, vol. 2. Pearson, Melbourne, pp. 963–1004.

Crisp, J., Douglas, C., Rebeiro, G., et al., 2021. *Potter & Perry's fundamentals of nursing*, 5th ed. Elsevier, Sydney.

McKenna, L., Wood, P., Williams, A., et al., 2019. Scope of practice and workforce issues confronting Australian Enrolled Nurses: A qualitative analysis. *Collegian* 26(1), 80–85.

McTier, L., Botti, M., Duke, M., 2015. Patient participation in pulmonary interventions to reduce postoperative pulmonary complications following cardiac surgery. *Australian Critical Care* 29(1), 35–40.

Nursing and Midwifery Board of Australia (NMBA), 2020. Decision-making framework for nursing and midwifery. Available at: <https://www.nursingmidwiferyboard.gov.au/Codes-Guidelines-Statements/Frameworks.aspx>.

Rebeiro, G., Jack, L., Scully, N., 2021. *Fundamentals of nursing: Clinical skills workbook*, 4th ed. Mosby Elsevier, Sydney.

The Royal Children's Hospital Melbourne, 2020. Central venous access device management. Available at: <https://www.rch.org.au/policy/public/Central_Venous_Access_Device_Management/>.

Tollefson, J., Hillman, E., 2021. *Clinical psychomotor skills: Assessment tools for nurses*, 8th ed. Cengage Learning, Melbourne.

Online Resources and Recommended Reading

Chest, Heart & Stroke Scotland. Living with a chest condition: <https://www.chss.org.uk/chest-information-and-support/living-with-your-chest-condition/airway-clearance-techniques/>.

Carrington, E. Active cycle of breathing technique. A patient's guide: <https://www.nnuh.nhs.uk/publication/active-cycle-of-breathing-technique-v4/>.

I COUGH UK: <https://www.youtube.com/channel/UCvOamR8Sb4RXENr56fvRehA>.

Underwood, F., Sareen, A., Klosowska, M., et al. Active cycle of breathing technique: <https://www.physio-pedia.com/Active_Cycle_of_Breathing_Technique?utm_source=physiopedia&utm_medium=search&utm_campaign=ongoing_internal>.

EMERGENCY CARE

Antony Robinson and Kate Stainton

Overview

Assessment of an individual can identify an impending clinical emergency. The deteriorating clinical situation could involve any number of body systems, chronic conditions or disease processes. The ABCDE assessment algorithm (**A** airway, **B** breathing, **C** circulation, **D** disability, **E** exposure) is a systematic method of universal assessment that can be utilised to efficiently assess any individual. The purpose of the ABCDE assessment is to identify—and start treating—life-threatening problems in the order that they are most likely to harm the individual (Drost-de Klerck et al 2020). For each step of the ABCDE assessment, use a look, listen and feel approach to gather information. Then consider what the gathered information could mean and what interventions might be appropriate.

A cardiac arrest is an example of a critical event that requires prioritised assessment and intervention for a successful outcome. Identification of an unresponsive individual using the acronym DRS ABCD (**D** danger, **R** response, **S** send for help, **A** airway, **B** breathing, **C** circulation, **D** defibrillation) should be followed (Australian and New Zealand Committee on Resuscitation [ANZCOR] 2021e).

The key elements of detection of the deteriorating person are the initial identification of the deterioration, escalation of care, effective communication and prevention of further deterioration.

A clinical emergency can occur at any time of day, in any location, or even more than one can occur simultaneously. Early detection of deterioration is key to good clinical outcomes. The skills required to achieve this include being able to accurately assess, document, communicate, prioritise and escalate care in a systematic and coordinated manner while responding to the needs of the individual's changing condition.

Continued professional development encourages all staff at all levels to participate in active learning. Self-directed learning allows staff to focus on their individual areas of clinical practice that can assist in development and enhancement of clinical skills, while mandatory training ensures that all staff within a particular institution follow policy and update their skills based on changes to legislation, policy, evidence and technological advances. Technology is an increasingly important aspect of the care that nurses provide. It can enhance assessment and communication; with any skill, nurses must ensure they are competent in the use of the new technology so that its use is not to the detriment of the individual. It is vital that nurses remember that people are at the centre of all the care they provide; therefore, the care needs to be person-centred. Nurses need to effectively communicate with individuals and their families; even more so when unexpected events occur. Mandatory basic life support (BLS) and cardiopulmonary resuscitation (CPR) training give all staff an opportunity to practise and refine skills in a non-urgent arena.

 CASE STUDY 43.1

As you walk into Mr Wilson's room and say good morning, you notice he doesn't give you the cheery greeting you are used to hearing from him, and he looks quite unwell. You decide to start an ABCDE assessment:

A—Mr Wilson's airway looks normal, with no foreign bodies or liquids and no swelling. His voice sounds normal.

B—You conduct a RATES assessment:

  Respiratory rate—33 breaths/min

  Air entry—bilateral normal breath sounds

  Trachea—midline

  Effort—no accessory muscle use

C—Mr Wilson's pulse feels week. The heart rate is 111 beats/min. You find his blood pressure is 88/47 mmHg.

D—Mr Wilson is responding to voice (aVpu).

E—You don't see any rashes, trauma or signs of bleeding. Temperature is 38.7°C.

1. Which important vital sign has not yet been assessed?
2. What could be causing this clinical picture? Think of three important causes.
3. What interventions would you consider for B and C?
4. While you are working with the team to assist Mr Wilson, you notice his eyes roll back, and he slumps back in the bed. What will you do?

CRITICAL THINKING EXERCISE 43.2

Safety is important during a resuscitation. Imagine you discover an individual who has suffered a cardiac arrest while sitting out of bed in a chair. How will you resuscitate this individual and keep them, yourself and the team safe?

CLINICAL SKILL 43.1 Cardiopulmonary resuscitation/basic life support (BLS)

Please adhere to the policy and procedures of the facility/organisation prior to undertaking the skill. Ensure this skill is in your scope of practice.

NMBA Decision-making Framework considerations (refer to NMBA Decision-making framework for nursing and midwifery 2020):	Equipment:
1. Am I educated? 2. Am I authorised? 3. Am I competent? If you answer 'no' to any of these, do not perform that activity. Seek guidance and support from your teacher/a nurse team leader/clinical facilitator/educator.	Airway equipment (bag-valve-mask, pocket mask) PPE (goggles, disposable gloves, gown and face shield) Resuscitation trolley (if available) Automated external defibrillator

 PREPARE FOR THE SKILL

(Please refer to the Standard Steps on p. xii for related rationales.)
Mentally review the steps of the skill.
Discuss the skill with your instructor/supervisor/team leader, if required.
Confirm correct facility/organisation policy/safe operating procedures.
Validate the order in the individual's record.
Identify indication and rationale for performing the activity.
Assess for any contraindications.
Locate and gather equipment.
Perform hand hygiene.
Ensure therapeutic interaction.
Identify the individual using three individual identifiers.
Gain the individual's consent.
Assess for pain relief.
Prepare the environment.
Provide and maintain privacy.
Assist the individual to assume an appropriate position of comfort.

 PERFORM THE SKILL

(Please refer to the Standard Steps on p. xii for related rationales.)
Perform hand hygiene.
Apply PPE: gloves, eyewear, mask and gown as appropriate.
Ensure the individual's safety and comfort throughout skill.
Promote independence and involvement of the individual if possible and/or appropriate.
Assess the individual's tolerance to the skill throughout.
Dispose of used supplies, equipment, waste and sharps appropriately.
Remove PPE and discard or store appropriately.
Perform hand hygiene.

Skill activity	Rationale
Danger	
Recognise an emergency situation. Identify potential/real dangers. Ensure area is safe.	Ensures the environment is safe to attend BLS for self and others involved, including the individual.
Response	
Assess individual's conscious status by appropriate tactile and verbal stimulus (using a simple command [i.e. gently shaking and speaking loudly, giving simple commands such as 'Open your eyes, squeeze my hand']. Then grasp and squeeze the individual's shoulders firmly). Identify whether the individual is rousable or unconscious.	Assesses whether the individual is conscious or unconscious, and CPR is commenced appropriately. Using simple commands, and not shaking the individual, helps to maintain spinal precautions and prevent any further injuries.

Continued

CLINICAL SKILL 43.1 Cardiopulmonary resuscitation/basic life support (BLS)—cont'd

Send

Identify how to send for help/trigger the alarm within the workplace. Describe the local clinical emergency response system protocols. Note the time. Identify the explicit relevant numbers used within the workplace for emergencies. If in a community setting, call emergency services.	Allows support to be activated and provides assistance and help with the individual. Allows for expert support to arrive quickly.

Airway

Assess airway for obstruction. Clear airway (describing different methods [i.e. suction/head turn, or roll individual onto their side]. Maintain C-spine precautions. Perform chin lift, jaw thrust or head tilt manoeuvre to open airway.	Assessing airway and removing debris allows for a patent airway and ensures oxygen/rescue breaths can effectively be administered to the individual. Only roll the individual if airway obstruction is seen; reduces time to start compressions, if required.

Breathing

Maintain open airway. Assess breathing for maximum 10 seconds. Look, listen and feel technique performed. Look for chest rise and fall. Listen for outflow of air from mouth and/or nose. Feel outflow of air and chest movement.	Minimises the amount of time to assess individual's breathing, decreases the amount of downtime and oxygen-poor system. Reduces risk of hypoxia. Look, listen and feel technique is easy to perform and assesses breathing simultaneously.

Circulation

In the absence of normal breathing commence CPR. For effective chest compressions the individual should be placed in a flat position, with a hard surface underneath. Commence compression using both hands on the centre of the chest. Correct hand position, one hand in centre of chest (heel of the hand) and the other hand on top. Maintain correct posture/alignment (arms straight and shoulder over chest, using hips as pivot point). Perform cardiac compression to one-third of the chest depth with a rate of 100–120/min. At 30 compressions, give two rescue breaths (1 second per breath) using appropriate workplace equipment. If unwilling/unable for perform rescue breaths, continue chest compressions only. Demonstrate appropriate mask positioning, showing good seal (two-person technique if required). Maintain cardiac compressions/rescue breaths at a ratio of 30:2. Demonstrate or state when the person performing compressions should be rotated (every 2-minute cycle, when two or more rescuers or signs of fatigue).	To provide effective cardiac compressions, hand placement is essential. One hand over the other, arms straight and shoulders over chest decreases the risk of fatigue and creates a greater chance of completing CPR for a 2-minute cycle. One hand wrapped around the dominant wrist is preferable. Compressions to one-third of the chest allow for effective pressure on the heart to pump blood around the body and deliver oxygen to vital organs. A hard surface increases compression depth; only place on hard surface if adequate staff present to do so efficiently, reducing lost compression time. A ratio of 30 compressions to two breaths maintains sufficient oxygen in the bloodstream to be pumped around the body. Proper mask positioning will ensure full delivery of oxygen or rescue breaths.

CLINICAL SKILL 43.1 Cardiopulmonary resuscitation/basic life support (BLS)—cont'd

Defibrillation

Attach an automated external defibrillator (AED) as soon as able, turn on and follow voice prompts. Communicate safety considerations—pad placement (not over pacemaker), individual unconscious, not in contact with fluid, chest clear and dry (shave and dry chest before applying pads firmly if good contact is required between pads and individual), pads rolled onto chest, remove metal/medication patches. Demonstrate correct pad placement, sternum right parasternal 2nd intercostal space, apex: mid-axillary 6th intercostal space. Or anterior–posterior positioning. If shock advised: Scan the environment and individual for danger, ensure all persons are clear of individual and environment; verbalise before administering the shock to the individual. State safety considerations (oxygen removed, nil contact with metal, and individual is unresponsive at time of shock delivery). Safely administer shock as per AED prompts. When safe, immediately recommence CPR, post-delivery of shock. Continue to follow voice prompts until help arrives.	Immediately attach the AED when able (*while CPR is in progress*) to determine if individual needs to be shocked. The sooner the shocks can be administered, the better the outcome. Attaching the AED allows the machine to quickly identify a shockable rhythm and provide prompts. Rapid defibrillation is associated with long-term survival. Understanding the safety consideration for persons involved and the individual will ensure minimal risk of potential injuries/dangers. Correct pad placement ensures that the shock(s) are delivered more effectively. Consider safety precautions—environment is clear, persons involved are clear, oxygen is removed—to minimise the risk of potential risks/dangers. Oxygen removal also reduces risk of fire/explosion during defibrillation. Recommence CPR when safe, post shock delivery, to minimise the amount of time between effective CPR applications.

Communication

Communicate to rapid response/ALS/ambulance team in ISBAR format. State when it is appropriate to cease BLS/CPR (response of life, medical officer pronounces time of death, physically impossible to continue, danger stopping any further rescue attempts). Communicate progress with relatives/significant others where appropriate.	Effective communication to further support services will help continue effective treatment of the individual. Understanding when it is appropriate to cease CPR/BLS avoids unnecessary length of CPR and decreases chance of injury to persons involved.

 AFTER THE SKILL

(Please refer to the Standard Steps on p. xii for related rationales.)
Communicate outcome to the individual any ongoing care and to report any complications.
Restore the environment.
Report, record and document assessment findings, details of the skill performed and the individual's response.
Report, record and document any abnormalities and/or inability to perform the skill.
Reassess the individual to ensure there are no adverse effects/events from the skill.

If the event occurs in a healthcare facility, document in healthcare record onset of arrest, medication and other treatments given, procedure performed and individual's response, plan of care (i.e. transferred to ICU). Include names and roles of staff present.	Informs all healthcare professionals of what occurred and allows for appropriate care to be planned and implemented. Accurate documentation is informative and supports the implementation of ongoing planning and care.

(ANZCOR 2021e; ARC 2024; Rebeiro et al 2021)

OBSERVATION CHECKLIST: CARDIOPULMONARY RESUSCI-TATION/BASIC LIFE SUPPORT (BLS)

STUDENT NAME: _____

CLINICAL SKILL 43.1: Cardiopulmonary resuscitation/basic life support (BLS)

DEMONSTRATION OF: The ability to effectively provide basic life support and cardiopulmonary resuscitation on an individual

If the observation checklist is being used as an assessment tool, the student will need to obtain a scale of independence for each of the performance criteria/evidence.

Independent (I)

Supervised (S)

Assisted (A)

Marginal (M)

Dependent (D)

COMPETENCY ELEMENTS	PERFORMANCE CRITERIA/EVIDENCE	I	S	A	M	D
Preparation for the activity	Identifies indications and rationale for performing the activity Identifies potential/real dangers Ensures area is safe Locates and gathers equipment Considers privacy and appropriateness of setting Considers advance care directive Positions individual in most appropriate position					
Performs activity informed by evidence	Assesses individual's conscious status using appropriate tactile and verbal stimuli Identifies whether individual is rousable/unconscious Identifies how to send for help/trigger the alarm within the workplace Notes the time Assesses airway for obstruction. Clears airway (describing different methods—suction/head turn—or rolls individual onto their side. Maintains C-spine precautions) Performs chin lift, jaw thrust or head tilt manoeuvre to open airway Maintains open airway Assesses breathing for maximum 10 seconds Performs look, listen and feel technique Commences compression using both hands on the centre of the chest Maintains correct hand position and posture Performs cardiac compression to one-third of the chest depth with a rate of 100–120/min Gives two rescue breaths (1 second per breath) at 30 compressions, using appropriate workplace equipment Demonstrates appropriate mask positioning Maintains cardiac compressions/rescue breaths at a ratio of 30:2 Attaches automated external defibrillator (AED) as soon as able, turns on and follows voice prompts Communicates safety considerations Demonstrates correct pad placement Ensures safety and considerations if shock advised Safely administers shock as per AED prompts Immediately recommences CPR post delivery of shock when safe					

COMPETENCY ELEMENTS	PERFORMANCE CRITERIA/EVIDENCE	I	S	A	M	D
Applies critical thinking and reflective practice	Demonstrates or states when the person performing compressions should be rotated Demonstrates how to delegate tasks to other team members offering assistance Demonstrates or states the most preferable position to perform cardiopulmonary resuscitation Is able to link theory to practice Demonstrates current best practice in the care provided Assesses own performance					
Practises within safety and quality assurance guidelines	Removes all dangers Identifies correct manual handling procedures Dons appropriate PPE as per infection control protocols Adheres to infection control/ANTT principles Continues chest compressions only if unwilling/unable for perform rescue breaths Cleans and disposes of equipment and waste appropriately					
Documentation and communication	Demonstrates how to communicate to rapid response/advanced life support/ambulance team States when it is appropriate to cease basic life support/CPR Documents event, including time of incident, interventions, outcomes Restocks trolley and equipment post event					

Educator/Facilitator Feedback:

Educator/Facilitator Score: Competent   Needs further development

How would you rate your overall performance while undertaking this clinical activity? (use a ✓ & initial)

Unsatisfactory   Satisfactory   Good   Excellent

Student Reflection: (discuss how you would approach your practice differently or more effectively)

EDUCATOR/FACILITATOR NAME/SIGNATURE:

STUDENT NAME/SIGNATURE: **DATE:**

References

Australian and New Zealand Committee on Resuscitation (ANZCOR), 2021e. Guideline 8 – Cardiopulmonary Resuscitation (CPR). Available at: <https://www.anzcor.org/home/basic-life-support/guideline-8-cardiopulmonary-resuscitation-cpr/>.

Australian Resuscitation Council (ARC), 2024. Guideline 11.1. Introduction to and principles of in-hospital resuscitation. Available at: <https://resus.org.au/download/guideline-11-1/>.

Drost-de Klerck, A., Olgers, T., Van De Meeberg, E., et al., 2020. Use of simulation training to teach the ABCDE primary assessment: An observational study in a Dutch University hospital with a 3–4 months follow-up. *BMJ Open* 10(7):e032023. Available at: <https://doi.org/10.1136/bmjopen-2019-032023>.

Nursing and Midwifery Board of Australia (NMBA), 2020. Decision-making framework for nursing and midwifery. Available at: <https://www.nursingmidwiferyboard.gov.au/Codes-Guidelines-Statements/Frameworks.aspx>.

Rebeiro, G., Wilson, D., Fuller, S., 2021. *Fundamentals of nursing: Clinical skills workbook*, 4th ed. Elsevier, Chatswood.

Index

A

Abbey Pain Scale, 451, 453–455t, 453–455b
ABG. *see* arterial blood gases
ABHR. *see* alcohol-based hand rub
ACSQHC. *see* Australian Commission on Safety and Quality in Health Care
activity preparation
  in admission and discharge process, 115b, 115t
  in anti-embolic stocking application, 346b, 346t
  in assisting with oral hygiene, cleaning teeth and dentures, 154b, 154t
  in assisting with transfer, 337b, 337t
  in blood glucose measurement, 488b, 488t
  in blood pressure measurement, 89b, 89t
  in body temperature assessment, 101b, 101t
  in cardiopulmonary resuscitation/basic life support, 524t, 526t
  in central venous access device, 508b, 508t
  in changing an ostomy appliance, 445b, 445t
  in chest tube/drainage and dressing change care, 319–320b, 319t
  in clinical handover, 35b
  in documentation, 16b, 16t
  in donning and doffing PPE (gloves, gown, mask, eyewear), 128b, 128t
  in drain tube removal, 379b, 379t
  in drain tube shortening, 375b, 375t
  in eating and drinking assistance, 385–386b, 385t
  in emptying urine drainage bag, 422b, 422t
  in enteral feed, 397–398b, 397t
  in establishing intravenous (IV) therapy, 206b, 206t
  in exercises, preoperative and postoperative, 515b, 515t
  in eye irrigation, 467b, 467t
  in eye pad application, 463b, 463t
  in falls risk assessment, 54b, 54t
  in female urinary catheterisation, 427–428b, 427t

activity preparation *(Continued)*
  in fluid balance charting, 330b, 330t
  in focused pain assessment, 456t, 458t
  in hand-held inhaler and spacer, 278b, 278t
  in handwashing/hand hygiene, 124b, 124t
  in health teaching, 5b, 5t
  in incentive spirometry, 297–298b, 297t
  in indwelling urinary catheter removal, 438–439b, 438t
  in infusion and bolus administration, 221b, 221t
  in instilling ear drops, 260b, 260t
  in instilling eye drops or ointment, 255b, 255t
  in intravenous (IV) blood administration, 232b, 232t
  in intravenous cannula removal, 226b, 226t
  in intravenous management, 212b, 212t
  in male urinary catheterisation, 433–434b, 433t
  in medication administration via enteral routes, 187b, 187t
  in medication administration via nebuliser, 272b, 272t
  in mental health assessment, 48b, 48t
  in mid-stream urine collection, 408–409b, 408t
  in mobility assessment, 68t
  in nasal sprays and drops administration, 284b, 284t
  in nasogastric tube insertion, 391–392b, 391t
  in nasopharyngeal (nasal) or nasopharynx (throat) swab collection, 305–306b, 305t
  in neurological assessment, 475–477b, 475t
  in neurovascular assessment, 481–482b, 481t
  in nursing informatics competency, 24b, 24t
  in nutritional assessment/weight, height and BMI, 64b, 64t
  in occupied bed making, 173b, 173t
  in open gloving, 132b, 132t
  in oral medication administration,

activity preparation *(Continued)*
  181b, 181t
  in oronasopharyngeal suction, 309–310b, 309t
  in oxygen saturation measurement, 81b, 81t
  in oxygen therapy-nasal, mask, 323b, 323t
  in palliative care, 495b, 495t
  in performing a bed bath, 146b, 146t
  in performing an eye toilet, 150b, 150t
  in performing ECG, 293–294b, 293t
  in performing special mouth care, 158b, 158t
  in positioning individuals in bed, 342b, 342t
  in postoperative bed making, 168b, 168t
  in pressure injury risk assessment, 44b, 44t
  in pulse assessment, 94b, 94t
  in rectal suppository or disposable enema insertion, 193b, 193t
  in respiration assessment, 76b, 76t
  in routine urinalysis, 404b, 404t
  in sheath/condom drainage device application, 417–418b, 417t
  in shower or bath assistance, 140b, 140t
  in skin tears assessment and management, 362b, 362t
  in sputum collection, 301–302b, 301t
  in stool assessment/collection, 449b, 449t
  in subcutaneous and intramuscular injections administration, 200b, 200t
  in subcutaneous (subcut) medication administration, 239b, 239t
  in sutures and staples removal, 371b, 371t
  in toileting assistance, 413b, 413t
  in topical medication administration, 244b, 244t
  in tracheostomy suctioning and tracheal stoma care, 314–315b, 314t
  in transdermal medication application, 249b, 249t
  in unoccupied bed making, 163b, 163t
  in vaginal medication administration, 266b, 266t